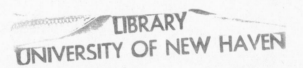

The

Social Setting

of

Mental Health

The
Social Setting
of
Mental Health

EDITED BY

Alfred Dean

Alan M. Kraft

Bert Pepper

Basic Books, Inc., Publishers   *New York*

Library of Congress Cataloging in Publication Data

Dean, Alfred, 1933–
    The social setting of mental health.

    Includes index.
    1. Social psychiatry. 2. Therapeutic
community. 3. Mental illness—Diagnosis.
4. Mental health services. I. Kraft, Alan M.,
1925–   joint author. II. Pepper, Bert,
1932–   joint author. III. Title. [DNLM:
1. Mental health—Essays. 2. Psychiatry,
Community—Essays. WM30 S6773]
RC455.D38   362.2'04'2   76–3487
ISBN 0–465–07918–0

CONTENTS

PART II

THE TREATMENT SETTING AS
A SOCIAL SYSTEM

PART III

ISSUES OF DEVIANCE, LABELING, AND
SOCIAL CONTROL

PART IV

THE MENTAL HEALTH
SYSTEM IN SOCIETY

Contents

The

Social Setting

of

Mental Health

CHAPTER 1

Introduction

Roy W. Menninger

"No man is an island"—hardly a contested statement, since the daily experience to each of us is a continuing reminder of the myriad connections which tie us to institutions, to groups, and to other people. Our lives, our worlds, are defined by our relationships to others, both as individuals and as groups. Out of this complex matrix of interactions and relationships come forces which affect our values, our behavior, even our sense of who and what we are.

Yet each of us in the mental health professions, particularly those with a background in psychiatry and psychology, have emerged from training systems dominated by an individualistic orientation so intense and so comprehensive as to permit—or even make inevitable—the ready assumption that the individual *is* an island unto himself—that his behaviors, his problems, his concerns can be understood almost exclusively in terms of data about his own mental and emotional processes.

Arising from a medical tradition, psychiatry has emphasized the diagnosis and treatment of the individual, sought causes of illness within the individual, and developed methods of amelioration essentially focused on the individual. Only slowly have group treatment methods come to be seen as both effective and relevant. And family therapy, an intervention focused on the primary group in which the disturbance of the individual is presumed to have developed, has been very slow to achieve general acceptance from an individual-oriented profession.

The brilliance of Freud's insights and their explanatory power established the significance of intrapsychic life. His concepts of conflict, of anxiety, of the unconscious, and of symbolic transformation helped explain behavior in a manner that gave legitimacy and effectiveness to psychiatry, and rescued it from the hands of the alienists who were mere custodians of the insane, the unwanted, and the unacceptable. This perspective of the individual, motivated by internal drives and conflicts, has become so ingrained in the very nature of dynamic psychiatry that it is no longer possible to think of psychiatry without it.

But the very success of our understanding of intrapsychic life has retarded a logical evolution toward still more comprehensive theories which relate the intrapsychic world of the individual to the interactive world of the environment. Moreover, the advantages of a dynamic theory which is both illuminating and effective have combined with the advantages of working with a single individual in the privacy and sanctity of the consulting room to make it less obvious that large parts of the person's environmental world were being excluded or discounted. It is even possible to suggest that these "islands" of therapeusis have been effective precisely because issues were thereby simplified and attention restricted to a more manageable number of problems, eliminating the "blooming, buzzing confusion" that surrounds each of us. And perhaps especially important, this isolation of treatment permitted a sharp focus on the individual's need to regain control of himself before he could attempt to deal effectively with the environment.

But again, the very success of this perspective has slowed an examination of the significance of these external forces on the individual, has made it harder to know how important they may be as etiologic agents, let alone how they may be shaped to therapeutic ends. This perspective has substantially blunted the development of a broad understanding of the nature of man as a social being as well as a psychodynamic organism.

It is not that we are ignorant of this perspective, nor that we do not use it. Indeed, virtually every clinician can cite examples in which the nature of the individual problem did not become clear until the dynamics of the larger social system—the "environment"—were examined. For example, the precipitously destructive behavior of ward patients is a mystery until a covert conflict among the staff is exposed and clarified; or the motivation of an adolescent to run away may be obscure until the surrounding family dynamics are examined; or the nonparticipation of a normally active group member may be incomprehensible unless the threatening competitive dynamics within the group become evident; or the failure of a presumably effective individual may be hard to understand until the double-bind characteristics of the role he was expected to fill are clarified. Examples are so numerous that the relevance of this larger perspective to our understanding of the individual is not hard to establish. What is lacking in our professional education is systematic exposure to the concepts, the theory, the structure of disciplines of knowledge other than our own. It would appear that the requirements for and advantages of becoming skillfully trained in individual treatment methods have downgraded the real significance of this broader perspective, and discouraged its systematic introduction into the training of most mental health professionals.

This is no longer merely a matter of academic emphasis, a perspective to consider for its intellectual advantages, for the environment itself has changed; it will no longer tolerate our indifference to it. It is not now possible to discount those who emphasize the significance of social roles, of relationships to social institutions or the cultural milieu, as "environmentalistic" and somehow deviant. It is no longer possible to define the work of clinical psychiatry or psychology, let alone social work, as limited to the treatment of the ill, for we find that the very definition of "illness" has lost the solid quality of "hard" knowledge that our diagnostic labels once appeared to give it. It is no longer clear just who is to provide those interventions we once comfortably and confidently called "treatment," nor is it self-evident who is to bear the costs of our work.

In short, our professions are not islands unto themselves, any more than are the patients who have sought our help and attention. We are part of a shifting context, affected professionally by the very social processes which we so readily acknowledge and manage in our social worlds, yet wish to ignore in our work. To feel overwhelmed is easy, perhaps even natural, but to stop there is neither personally adaptive nor especially effective in managing the changes which demand our attention.

It is precisely at this point that the perspectives, the methods, the concepts, and even the theories of sister disciplines can help us, but only as we in the mental health field are willing to engage the data from other disciplines, listen to the practitioners from other disciplines, and undertake the difficult but vital task of relating their perspectives to our own. We do not believe that man is an island unto himself; for all their success, our exclusively individually focused theories are not enough, and we know this well. Advancing the frontiers of our knowledge is a value to which almost all of us subscribe, but this advancement can occur only with the translation of our dissatisfaction and discomfort into efforts which achieve a broader, more comprehensive understanding of man *and* social context.

In his search for this broader understanding it is easy for the clinician to set forth with high hopes that understanding is not far off—only to become mired amidst concepts so abstract, language so foreign, teachers so unfamiliar that retreat to older patterns of professional behavior, with the comfort of a sour-grapes superiority, is the only alternative. Few of us have models for the difficult task of pursuing this kind of knowledge, and for this our centers of mental health education are largely to blame. But even they are handicapped by the lack of guides and guidelines in this uncharted area.

This book is an artful and provocative guide which deserves the attention of any mental health clinician, no matter what his discipline of origin. The editors, exemplifying the cross-disciplinary perspective they ask us to develop, are eminently well qualified: a sociologist, a state mental health commissioner, and a psychiatrist-educator. They have culled the literature for articles which highlight the intersections of sociological theory with psychiatric knowledge and practice, and have focused upon each of the issues. As is proper, this volume offers new perspectives, and will therefore have a disconcerting effect on the reader who has unwittingly settled for narrower "explorations" of the phenomena his patients present. More than this, the editors have utilized a dialectical approach to the "truth"—persuasive accounts in conflict with each other—so that the reader is required to engage in the challenging task of defining his own resolution of the issues discussed without the dubious benefit of a single predigested posture. This hardly makes for pleasant bedtime reading—but this book is guaranteed to speak to some of the issues which have been keeping many of us awake at night.

CHAPTER 2

Intentions

Alfred Dean, Alan M. Kraft, and Bert Pepper

Among the important cross-currents of thought in the mental health field is the recurring theme of the relevance of the social sciences to theory and clinical practice. Within a relatively short span of time, sociology and social psychology have moved from a peripheral position to a central one, as basic sciences for medicine, psychiatry, clinical psychology, psychiatric social work, and psychiatric nursing. The social sciences increasingly have come to be regarded, along with the biological and psychological sciences, as the fundamental building blocks for understanding human behavior.

This book was conceived by the three of us as we collaborated in teaching a course about the intersections of the social sciences with psychiatry. In the process of our teaching experience we were impressed with the need for a book which could guide the reader through an intellectual exploration beginning with basic social science concepts and data, leading him through a selection of ideas and information which are significant to clinical experience.

This book is a by-product of a course for psychiatric residents. As a consequence of our own teaching and learning with residents, and after discussing with other mental health educators the problem of presenting these subjects, we have come to believe that this kind of collection of ideas and information is long overdue in the education of the various mental health professions. It is clear that instructional materials and approaches have lagged behind the need for them. The selections in this book are the distillate of a much larger number of readings for some subject areas. In addition, we have written chapters specifically for the book. We have found these new and reprinted chapters to be most useful as building blocks and stimuli for thoughtful discussions.

The volume was designed to be a vehicle for a seminar. It contains important articles which are connected by introductory and explanatory material, topically arranged by sections so as to catalyze discussion and further exploration. Introductory chapters to the parts deal with major subject areas. Each reading is introduced by a discussion of the central subject themes, followed by a commentary on key points and questions designed to enhance and provoke meaningful, thoughtful discussion. The organization thus provides structure as well as content for a seminar.

This book is not intended to be an exhaustive collection. We have been selective in three ways. First, we have selected the best readings we could find which deal with the subjects chosen for study. Second, we have chosen certain concepts which are seminal and which build on each other. Third, we have excluded other important subjects which are usually covered in the mental health training curricula. The decision to exclude was difficult but necessary. Consequently, the reader will find little or no material concerned with such important subjects as transcultural psychiatry, drug abuse, delinquency, crime, violence, racism, and communications theory.

The selected topics represent some of the most provocative, controversial, and consequential issues in contemporary psychiatry. They can hardly be ignored by any serious worker in the field. If the material presented offers added perspectives, facilitates a clear understanding of those issues, and serves as a foundation for further learning, our intent will have been served.

We have found the teaching of the seminar and the preparation of this volume to be rewarding, satisfying, and of material assistance to each of us in integrating our own knowledge and experiences in social science and psychiatry. We hope this book will prove to be of similar benefit to each reader.

CHAPTER 3

Orientation

Alfred Dean, Alan M. Kraft, and Bert Pepper

The Sociology and Social Psychology of the Individual Patient

The junior resident in psychiatry had listened to his young female psychotherapy patient remark repeatedly: "But Doctor, you just don't *understand* me!" His working hypothesis was that this was testimony to her inability to face her unconscious conflicts. Fleetingly at first, this was challenged by the thought that she might in part—but *significant part*—be right. He reflected on the possible barriers to his understanding: little more than a year of psychiatric training, and perhaps of equal importance, their substantially different backgrounds. He was a single young man, long wrapped in professional education, rooted in rural Vermont, by birthright an "Old American." In contrast, the olive-complexioned, dark-haired girl had been born and raised in upstate New York, but her social origins were derived more from the figure of her Italian immigrant father.

On the other hand, he had recurrent facts to work with: the father's controlling behavior—holding a short leash on her contacts with boys and expecting her home by 11:00 P.M.; the girl's obvious attachment to her father; her anguish about their frequent arguments over what was good and right; her wish for his approval. She was concerned about similar arguments between her mother and father as well. How characteristic of adolescents!

In a reading seminar one of the papers selected to illustrate the concept of culture happened to be Campisi's detailed description of "The Italian Family in the United States" (see Chapter 10). By richly exposing the *socially patterned conflicts* experienced by both the patient and her parents, this paper struck home to the psychiatrist.

After reading and discussing this new sociological perspective, the resident psychiatrist began to appreciate that his patient's family's behavior was not entirely idiosyncratic, but was in many ways characteristic of a particular group of people with similar social experience. Importantly, he gained fresh insight into how an additional conceptual framework may help to place facts in a multidimensional perspective.

The preceding vignette of a real situation was presented to illustrate one major educational aim of this book—to examine the clinical application of sociological data and concepts in the treatment of the individual patient. While the traditional concepts of intrapsychic processes are relevant to an understanding of the patient, they require integration with the less familiar but equally appropriate concepts of the social sciences. The primary task of the clinician is to help in the understanding and resolution of the patient's conflicts and problems. An appreciation of the patient's behavior, thoughts and feelings, historical experiences, and current life situation may be enhanced significantly by increased knowledge of their cultural and social context.

For students of John Donne, the concept that "no man is an island" may represent a lofty existential sentiment, but to students of human behavior it might well stand as a poetic phrasing of a first principle of human nature—that man is everywhere an interdependent animal. To declare further that he lives with, by, and even *for* the groups to which he is attached "like a piece of the continent" is in keeping with matters of scientific observation rather than sheer utopian rhetoric. To students of man's states of "dis-ease" (or "ease"), a comprehensive understanding of the patient requires knowledge of group properties and social psychological processes. The case of the Italian American girl would provide a poor lesson if it left us with the idea that only patients from unfamiliar backgrounds belong to groups which require our understanding; rather, this is true of all our patients.

The Status of the Social History. Perhaps there is a seeming redundancy in addressing the need for clinical application of sociological concepts, since the "social history" is part of a longstanding tradition in medicine in general and psychiatry in particular. Any experienced clinician can cite numerous cases which testify to the importance of the social history, just as clinical experience and research testify to the importance of interviewing techniques. Yet while medicine has generally insisted on refining the logic, techniques, and empirical knowledge which serve as foundations for diagnosis and treatment, it has virtually been content to leave the procedures of the social history and the interview in the status of a vague and undefined art. As a result, the content, form, and methods of *social diagnosis* are ambiguous in concept and uncertain in practice. Consideration of the reasons for this state of affairs would require a long aside. Suffice it to say that the application of relevant social scientific data and concepts to the social history and to treatment in mental health has lagged behind the growth of available knowledge.

History does not speak for itself. The format and conceptual framework of the social history, which indicate what data should be collected—and which provide a scheme for data analysis—are decisive. In the following chapters a number of basic social science concepts are considered, with the view that they will facilitate a firmer examination reader to develop a rich and useful format of his/her own. To antici- of the sociocultural inner and outer worlds of patients by assisting the pate the central concerns of this book, we suggest that an under- standing of the case cited above is amplified by an appreciation of the Old World *culture* to which the patient had been *socialized;* the *struc- ture* of the Italian family; the dynamics of *culture contact* and *change;* the patterns of *social stratification* and *mobility* in both societies; and the organization of *familial roles.* Adapted to fit a different environ- ment, the Old World Italian family was easily transported, but uneasily transplanted in the New World. Each member of the family assumed different roles which were in transition, resulting in socially patterned conflicts, strains, stresses, and dilemmas. To a significant degree, the social system had precast the forms of individual disturbances.

Social Analysis and Psychoanalysis. The web of anxiety, con- flict, and stress—which is generic to functional psychological distur- bances—inevitably implicates interactions between the social system and the biological and psychological systems. This truth was recog- nized in the earliest clinical studies and theoretical formulations of dynamic psychiatry. Simply illustrated, it was no accident that the dynamics of sexual conflicts were identified in the context of mid- Victorian Vienna. Freud's three-dimensional model of personality—id, ego, and superego—was an explicit attempt to link each of these sys- tems, as well as "inner" and "outer" reality. Similarly, Freud noted in some of his early writings that the sexual drive was subjected to different social forces in various social classes of his society.

Such observations were consistent with his view that a general theory of psychodynamics was necessarily a psychology of the normal as well as the abnormal—and a "social psychology" as well. The general principle exposed here is that psychological disturbances or syndromes reflect their sociocultural context—a principle recognized in the epidemiology and etiology of medical as well as psychiatric disorders. In keeping with this principle, a variety of neo-Freudian observations and theories—such as those of Horney, Sullivan, and Wheelis—subsequently proposed more specific sociopsychiatric theo- ries of psychological disturbance. That principle also inclines us to regard our illustrative case not as a special syndrome of acculturation, but, to use Meyer's penetrating phrase, as one "experiment in na- ture." [1] By the same token we are invited to explore, as best we can, the specific social psychological dimensions which may be implicated in the lives of each of our patients.

Clinical Use of Social Psychological Data in Understanding Groups

The point has been made that social science data are important for the understanding of the individual patient, and that such data must be integrated with biological and psychological information. The same may be said for understanding man in naturally occurring group settings, such as family or work groups, and in groups created for therapeutic purposes, such as therapy groups and therapeutic communities.

As the clinician shifts focus from dyadic to group relationships, the interrelationships among individuals become more complex and therefore more difficult to understand and work with. Comprehension of behavior in a group not only requires an understanding of the individuals, but also of the relationship *among* the people in the group. Just as dyadic relationships have certain common qualities, regardless of the individuals involved, so do group relationships. The social sciences are engaged in the study of the behavior of humans in groups. The breadth of social science studies ranges from very large groups, such as societies and nations, to very small groups, such as families. The interests of social scientists vary in perspective from the behavior of collectivities, without regard to individual differences among people, to the interdependent relationship between personal (psychological and biological) needs and interests and the needs and interests of the group.

An example of the former—studying group phenomena without regard for individual differences—is the work of Durkheim,[2] a sociologist who studied the phenomenon of suicide. He approached the problem of suicide as a societal event: Certain numbers of people, in response to social forces, take their lives. His focus was *not* on the question "Why did this individual rather than that individual end his life?" Rather, he inquired about the dynamic forces in a society which affect the rate and nature of suicide.

An example of a social psychologist who is concerned with the relationships between individual psychology and the needs of groups is Levinson (see Chapter 6). He examined the complex interplay of forces as an individual fulfills a social role. Social roles are behaviors prescribed by groups for individuals who, to a greater or lesser extent, find these roles to be gratifying and suited to their abilities and needs.

These two perspectives need not be competitive; in fact, they can complement each other. One may study the phenomenology of auto accidents by discovering where accidents occur and under what circumstances and conditions, such as weather, light, or types of cars. From such a study one might find patterns of mishaps—a particular kind of roadway intersection, a particular time of day or night, the frequency of drunk drivers. One could also profitably examine the same phenomena by studying the individuals who have accidents, to learn about their personal characteristics and discover patterns among them.

Whether a clinician is engaged in group therapy, a home visit, or family therapy, is acting as leader of an interdisciplinary team, or is responsible for developing a psychiatric program for a specific population, he/she will have to call on a repertoire of knowledge and skills. In each of the examples cited, the social sciences might be considered one of several basic "legs" upon which the practitioner will be standing. Each of these practices requires some fundamental knowledge of groups, ranging in size and type from families to work groups to communities. It is essential that the practitioner understand the concepts and phenomena of socialization, roles, values, stratification, and deviance.

Deviance and Labeling. The phenomena of deviance and labeling are dealt with at some length in Part III. However, at this point it may be useful to introduce them briefly, as they relate to clinical practice.

As long as everyone in a family behaves in an expected and acceptable way, each member of the family can depend on the predictability of each other's behavior. But if father sporadically and unpredictably takes off on drinking binges, misses work, and disappears for days on end, then the family's balance of forces is disturbed. The family members must now come to grips with father's behavior. In order to reassure themselves that the family group as a whole is still stable and functioning, they may first define father as "deviant": not behaving like other fathers in their community, and, indeed, not behaving "like himself." Beyond this, they may attach a specific "deviance" label to him, depending on their feelings toward him and their cultural set toward the use of various available labels. The label chosen may, in turn, direct their response toward him. If he is labeled "sick" they are more likely to be sympathetic and helpful than if he is considered merely irresponsible and selfish.

In general, a person who breaks society's rules of behavior is labeled "deviant." "Explanations" for deviance also develop. The "sick" label is an example of this. This is a corrective step by which the person is given special positive status and becomes the recipient of special help. Another example is referring to a person who is out of contact with ordinary reality as having been "touched by God." Of course, some labels are clearly pejorative and are used to legitimize exclusion from society; "criminal" and "bad" are everyday examples.

The person who has been labeled deviant is often emotionally troubled. In this sense, psychiatry is a medical specialty which deals with various forms of social deviance. Patients have often broken some generally accepted rule of behavior which marks them as deviant, and then have been labeled—often by others, sometimes by themselves—as "mentally ill."

We have mentioned that our responses to rule-breaking behavior are themselves dependent in part on cultural patterns. The current controversy about labeling persons who are alcoholic can be viewed as a contemporary example of this process. It has been common practice for the police to arrest people who are apparently homeless and intoxicated on public streets. City court dockets are overcrowded with such people, who are often charged with public intoxication, disturbing the peace, loitering, or similar offenses. Yet recently, perhaps representing changing cultural attitudes on the matter, some courts and state legislatures have ruled that alcoholism is to be labeled an illness and is therefore a treatable, rather than punishable, form of deviance.

In group therapy, when the group is composed of a small number of individuals, each of whom has been labeled as "deviant" by his family, friends, work associates, or the community at large, it is an impressive phenomenon that within the group there quickly develops an expectation of "normal" behavior. The individual who breaks its rules stands at risk of being labeled "deviant" by the group. This phenomenon demonstrates the ubiquitousness of the term and its function in maintaining group integrity.

The Treatment Setting as a Social System. Since World War II a great deal of attention has been focused on the social setting in which psychiatric treatment takes place. The psychiatric hospital has been the subject of many studies which examine the nature of the social system of the hospital, relationships between staff and patients, and effects of one upon the other. The concept of making sophisticated use of the social relationships within a treatment setting has led to the notion of the *therapeutic community.* This linking of social science information and clinical management has had a profound effect on the treatment of the hospitalized seriously ill. It has provided a theoretical framework for understanding and manipulating the social environment of patients. Additionally, it has encouraged the development of interdisciplinary teamwork, since it led psychiatric personnel to consider *all* activities and events in a patient's life as being potentially helpful and important.

The Role of Social Science in Mental Health Education. The social sciences (sociology, cultural anthropology, social psychology) may well be considered basic sciences for the mental health specialties. They complement the other basic sciences of psychology, biochemistry, genetics, and psychophysiology. It is important that they not be considered competing fields of knowledge. The clinician is faced with the task of integrating the knowledge of these disciplines, not of choosing among them. This is an extraordinarily difficult task because the mental health field has been one in which practitioners have frequently subscribed to "a school of thought" which is under attack by other schools and which itself rejects the views of other schools. It has been characteristic of the "true believer" that he/she would not seriously consider other kinds of data and theory, but consider only those events which fit his/her theoretical framework, and treat only those people who lend themselves to that particular approach. Fortunately, the mental health disciplines are presently moving beyond this stance, and there are increasing attempts to integrate biological, psychological, and social science data in clinical work and in research.

It is in the spirit of this position that the present book is offered. Social science cannot stand alone as a basis for clinical practice. The ideas, theories, criticisms, and experiences presented in this volume are offered as data for integration with psychological and biological data.

This chapter has already stated two of the basic goals of the book: The first is to provide a foundation of basic sociological knowledge for the mental health clinician; the second, to assist in integrating this information into his/her psychotherapeutic armamentarium, making it readily available as he/she deals with patients, individually and collectively.

The Sociology of the Mental Health System

A third basic goal of this book is to explore some of the ways in which the social system shapes, impinges upon, and influences the mental health system, thereby using it to meet social needs and weave it into the total social tapestry.

Mental health programs are changing rapidly, and current demands of society supply the major impetus for the speed and direction of these changes. The use of this perspective makes it possible to attend to apparently independent and unrelated events and comprehend them as parts of a pattern. The sharp decrease in average length of hospitalization for first admissions to state hospitals, the current role of the courts in right-to-treatment suits, and the rapidly changing relationships between psychiatry and the other mental health professions are in significant part *responses to related social pressures*. An instructive approach to understanding the relationships between these and other changes in the mental health field, and perhaps to predicting future changes, may come from considering mental health as a subsystem of the overall social system (society). In this way we may further appreciate the reasons for changes in our state mental hospitals (shortening of length of stay, unlocking of doors, integration of staff and services with community programs); the development of alternatives to psychiatric hospitals (day hospitals, comprehensive community mental health centers); blurring and modifying of professional roles; the development of the unified interdisciplinary mental health team; and the emergence of alternative conceptual models (social, deviance, developmental-educational) which challenge the *medical model*.

We offer the concept of the sociology of mental health as an alternative perspective to the oft-stated view: "There is too much political influence and governmental interference in our field. We professionals must resist the demands of special interest groups." Social pressures have always impinged upon every aspect of mental health care. Today —and 100 years ago as well—social inputs have been major determinants in deciding:

1. Who is ill?
2. What is defined as mental illness?
3. Who shall treat?
4. Who shall receive treatment?
5. Who shall receive *what kind* of treatment?
6. Where, when, and how will treatment be provided?
7. What kinds of behaviors will be tolerated in the open community?
8. What behaviors will not be tolerated—who will be extruded?

If we grant that society shapes the definitions and functions of the mental health system, it may be useful to list a series of linked and simultaneous aspects of this relationship:

1. The sociology of psychiatrists and other mental health professionals.
2. Social uses of mental health services.
3. Roles of the professional: at work, in the community at large.
4. Social support for the maintenance and improvement of the mental health system, including funding of training and of services.
5. Changes in society at large, and consequent new demands on the mental health system—"new priorities for mental health."

While a full elucidation, exploration, and integration of these items would require a book of its own, a preliminary analysis is offered below.

The Sociology of Psychiatrists and Other Mental Health Professionals. The first major American investigative report on this subject, now a foundation block of psychiatric epidemiologic research, was *Social Class and Mental Illness: A Community Study.*[3] This book by August B. Hollingshead (a sociologist) and Frederick C. Redlich (a psychiatrist) was published in 1958, but reported research efforts which had been planned in 1948 and carried out in the intervening decade. The research was essentially designed to examine the New Haven, Connecticut, population and its mental health system. It concerned itself with the distribution of mental illness and with the ways that patients were treated by psychiatrists.

The sociology of psychiatrists received significant attention as part of a review of psychiatric facilities, particularly those in private practice. For descriptive purposes Hollingshead and Redlich divided all psychiatrists into two groups: the A-P group (those with an analytic and psychological orientation) and the D-O group (those with a directive and organic orientation). The A-P's basically practiced psychoanalysis or psychodynamically oriented psychotherapy. They were little involved in general medicine, did not make much use of somatic or drug therapies, generally did not belong to the medical society or read medical journals, and were characterized as being more introspective and psychologically sensitive than the D-O psychiatrists. In contrast, the D-O group tended to follow a more medical model, wore white coats, and did not much use psychoanalytic theory or method, preferring to utilize support, guidance, and suggestion, coupled with drugs and shock therapies.

Those of us (Alan Kraft, Bert Pepper) who were already in psychiatry at the time *Social Class and Mental Illness* was published recall reading the above and experiencing an "Aha!" reaction. While perhaps no one felt that he fitted completely into either of these dichotomous groups, most felt that the groupings and descriptions were substantially accurate. Even more provocative were the correlations between these typologies of psychiatrists and their social antecedents and roles. In a succeeding section of the book, entitled "Psychiatrists and the Social Structure," [4] it was indicated that entry into psychiatry in the first instance, and then into one of the two described groups, was not as much a matter of free will as we might have liked to think. The data offered suggested strongly that these decisions were consequences of social forces beyond the control of the individual. Our confidence in free will was a bit shaken, for example, when it was pointed out that 44 percent of the D-O's came from old American stock, in contrast to only 8 percent of the A-P group. This indicated that one's theoretical orientation about mental illness was linked to the number of generations that one's forebears had lived in the United States.

Similarly, religion and associated cultural influences played a major role in determining psychiatric orientation: 83 percent of the A-P group came from Jewish homes, in contrast to only 19 percent of the D-O group. Statistically, this is a highly significant difference. Further, 58 percent of the A-P group who came from Jewish homes reported no contact with organized religion at the time of the study, suggesting that it was more a matter of cultural than formal religious influences which directed these individuals toward A-P psychiatry.

Other sociologically significant differences separating A-P from D-O psychiatrists included differences in upward mobility, mate selection by religious background, participation in community activities, and even differences in the extent of community participation on the part of their wives. In part, Hollingshead and Redlich analyze the traits of the A-P group as follows: "Like all phenomenally upward mobile persons, those who have achieved their present class positions largely through their own efforts and abilities have passed through a social, possibly also a psychological, transformation. Their pursuit of the American ideal of personal success and self-advancement has taken them away from the subcultures they learned as children." [5]

There have been significant changes in the sociological characteristics of psychiatrists, especially in their interest areas, since the above-cited work was written. As remarked by Alan Kraft in 1971: "In the 1960s there developed another grouping of psychiatrists that might be labeled S-C (social-community psychiatrists)." [6] Kraft noted that as a result of the impetus of the report of the Joint Commission On Mental Illness and Health, the succeeding message to a joint session of Congress by President Kennedy, and federal legislation creating and funding community mental health centers, community psychiatry became "the third major ideology in psychiatry." He went on to note that the leaders of the new S-C psychiatry were drawn largely from the A-P group. This last point might be puzzling, except for what we had learned from Hollingshead and Redlich: Since the A-P's are upwardly mobile, socioculturally "fluid," and devoted to the relatively new ideology of psychoanalysis, it might have been anticipated that young and ambitious A-P's might be powerfully attracted to a newer ideology. In contrast, it would be less likely that D-O's, already rooted in the country, its culture, land, and medical ideology, would be as wont to embrace new concepts which challenge traditional D-O values.

Other Mental Health Professionals. In the 1950s the term *mental health professional* referred first to psychiatrists, and next to psychologists and social workers. Earnest debate then followed about the possible importance of *"paramedical assistants"* or *"nonmedical sub-*

professional aides" in *assisting the psychiatrist in his work.* Hollingshead and Redlich, reflecting their times, devoted much analysis to the
psychiatrists in practice in New Haven, but did not study social workers,
psychologists, psychiatric nurses, aides, mental health assistants, administrators, sociologists, and others who today are counted among the
members of the *mental health interdisciplinary team.* The whole story
of the social forces which have opened up the field of *psychiatry* into
the field of *mental health* is fascinating, and still unfolding. At this
point we can observe only that admission of these "nonmedical
others" to the heretofore relatively closed shop of psychiatry did not
come about simply because of new scientific knowledge, new treatment
techniques, new interest or willingness on their part to undertake major
responsibilities in the treatment of the mentally ill, or an entirely voluntary welcome into the club by the profession of psychiatry. To begin to
understand why interdisciplinary *mental health* has challenged unidis-
ciplinary *psychiatry,* we must return to a brief elucidation of the schema
offered earlier in this chapter.

   Social Uses of Mental Health Services. Social forces operate to
create opportunities for psychiatrists and other mental health professionals to come into existence, in order to carry out the social uses of
psychiatry. These uses expanded greatly during World War II (1941–
1945) and thereafter. As general attitudes have changed regarding society's duties and responsibilities toward its citizens—for example,
health care being considered a right for all rather than a privilege for
the few—we have experienced new demands for mental health manpower. Not only the community mental health center program, but also
the Great Society and War on Poverty programs of the 1964–1968 period contributed to these increased expectations. The trend continues.
Right-to-treatment and *right-to-education cases* are increasing demands
for mental health manpower in the 1970s. The class action cases and
judicial decisions which require these changes may be viewed as the
judiciary impinging on the mental health system. *We* see them more
broadly as the judiciary itself acting as an agent and expression of
changing societal forces, stating society's current expectations. *Society
is now defining new uses of mental health services,* as expressed and
specified in legislation and court decisions.

   Roles of the Professions. In order to carry out these new uses of
mental health programs, the mental health field assigns new tasks and
roles to new and old professions. Moving on to the fourth item in our
scheme, these societal demands are reinforced and supported by the
provision of resources—educational, institutional, and financial—to
new mental health professions and programs.

   From a behaviorist perspective, society provides "positive reinforcement" to persons and programs carrying out the new missions, thus
creating the opportunity for upward socioeconomic mobility. If the
above chain is given credence, this scheme may be of some use in predicting future developments in the mental health field: We must look at
unfolding changes in our society at large, and try to anticipate which

of them may be assigned for implementation to our mental health subsystem.

We will address this issue again—as we take up changes in society at large, and consequent new demands on the mental health system—in Chapter 29.

NOTES

1. As exemplified in the pioneering work of Adolf Meyer, American psychiatry historically recognized psychiatric disorders as implicating biological, psychological, and social factors in interaction. Meyer emphasized the use of the social history and life-situational analysis. Contemporary interdisciplinary psychiatry thus pursues an old rather than new perspective, but one which has lagged in its development. See Alfred Lief, *The Commonsense Psychiatry of Dr. Adolf Meyer* (New York: McGraw-Hill, 1948).

2. Emile Durkheim, *Le Suicide* (Paris: F. Alcan, 1897); trans. George Simpson (New York: Free Press, 1947).

3. August B. Hollingshead and Frederick C. Redlich, *Social Class and Mental Illness: A Community Study* (New York: Wiley, 1958).

4. Ibid., pp. 161–165.

5. Ibid., p. 165.

6. Alan Kraft, "Psychiatry in the Community," *Bulletin of the Menninger Clinic* 35, no. 6 (November 1971): 416–421.

PART I

BASIC SOCIOLOGICAL CONCEPTS

CHAPTER 4

Basic Sociological Concepts

Alfred Dean

Like Darwin's Galapagos, nature can stage some remarkable exhibits of adaptational processes to the searching observer. Nowhere are they more strikingly revealed than in the processes of disease. This chapter begins to specify the *social* dimensions of human adaptation.

From the beginning of time, man's attempt to comprehend and cope with life have led him to both fact and fancy. The libraries, laboratories, and technologies around us belie how recently man discovered that special approach to knowledge termed "science." Within the brief biography of science, the concept that man's behavior and social systems could also be placed under the microscope has scarcely been recognized and pursued. Much has been accomplished within virtually the span of a man's life.

True, the social sciences have not gone to the moon. Yet in word and deed they are so much in the mainstreams of our everyday life that our readers will vary only in the depth of their acquaintance with them. Of this more must be said.

There is a misleading familiarity to social science concepts, as Peter Berger indicates:

> The sociologist moves in the common world of men, close to what most of them would call real. The categories he employs in his analyses are only refinements of the categories by which other men live—power, class, status, race, ethnicity. As a result, there is deceptive simplicity and obviousness about some sociological investigations. One reads them, nods at the familiar scene, remarks that one has heard all this before and don't people have better things to do than to waste their time on truisms—until one is suddenly brought up against an insight that radically questions

everything one had previously assumed about this familiar scene. This is the point at which one begins to sense the excitement of sociology.[1]

Berger also notes that certain sciences, such as astronomy or bacteriology, may fascinate us because they provide glimpses of unfamiliar and exotic things. Like a space odyssey, they convey the dramatic sense of new worlds seen by extraordinary means. Of the social sciences he writes:

> The excitement of sociology is usually of a different sort. Sometimes, it is true, the sociologist penetrates into worlds that had previously been quite unknown to him—for instance, the world of crime, or the world of some bizarre religious sect, or the world fashioned by the exclusive concerns of some group such as medical specialists or military leaders or advertising executives. However, much of the time the sociologist moves in sectors of experience that are familiar to him and to most people in his society. He investigates communities, institutions and activities that one can read about every day in the newspapers. Yet there is another excitement of discovery beckoning in his investigations. It is not the excitement of coming upon the totally unfamiliar, but rather the excitement of finding the familiar become transformed in its meaning. The fascination of sociology lies in the fact that its perspective makes us see in a new light the very world in which we have lived all our lives.[2]

Concepts and theories are sometimes erroneously viewed as the weak, fuzzy, and unproven ideas of a "soft" science, eventually to be displaced by concrete facts. Actually, concepts are indispensable elements of all knowledge, whether sophisticated or crude. They serve to organize, "explain," and predict facts. The genius of concepts and the larger theories of which they are a part may be expressed in the converse of the Missourian vantage point that "seeing is believing"; namely, "to believe is to see." [3]

Like the discovery of previously unknown facts, the invention of new ideas may result in a breakthrough in the development of systematic knoweldge. The falling apples, slips of the tongue, and strange customs were matters of ordinary observation; the concepts of gravity, unconscious process, and culture brought a new light to these and related observations.

We will give careful attention to defining, explaining, and illustrating several *key concepts* which offer a distinct sociological perspective of the individual and the group. Like a Rosetta stone, they also open up the wider language of social science. Hopefully, as in the meeting of people, the preliminary introductions in this chapter will enhance the communications which follow. A relationship must wait upon further encounters. A relationship also depends upon a basic trust, and here we would like to ask the reader to give the following basic sociological concepts a considered but unanxious review. They will be given further illustration, clarification, and application in later chapters. In the process the reader will acquire a sense of familiarity, comfort, and value in them. They will, as it were, shed the properties of new acquaintances to assume those of old friends.

Culture

Edward B. Tylor supplied social science with its most classic definition of culture: "That complex whole which includes knowledge, belief, art, morals, law, custom, and any other capabilities and habits acquired by man as a member of society." [4] Tylor's omnibus definition of culture emphasizes the great variety of "ingredients" or elements of human life which individuals acquire as a "social heritage." From abstract ideas to tangible tools, *these elements are cultural to the extent that they are learned, shared, and transmitted in human groups.*

The extent to which culture regulates group processes and influences individual behavior (in its broadest sense) is truly enormous. Many observations, concepts, and theories pertaining to culture are relevant to the theory and practice of psychiatry. Let us extend some central observations.

The existence of culture reflects a basic principle of group life: *Wherever individuals interact recurrently and are interdependent, culture develops.* Culture is a monument to the most elementary and consequential twin facts of collective life—it requires *consensus* and *cooperation.* The specific "contents" or forms of culture vary remarkably, but the existence of culture is a universal feature of human groups, from two-person friendships to societies of several hundred million.

Culture is the foundation of social order. It introduces regularity and predictability into social life. Some of the most important elements and processes of social systems are cultural. We will consider some of them briefly.

Norms. These are essentially cultural rules for appropriate social behavior. Norms *prescribe* how one should behave or *proscribe* how one should not behave in specific situations. The bromide, "When in Rome, do as the Romans do," testifies to popular recognition of cultural variation in norms and of the consequences of norm breaking (deviance).

Cross-cultural normative variations have been so great as to have been real eye-openers for early explorers, traders, and missionaries. Anthropologists have documented them almost endlessly, as if incessantly amused by the wondrous array of social standards. So great, indeed, is the array as to cast serious doubt on the very concept of "human nature," illustrating that the globe-trotting voyeurism of anthropologists has not been entirely frivolous.

Several thousand societies in time and space have constituted natural laboratories for the study of human behavior and human groups. The sheer documentation of variations in economic, political, religious, and familial behavior is of great value in examining the relationships among biological, psychological, and sociological factors. These observations have challenged numerous culture-bound theories in biology, psychology, and psychoanalysis.

Most norms are informally held and enforced, as by "public opinion." In contrast, *laws* are *legal norms* which are written, codified, and subjected to a specialized organization of adjudication and enforcement. Norms vary in the degree of importance, strength of feeling, and severity of sanctions attached to them. Every society has a set of core moral norms or *mores* which are highly resistant to change. *Folkways* are "lesser" norms, such as rules of etiquette.[5]

Values. Rules for behavior in society, even less than those of games of amusement, are not inherently charming or compelling. Conformity to norms is neither guaranteed nor persuaded by the sheer existence of rules. By attaching conceptions of "good" and "evil" and "right" and "wrong" to the rules, groups take a powerful step toward insuring individual commitment to group standards. Every society develops cultural values which serve to explain, justify, legitimize, and rationalize cultural norms. The power of values is that they mobilize deeply experienced sentiments and feelings.

Values are conceptions of what is good, valuable, or desirable. They have the following properties:

1. They have a conceptual element; they are more than pure sensations, emotions, reflexes, or so-called needs. Values are abstractions drawn from the flux of the individual's immediate experience.
2. They are affectively charged; they represent actual or potential emotional mobilization.
3. Values are not the concrete goals of action, but rather the *criteria* by which goals are chosen.
4. Values are important, not "trivial" or of slight concern.[6]

Anthropologists have observed that values are culturally defined and patterned in every society, but show remarkable variation between societies. Scientifically speaking, values display relativity and may seem philosophically arbitrary. However, in any given culture they tend to be regarded as natural, immanent, or absolute truths. In American culture equality, freedom, and individualism are choice examples.

The core values and beliefs of a society give meaning and motivation to both the individual and the social order. It matters little or not at all whether cultural values and beliefs are in some sense "valid" or "true," for, in the words of W. I. Thomas, "What is defined as real is real in its consequences."[7]

The Value-Belief Complex. Cultural values and beliefs are central elements in the structure and functioning of human groups and have a powerful impact upon individuals. At the group level, values and beliefs serve to *legitimize, explain,* or *justify existing social arrangements* such as constitutional democracy, monarchy, capitalism, socialism, communism, or the like. Similarly, social movements which press for a change in the social structure from revision to revolution are mobilized and legitimized by an appeal to emotionally charged values and beliefs. The value-belief complex of a society may thus be regarded as an ideology for the social system.

In one of the most systematic efforts to study the role of values in American society, for example, Robin Williams, Jr., identifies the following major "value-orientations":

1. Achievement and success.
2. Activity and work.
3. Moral orientation.
4. Humanitarian mores.
5. Efficiency and practicality.
6. Progress.
7. Material comfort.
8. Equality.
9. Freedom.
10. External conformity.
11. Science and secular rationality.
12. Nationalism—patriotism.
13. Democracy.
14. Individual personality.
15. Education.[8]

Perhaps we are sufficiently culture bound to find difficulty in recognizing the relativity and subtlety of these values, and therefore should consider them further. America's premium on individual personality, individualism, and individual freedom, so explicit and concrete in the Declaration of Independence, the Bill of Rights, and the Constitution, evolved out of the painful social history of the Old World and the fresh, vast frontier of the New World. In this value system or *ethos* it has ordinarily not been possible to advocate frankly or persuade the suppression of individual freedoms in the interest of the "state." [9]

Unlike contemporary China, Cuba, or the Soviet Union, concepts of the "superiority of the state" and subordination of individual interests to those of the state are alien and anathema to Americans. *Individual* can be capitalized, but not *state*. Individual personality was not remarkably valued in many cultures, such as traditional China or India. It should be noted that collectivism, so foreign to American ideology, is not peculiar to what we now regard as the Communist societies.

The American value on education is partly reflected in our preoccupation with our schools and in norms which pressure Americans to seek an ever-higher level of training. This value is decidedly governed by utilitarianism. It is historically linked to religion, government, and the economic order, and is personified by the "three R's."

Ability to read the Scriptures was viewed as essential to the formation of Christian values and provided explicit justification for the creation of the first public school act in Massachusetts. Later, within the perspective of Jeffersonian democracy, an educated electorate was viewed as essential to the functioning of our representational and constitutional system. Education was also valued as a means of enabling the individual and society to engage in economic activities. Our emphasis on education is related to our emphasis on social mobility. As C. Wright Mills has written in *White Collar*, our colleges have become the great social elevators of our time.[10]

The American "faith in education," as Williams terms it, is a widespread, somewhat naïve conviction that education will solve society's most stubborn problems of poverty, racism, disease, and even war. This faith is perhaps closely related to the American "belief" in science and secular rationality, although recent disenchantment with science and technology has enabled us to identify them as values and philosophies not unlike other sacred, religious, or philosophical systems.

At the individual level, the significance of values has been long recognized by both social science and psychiatry. Durkheim wrote early in the twentieth century: "When our conscience speaks, it is society which speaks, not us." [11] This concept is similar to Freud's concept of the superego.

Values serve as standards for behavior. They regulate the selection of goals and means as well as being criteria of self-evaluation. In brief, they shape and organize the basic psychobiological functions of motivation, perception, behavior, and feeling.[12]

Status and Role

Status refers to a label attached to a position in a social system, such as "medical student," "husband," "president." The specific labels and positions vary remarkably from society to society and among various subgroups. However, the fact of labeled social positions (formal or informal) is universal, and is so well known by everyone as to seem trivial (which, after all, testifies to the "purpose" of social positions). Upon close examination, however, social roles are seen to be rather complex. They have been the object of study for fifty years and remain a fertile area for further inquiry.[13]

A social position may be regarded as a basic building block in the structure of human groups, which are organized systems of interrelated social positions. In a sense, a group's social network of positions may be thought of as its "anatomy." As in the human animal (or any other living form), the *function* of any part must be fundamentally understood with reference to other parts, the vital life processes of the total system, and system-environment relationships. A heart pumping is like a social status engaging its task. It is in this sense that Linton speaks of *roles* as the *"dynamic aspect* of status." [14] (Italics added.)

To label is to categorize. Social statuses are first and foremost social categories. The object of classification is to create uniformities for some purpose. It is no accident that formal or informal *uniforms* are typically associated with specific statuses. As the form of the heart is genetically programmed, so groups tend to establish a standardized script or *role* for individuals who occupy any given social position. While it may violate our sense of uniqueness, freedom, autonomy, or independence, it remains true to a significant degree in *every* enduring social group that we are cast and we cast others into roles: "All the world's a stage, and all the men and women merely players."

The scripts for social roles are culturally patterned or standardized by means of *norms* (rules for behavior) which prescribe or proscribe *what individuals in a given status should or should not do.* In essence, roles consist of consensually validated *expectations for behavior* attached to social positions. Like other aspects of culture, role expectations are learned, shared, and transmitted in human groups.

Role expectations and the criteria by which they are assigned to members of a society vary cross-culturally. Age and sex are universal criteria for role assignment. Age and sex roles, because they are close to everyone's experience and are currently being subjected to profound debate, conflict, and change in American culture, illustrate clearly the realities of social roles.

Historically, women have usually been expected to be wives and mothers, preferably in that order. The division of labor in the home, such as cooking, cleaning, shopping, and child care, was sharply delineated along male and female lines. Women held lower status than men and were expected to be submissive to the authority of their husbands. Similarly, children have been expected to be submissive, dependent, and asexual.

Age and sex roles are examples of *ascribed roles,* assigned on the basis of some characteristic which is essentially arbitrary, in contrast to *achieved roles,* which are based on competition. Other ascribed roles, such as those based on race, family origin, caste, or class, illustrate how social roles influence the social expectations, pressures, and options experienced by individuals virtually from the moment of birth. Indeed, the power and provocativeness of the role concept is that it reveals the links between the individual and the group. It is a concept which bridges biological, psychological, and social systems.

Several mechanisms serve to promote conformity to roles and the functioning and integration of role systems. Socialization into roles is, of course, one such mechanism. Structurally, roles involve *rights as well as obligations.* Thus whatever a women is obliged to do as a wife and mother, she has, as well, publicly supported rights of protection, support, affection, and so on. In such terms, no role can be understood without reference to its *complementary roles.*

Every role is invested with legitimate power and authority, the nature, use, and limits of which are culturally defined. Similarly, role relationships are *systems of exchange.* If one person fails to fulfill his obligations, he may be denied the rewarding rights to which he is entitled. It is thus that Parsons refers to the "double contingency" of role expectations.[15] Reciprocity, as is so graphically illustrated in gift giving, is a well-recognized principle of social relationships.

Primary Groups

Charles Horton Cooley, a pioneering social psychologist, was one of the first to recognize that certain small, intimate groups had a particularly powerful impact upon individuals, and also served some rather special functions for society.[16] It was partly because of the preeminent roles of such groups that he termed them *primary* groups. Cooley writes:

> [Such groups are] characterized by intimate face-to-face association and cooperation. They are primary in several senses, but chiefly in that they are fundamental in forming the social nature and ideas of the individual. The result of intimate association, psychologically, is a certain fusion of individualities in a common whole, so that one's very self, for many purposes at least, is the common life and purpose of the group. Perhaps the simplest way of describing this wholeness is by saying that it is a "we"; it involves the sort of sympathy and mutual identification for which "we" is the natural expression. One lives in the feeling of the whole and finds the chief aims of his will in that feeling. . . .[17]

The prototype of the primary group is the family, or perhaps our idealized conception of it. Other groups also exemplify the qualities identified by Cooley: friendships, informal cliques, clubs, gangs, neighborhoods, even small communities and societies. Let us consider some of the properties of such groups more carefully.

Size. It is a matter of common experience as well as scientific documentation that the size of a group significantly influences the interaction and social relationships which occur within it. This proposition is perhaps most dramatically illustrated by the changes introduced by changing even a two-person group into a three-person group.

Smallness in size is at once an element of the "primariness" of the group in conveying its special exclusiveness, boundaries, or cohesiveness, and at the same time a factor which influences other elements of primary relationships. Restricted size and composition of a group may serve as a special symbol of its distinct identity and solidarity. Similarly, the size of the group may influence the possibilities for intimacy and person-centered interactions. That such dynamics are recognized by laymen, and are deliberately manipulated, receives testimony in such groups as the United States Marine Corps and the Green Berets, and in the restrictive clauses of country clubs or colleges.

Intimacy. Intimacy refers in part to the fact that primary relationships deal with matters ordinarily considered personal and private. Such matters may be financial, political, religious, or personal problems, dreams, fears, or experiences. Otherwise stated, *communication in the primary group is deep and extensive.*

It is also true, of course, that primary relationships are often intimate in the narrower sense of involving physical contact, sexual or affectional interactions, sharing of personal property, or relaxation of norms of modesty. In the broadest sense, then, intimacy refers to physical, social, and psychological closeness.

"Face-to-face association." This is one of the most provocative, ambiguous, and controversial phrases that Cooley used to characterize the primary group. We take it to have various implications. In the literal sense, the primary group permits, indeed values, direct, person-to-person interaction. This is in contrast to groups in which communication is indirect through other persons or correspondence, or where sheer

size or *organization* does not enable or permit face-to-face interaction among the full range of group members.

On the other hand, some *secondary* relationships may be face-to-face typically or occasionally, such as the clerk-customer relationship.[18] Direct contact does not guarantee the existence or development of a primary relationship, although it may facilitate it. Practical men of affairs, such as politicians and salesmen, as well as social scientists have recognized the power of face-to-face interaction.

The example of the clerk-customer relationship reveals a metaphorical usage of the phrase "face-to-face" which is closely related to person-centered properties. That particular role relationship is a stereotype in which the individuals relate to each other not so much as individuals as "social actors." The faces of each are "personae"—social masks. The attention which each pays to the other is usually contrived and manipulative.

Cooley drew many of his insights from literature, and he was fond of conveying them in the richly condensed patterns of literary expression. In such terms it may be noted that the face is a remarkably expressive and communicative surface. Since the time of Cooley a number of disciplines have discerned how complex, subtle, and effective personal communication can be. Cooley paid special attention to the dynamics of face-to-face interaction in his formulation of the "looking-glass self." [19] This concept emphasizes that we see ourselves in the eyes of others. Cooley states:

> As we see our face, figure, and dress in the glass, and are interested in them because they are ours, and pleased or otherwise with them according as they do or do not answer to what we should like them to be; so in imagination we perceive in another's mind some thought of our appearance, manners, aims, deeds, character, friends, and so on, and are variously affected by it. . . .[20]

Cooley regarded "self-ideas" as having three principal elements: "the imagination of our appearance to the other person; the imagination of his judgement of that appearance, and some sort of self-feeling, such as pride or mortification." [21] It should be vividly clear that these conceptualizations focus upon the nature and products of *interpersonal interaction*. The emphasis is upon *personal*, thereby demonstrating Cooley's preoccupation with the deep, "intimate," unique, and distinctly consequential nature of primary relationships. Indeed, his analyses are as graphically social *and* personal as one's own name: "Society exists in my mind as the contact and reciprocal influence of certain ideas named 'I,' Thomas, Henry, Susan, Bridget and so on. It exists in your mind as a similar group, and so in every mind." [22]

The reader may now recognize more fully that part of Cooley's special interests in primary groups stems from his view that they were fundamental in the shaping of personality. But also reflected is his simultaneous interest in how groups and sociocultural constructs develop. This linked, dual interest in the individual and the group within a conceptual framework of social interaction has been termed the *sym-*

bolic interactionist perspective. Psychiatry could well be expected to find these views compelling.[23]

Relatively unspecialized in purpose.   Many groups and their component role relationships, such as doctor-patient, employer-employee, student-teacher, have fairly limited purposes. Stated differently, role relationships vary from the *functionally specific* to the *functionally diffuse.* Primary groups tend to engage in a wide range of activities, involving multiple functions for individual members and for the group as a whole.

The functional diffuseness of the primary group is closely related to its ability to provide its individuals with their most extensive experience as multifaceted and "whole" persons. In contrast, when we relate to persons only as students, teachers, patients, or doctors, we come to know and evaluate only a limited part of the total person. Reciprocally, that person experiences a part of his total self. This is what is meant by *secondary roles* as being *segmented* in form and in self-presentation. It is partly for this reason that primary relationships are experienced as a valuable means for self-understanding, self-expression, and self-actualization.

Mutual identification.   Cooley emphasized that members of primary groups have strong identifications with each other and with the group as a whole. This quality of "we-ness" is perhaps essentially captured by the phrase, *a sense of kinship.*

However easily we may confirm subjectively this quality of "we-ness," it probably has its roots in complex psychosocial processes. In part it would seem to be a result of the most distinct characteristic of primary relationships: the extraordinary and multifaceted devotion to serving the welfare of each person and the group as a whole. The varieties of mutual concern, of giving and receiving, cover a broad canvas of biological, social, and psychological needs.

Protection, nurturance, support, affection, response, security, acceptance, understanding—these are a few of man's most unusual properties and potentialities which are cultivated, nourished, and sustained in these special groups. How easily the familiar obscures the remarkable.

Relatively permanent.   Cooley believed that primary groups tend to develop enduring bonds and enduring social relationships. In modern terms we might say that he expected them to constitute continuing reference groups and membership groups of individuals.[24]

In view of the fact that modern industrial societies are characterized by dislocation of individuals from their extended families, high rates of divorce, and parent-youth conflict, Cooley's characterization may seem unclear or inaccurate. If we regard Cooley's statement to mean that relationships to families tend to be characterized by continuing frequent interaction and continuity as an instrumental and socioemotional social system, it is clearly not fully accurate. Despite the barriers of space and time, however, we do know that the modern, urban, conjugal family continues to have strong emotional, identificational, social, and economic ties to the extended family.[25]

Socialization

> Why do the Chinese dislike milk and milk products? Why would the Japanese die willingly in a Banzai charge that seemed senseless to Americans? Why do some nations trace descent through the father, others through the mother, still others through both parents? Not because they were destined by God or Fate to different habits, not because the weather is different in China and Japan and the United States. Sometimes shrewd common sense has an answer that is close to that of the anthropologist: because they were brought up that way.[26]

In ordinary language, if not with disarming simplicity, Kluckhohn's preceding statement deftly captures the essential meaning of *socialization*, which refers, more technically, to the processes by which the culture of the group is transmitted to individuals. Broadly conceived, *socialization* may be viewed as a process of teaching and learning through which an individual acquires the norms, values, beliefs, and goals characteristic of a group.

The socialization of the infant or child is probably the richest and most revealing demonstration of the concept, dynamics, and consequences of socialization. From virtually any theoretical or empirical point of view, the infant is a culture-free, biologically driven, asocial, if not antisocial, organism. Progressively, parents or parent-substitutes, as agents of socialization, impress upon the child the culture of the group. Kluckhohn offers another cogent illustration:

> Some years ago I met in New York City a young man who did not speak a word of English and was obviously bewildered by American ways. By "blood" he was as American as you or I, for his parents had gone from Indiana to China as missionaries. Orphaned in infancy, he was reared by Chinese families in a remote village. All who met him found him more Chinese than American. The facts of his blue eyes and light hair were less impressive than a Chinese style of gait, Chinese arm and hand movements, Chinese facial expression, and Chinese modes of thought. The biological heritage was American, but the cultural training had been Chinese. He returned to China.[27]

The socialization of the infant and child is sometimes referred to as *primary* socialization because it involves the cultural and social patterning of biologically given, primary drives and potentialities of the human animal. Familiar examples include modification of such drives as elimination, eating and drinking, sleep, and sex.[28] Kluckhohn offers still another penetrating example:

> I once knew a trader's wife in Arizona who took a somewhat devilish interest in producing a cultural reaction. Guests who came her way were often served delicious sandwiches filled with a meat that seemed to be neither chicken nor tuna fish but was reminiscent of both. To queries she gave no reply until each had eaten his fill. She then explained that what they had eaten was not chicken, not tuna fish, but the rich, white flesh of freshly killed rattlesnakes. The response was instantaneous—vomiting, often violent vomiting. A biological process is caught in a cultural web.[29]

Primary socialization, as in parent-child interaction, is conspicuous, but it is often overlooked that socialization is a continuing, powerful, and consequential process *throughout the life cycle.* Even in the simplest of societies, not to mention those with elaborate industrial-urban characteristics, individuals move through different statuses, roles, and groupings. Becoming an adult, parent, or physician is each an illustrative event in which skills, attitudes, values, and beliefs are significantly shaped by "custom." [30]

Having outlined some of the basic characteristics of socialization, let us consider some of its *functional consequences* for individuals and groups. As a process of cultural transmission, socialization provides for the perpetuation of culture and the continuity of the group. It enables the group to function as an ongoing system, training individuals for instrumental tasks, fostering social cohesion, and serving integrative and socioemotional functions through the establishment of attitudes, beliefs, values, and behavior patterns appropriate to the performance of independent and interdependent roles. Socialization is thus a mechanism for role training. At the same time, socialization is a major mechanism of *social control,* serving to prevent or reduce the potential for role failure which would be occasioned by deviance.

Socialization also has a powerful impact upon the development of personality and its component content, structure, and processes. It is for this reason that studies of relationships among personality, culture, interpersonal interaction, and social systems are at once of basic interest to social scientists and the applied concerns of social psychiatry.

From the standpoint of the individual in the group, the content, form, and mechanisms of socialization represent objective realities with which he must cope in order to fulfill his biological, economic and/or sociological strivings for such things as food, protection, security, love, social acceptance, and income.

Stratification

While all concepts are abstractions, some are more easily grasped than others. The essential meaning of social stratification is usually appreciated quickly, perhaps because it is so tangibly a part of everyday life. So many key elements of American culture relate to stratification, as is so richly suggested by the idea of the "American Dream." Basically, the concept has reference to differentials in wealth, power, and prestige in human groups.

The centrality of this concept in social science is attributable to the remarkably broad range of individual, collective, and group behavior which is profoundly influenced by social stratification. Various measures demonstrate that it is associated significantly with educational aspirations and achievement, expectable lifetime income, reading patterns, political activity, sexual behavior, mate selection, recreational patterns, religious identifications, informal social relationships, participation in voluntary organizations, prejudice, and discrimination.[31]

Similarly, stratification is dramatically associated with significant differentials in life expectancy, infant mortality, and maternal deaths. Rather than being randomly distributed in populations, many diseases and disorders such as tuberculosis, malnutrition, coronary heart disease, and severe psychiatric disturbances are significantly correlated with socioeconomic status. Similarly, health-related beliefs, values, and behavior; the availability of health care services; and the types of treatment received are unequivocally associated with differentials in wealth, power, and prestige.[32]

An understanding of some of the most prominent social issues of our time, including health care delivery systems, racial conflict, poverty, illness, and the "cold war," requires a full appreciation of the dynamics of social stratification.

Thus far we have looked at the idea of social stratification in broad terms. A closer examination is required to refine our understanding of its various elements and processes. To Karl Marx, who formulated one of the classic and controversial concepts of social stratification, the phenomenon was exclusively a matter of economics.[33] Marx regarded social classes as groupings of individuals who shared similar positions in the economic order. In essence, one's social class depends upon the extent to which one has *capital*—wealth, property, or control over the means of production. Inevitably these groupings become *interest groups*, develop *class consciousness*, and engage in mortal combat. History and social science have served to clarify both the explanatory power and limitations of these concepts.

Who, for example, can deny that differentials in wealth are related to specific patterns of disease, access to health care, and a great variety of other "life chances," as Max Weber so aptly termed them? [34] Nutrition, housing, conditions of work, possessions, leisure, and recreation are all fundamentally a matter of money. Nevertheless, the arena of social stratification has diverse economic, political, and sociological factors in complex interactions; the economic factor is neither all-powerful nor adequate to explain them.

Max Weber recognized long ago that economic status, prestige ("social honor"), and power were not coterminous. He thus distinguishes among the following types of groupings: classes (economic), status groups (prestige), and parties (power).[35]

Prestige is an almost unbelievably powerful force in human affairs. What is prestigious is culturally defined. In various societies it can reside in the writing of poetry, civic service, the hoarding of property, the giving away of property, or the ability to humiliate one's rival by burning more possessions than he.

If prestige is culturally defined, it is transmitted in social interaction. How hollow a victory it would be to read rave reviews alone in your room. What "basic biological need" has not been subordinated to prestige? If it were prestigious to be poor, how many would throw away their finery?

If prestige is socially transmitted, it is self-esteem that is experienced. It is a significant transformation, but nothing is lost in the translation. How many psychiatric disturbances implicate problems of self-esteem? This one illustration of the proposition that self-concepts are developed and confirmed in social interaction is but a suggestion of the varieties of social and psychological processes involved in the theater of social stratification: ascribed status, achievement orientation, mobility aspirations, blocked mobility, anomie, alienation, and so on.

There are social classes in America, and class consciousness as well, but their nature and consequences are not reducible to economics. Income, education, and occupation all serve to establish one's social class, as do ethnicity, race, religion, and lineage.

One of the most significant features of socioeconomic status is that it seems to form a nucleus around which class cultures develop. These class-related cultures involve values, beliefs, norms, goals, family structure, and so on. It has been amply documented that class cultures cut across subcultural variations. For example, many of the cultural traits of black social classes—upper, middle, and lower—are similar or identical to those of the respective white social classes.[36]

"The past," said Shakespeare, "is prologue." So we may say of this formative examination of basic concepts. Chapters 5 through 10 provide for a further understanding of each of these concepts and point increasingly to their implications for the mental health field.

NOTES

1. Peter L. Berger, *Invitation To Sociology* (Garden City, N.Y.: Doubleday, Anchor Books, 1963), pp. 21–22.
2. Ibid., p. 21.
3. For an excellent discussion of the nature of scientific concepts, see William J. Goode and Paul K. Hatt, *Methods in Social Research* (New York: McGraw-Hill, 1952), pp. 41–55.
4. Edward B. Tylor, *Primitive Culture*, vol. 1 (London: John Murray, 1871), p. 1.
5. For a further discussion of norms see Robin M. Williams, Jr., *American Society: A Sociological Interpretation*, 2nd ed. (New York: Knopf, 1960), pp. 25–30.
6. Ibid., p. 400.
7. Edmund H. Volkart, ed., *Social Behavior and Personality: Contributions of W. I. Thomas to Theory and Social Research* (New York: Social Science Research Council, 1951), pp. 14–15.
8. Williams, *American Society*, pp. 397–470.
9. "Each society has its own characteristic quality, its own *ethos*, that springs . . . particularly from the beliefs and values around which the culture is integrated." John Biesanz and Mavis Biesanz, *Modern Society*, 3rd ed. (Englewood Cliffs, N.J.: Prentice-Hall, 1964).
10. C. Wright Mills, *White Collar* (New York: Oxford University Press, 1957).
11. Don Martindale, *The Nature and Types of Sociological Theory* (Boston: Houghton Mifflin, 1960), pp. 88–89.
12. See, for example, Dorothy Lee, "Are Basic Needs Ultimate?" in *Personality in Nature, Society and Culture*, ed. C. Kluckhohn, H. A. Murray, and D. Schneider, 2nd ed. (New York: Knopf, 1954), pp. 335–341.
13. The complexities of role systems may be suggested by the following questions: By what processes do social systems develop? What properties (such as au-

thority and prestige) do such positions have? What are the intended or unintended consequences of social positions for the social system—and the persons located in them? See, for example, William A. Rushing, *The Psychiatric Professions: Power, Conflict and Adaptation in a Psychiatric Hospital Staff* (Chapel Hill: University of North Carolina Press, 1964).

14. Linton's examination of status and role has become a classic. See Ralph Linton, *The Study of Man* (New York: Appleton-Century, 1936). For more recent studies of status and role, see Bruce J. Biddle and Edwin J. Thomas, eds., *Role Theory: Concepts and Research* (New York: Wiley, 1966).

15. Talcott Parsons, *The Social System* (New York: Free Press, 1951), pp. 39–45.

16. Charles Horton Cooley, *Social Organization* (New York: Scribner's, 1909), pp. 23–31.

17. Ibid., p. 23.

18. The term "secondary group" is sometimes used by sociologists to refer to groups which are not primary in nature.

19. Charles Horton Cooley, *Human Nature and the Social Order* (New York: Scribner's, 1902).

20. Ibid., p. 152.

21. Ibid.

22. Ibid., p. 84.

23. From the pioneering observations and theories of Charles Horton Cooley, George Herbert Mead, and William Isaac Thomas, to the present time, "symbolic interactionism," so-called, remains an important perspective in American sociology. For a basic introduction see Leonard Broom and Philip Selznick, *Sociology: A Text with Adapted Readings*, 4th ed. (New York: Harper & Row, 1968), pp. 90 ff. This tradition of inquiry substantially influenced early psychiatry and remains highly relevant. See Harry Stack Sullivan, *The Interpersonal Theory of Psychiatry*, ed. H. S. Perry and M. L. Gawell (New York: Norton, 1953), p. 16.

24. It has been observed that an individual's behavior and self-evaluations may have reference to groups of which he is not a member. See Herbert H. Hyman and Eleanor Singer, eds., *Readings In Reference Group Theory and Research* (New York: Free Press, 1968).

25. See, for example, Bert N. Adams, *Kinship In An Urban Setting* (Chicago: Markhan, 1968).

26. Clyde C. Kluckhohn, *Mirror For Man* (Greenwich, Conn.: Fawcett, 1949), p. 20.

27. Ibid., p. 21.

28. Due to the influence of Freud, many early studies of "culture and personality" in anthropology centered around the modification of primary drives. See, for example, Kluckhohn, Murray, and Schneider, eds., *Personality in Nature,* and J. Whiting and I. Child, *Child Training and Personality* (New Haven: Yale University Press, 1953).

29. Kluckhohn, *Mirror for Man,* p. 22.

30. For some studies of socialization into professions, see Robert K. Merton, George G. Reader, and Patricia C. Kendall, eds., *The Student-Physician* (Cambridge, Mass.: Harvard University Press, 1957), and Howard S. Becker et al., *Boys In White* (Chicago: University of Chicago Press, 1961).

31. For an excellent examination of correlates of social class, see Broom and Selznick, *Sociology.*

32. For some basic data and concepts relating socioeconomic status to illness and care, see Robert N. Wilson, *The Sociology of Health: An Introduction* (New York: Random House, 1970), pp. 70–110. In the mental health field, August B. Hollingshead and Fredrick C. Redlich, *Social Class and Mental Illness: A Community Study* (New York: Wiley, 1958), was of historic importance in rigorously documenting significant differences in the prevalence of treated psychiatric disturbance as well as patterns of treatment by social class. See also Jerome K. Meyers and Lee L. Bean, *A Decade Later: A Follow-up of Social Class and Mental Illness* (New York: Wiley, 1968), and B. P. Dohrenwend and B. S. Dohrenwend, *Social Status and Psychological Disorder* (New York: Wiley, 1969).

33. See, for example, Karl Marx, "Theory of Social Classes," in *Class, Status and Power,* ed. Reinhard Bendix and Seymour Martin Lipset (New York: Free Press, 1953), pp. 26–35.

34. Max Weber, "Class, Status, Party," in *Class, Status and Power,* ed. Bendix and Lipset, pp. 63–75.

35. Ibid.

36. For a basic introduction to the ways in which socioeconomic status and social classes are defined and measured, see Broom and Selznick, *Sociology,* pp. 153–

177. A more advanced, but highly readable and illustrative, book is Joseph A. Kahl, *The American Class Structure* (New York: Reinhart, 1957). For additional references to the nature and consequences of social stratification, see Bernard Barber, *Social Stratification* (New York: Harcourt, Brace, 1957); Milton M. Gordon, *Social Class In American Sociology* (Durham, N.C.: Duke University Press, 1958); Melvin L. Kohn, *Class and Conformity* (Homewood, Ill.: Dorsey Press, 1969); and Donald G. McKinley, *Social Class and Family Life* (New York: Free Press, 1964).

CHAPTER 5

Culture

INTRODUCTION

Margaret Mead once described Mirror For Man *as "the best contemporary introduction to modern anthropology." While the field has since broadened and deepened substantially, Kluckhohn's discussion of culture remains one of the clearest and most beautifully illustrated articles on that subject. With a master's virtuosity he conducts the reader from simple beginnings to advanced endings, from the conspicuous to the subtle. Along the way he exhibits the varieties, forms, functions, and implications of cultural elements. Beyond mastery, a virtuoso reveals a well-preserved, deep feeling for his subject. Perhaps that is why Kluckhohn's writing has continuing appeal to the scholar as well as to the newly initiated.*

The following excerpt further illustrates and extends our preceding treatment of the subject. As the title of the book implies, he shows how cross-cultural data sharply reveal the differences, similarities, and commonalities of human behavior and groups—much as the study of chemical elements, compounds, and reactions leads to the discovery of underlying principles.

This article considers a number of continuing, critical concerns of the mental health field, including distinguishing biological, psychological, and cultural determinants of behavior; the nature, directions, and weight of these interacting variables; the framework of adaptation and maladaptation; the foundations of emotional reactions and expression; the unconscious character of culture; and the applications of social science.

QUEER CUSTOMS

Clyde C. Kluckhohn

By "culture" anthropology means the total life way of a people, the social legacy the individual acquires from his group. Or culture can be regarded as that part of the environment that is the creation of man.

This technical term has a wider meaning than the "culture" of history and literature. A humble cooking pot is as much a cultural product as is a Beethoven sonata. In ordinary speech a man of culture is a man who can speak lanaguages other than his own, who is familiar with history, literature, philosophy, or the fine arts. In some cliques that definition is still narrower. The cultured person is one who can talk about James Joyce, Scarlatti, and Picasso. To the anthropologist, however, to be human is to be cultured. There is culture in general, and then there are the specific cultures such as Russian, American, British, Hottentot, Inca. The general abstract notion serves to remind us that we cannot explain acts solely in terms of the biological properties of the people concerned, their individual past experience, and the immediate situation. The past experience of other men in the form of culture enters into almost every event. Each specific culture constitutes a kind of blueprint for all of life's activities.

One of the interesting things about human beings is that they try to understand themselves and their own behavior. While this has been particularly true of Europeans in recent times, there is no group which has not developed a scheme or schemes to explain man's actions. To the insistent human query "why?" the most exciting illumination anthropology has to offer is that of the concept of culture. Its explanatory importance is comparable to categories such as evolution in biology, gravity in physics, disease in medicine. A good deal of human behavior can be understood, and indeed predicted, if we know a people's design for living. Many acts are neither accidental nor due to personal peculiarities nor caused by supernatural forces nor simply mysterious. Even those of us who pride ourselves on our individualism follow most of the time a pattern not of our own making. We brush our teeth on arising. We put on pants—not a loincloth or a grass skirt. We eat three meals a day—not four or five or two. We sleep in a bed—not in a hammock or on a sheep pelt. I do not have to know the individual and his life history to be able to predict these and countless other regularities, including many in the thinking process, of all Americans who are not incarcerated in jails or hospitals for the insane.

To the American woman a system of plural wives seems "instinctively" abhorrent. She cannot understand how any woman can fail to be jealous and uncomfortable if she must share her husband with other women. She feels it "unnatural" to accept such a situation. On the other hand, a Koryak woman of Siberia, for example, would find it hard to understand how a woman could be so selfish and so undesirous of feminine companionship in the home as to wish to restrict her husband to one mate.

A highly intelligent teacher with long and successful experience in the public schools of Chicago was finishing her first year in an Indian school. When asked how her Navaho pupils compared in intelligence with Chicago youngsters, she replied, "Well, I just don't know. Sometimes the Indians seem just as bright. At other times they just act like dumb animals. The other night we had a dance in the high school. I saw a boy who is one of the best students in my English class standing off by himself. So I took him over to a pretty girl and told them to dance. But they just stood there with their heads down. They wouldn't even say anything." I inquired if she knew whether or not they were members of the same clan. "What difference would that make?"

"How would you feel about getting into bed with your brother?" The teacher walked off in a huff, but, actually, the two cases were quite comparable in principle. To the Indian the type of bodily contact involved in our social dancing has a directly sexual connotation. The incest taboos between members of the same clan are as severe as between true brothers and sisters. The shame of the Indians at the suggestion that a clan brother and sister should dance and the indignation of the white teacher at the idea that she should share a bed with an adult brother represent equally nonrational responses, culturally standardized unreason.

All this does not mean that there is no such thing as raw human nature. The very fact that certain of the same institutions are found in all known societies indicates that at bottom all human beings are very much alike. The files of the Cross-Cultural Survey at Yale University are organized according to categories such as "marriage ceremonies," "life crisis rites," "incest taboos." At least seventy-five of these categories are represented in every single one of the hundreds of cultures analyzed. This is hardly surprising. The members of all human groups have about the same biological equipment. All men undergo the same poignant life experiences such as birth, helplessness, illness, old age, and death. The biological potentialities of the species are the blocks with which cultures are built. Some patterns of every culture crystallize around focuses provided by the inevitables of biology: the difference between the sexes, the presence of persons of different ages, the varying physical strength and skill of individuals. The facts of nature also limit culture forms. No culture provides patterns for jumping over trees or for eating iron ore.

There is thus no "either-or" between nature and that special form of nurture called culture. Culture determinism is as one-sided as biological determinism. The two factors are interdependent. Culture arises out of human nature, and its forms are restricted both by man's biology and by natural laws. It is equally true that culture channels biological processes—vomiting, weeping, fainting, sneezing, the daily habits of food intake and waste elimination. When a man eats, he is reacting to an internal "drive," namely, hunger contractions consequent upon the lowering of blood sugar, but his precise reaction to these internal stimuli cannot be predicted by physiological knowledge alone. Whether a healthy adult feels hungry twice, three times, or four times a day and the hours at which this feeling recurs is a question of culture. *What* he eats is of course limited by availability, but is also partly regulated by culture. It is a biological fact that some types of berries are poisonous; it is a cultural fact that, a few generations ago, most Americans considered tomatoes to be poisonous and refused to eat them. Such selective, discriminative use of the environment is characteristically cultural. In a still more general sense, too, the process of eating is channeled by culture. Whether a man eats to live, lives to eat, or merely eats and lives is only in part an individual matter, for there are also cultural trends. Emotions are physiological events. Certain situations will evoke fear in people from any culture. But sensations of pleasure, anger, and lust may be stimulated by cultural cues that would leave unmoved someone who has been reared in a different social tradition.

I have said "culture channels biological processes." It is more accurate to say "the biological functioning of individuals is modified if they have been trained in certain ways and not in others." Culture is not a disembodied force. It is created and transmitted by people. However, culture, like well-known concepts of the physical sciences, is a convenient abstraction. One never sees gravity. One sees bodies falling in regular ways. One never sees an electromagnetic field. Yet certain happenings that can be seen may be given a neat abstract formulation by assuming that the electromagnetic field exists. Similarly, one never sees culture as such. What is seen are regularities in the behavior or artifacts of a group that has adhered to a common tradition. The regularities in style and technique of ancient Inca tapestries or stone axes from Melanesian islands are due to the existence of mental blueprints for the group.

Culture is a *way* of thinking, feeling, believing. It is the group's knowledge stored up (in memories of men; in books and objects) for future use. We study the products of this "mental" activity: the overt behavior, the speech and gestures and activities of people, and the tangible results of these things such as tools, houses, cornfields, and what not. It has been customary in lists of "culture traits" to include such things as watches or lawbooks. This is a convenient way of thinking about them, but in the solution of any important problem we must remember that they, in themselves, are nothing but metals, paper, and ink. What is important is that some men know how to make them, others set a value on them, are unhappy without them, direct their activities in relation to them, or disregard them.

"Culture," then, is "a theory." But if a theory is not contradicted

by any relevant fact and if it helps us to understand a mass of otherwise chaotic facts, it is useful. Darwin's contribution was much less the
accumulation of new knowledge than the creation of a theory which
put in order data already known. An accumulation of facts, however
large, is no more a science than a pile of bricks is a house.

A culture constitutes a storehouse of the pooled learning of the
group. A rabbit starts life with some innate responses. He can learn
from his own experience and perhaps from observing other rabbits. A
human infant is born with fewer instincts and greater plasticity. His
main task is to learn the answers that persons he will never see, persons long dead, have worked out. Once he has learned the formulas
supplied by the culture of his group, most of his behavior becomes
almost as automatic and unthinking as if it were instinctive. There is
a tremendous amount of intelligence behind the making of a radio,
but not much is required to learn to turn it on.

The members of all human societies face some of the same unavoidable dilemmas, posed by biology and other facts of the human
situation. This is why the basic categories of all cultures are so similar.
Human culture without language is unthinkable. No culture fails to
provide for aesthetic expression and aesthetic delight. Every culture
supplies standardized orientations toward the deeper problems, such
as death. Every culture is designed to perpetuate the group and its
solidarity, to meet the demands of individuals for an orderly way of
life and for satisfaction of biological needs.

However, the variations on these basic themes are numberless.
Some languages are built up out of twenty basic sounds, others out
of forty. Nose plugs were considered beautiful by the predynastic Egyp-
tians but are not by the modern French. Puberty is a biological fact.
But one culture ignores it, another prescribes informal instructions
about sex but no ceremony, a third has impressive rites for girls only,
a fourth for boys and girls. In this culture, the first menstruation is
welcomed as a happy, natural event; in that culture the atmosphere
is full of dread and supernatural threat.

Every culture must deal with the sexual instinct. Some, however,
seek to deny all sexual expression before marriage, whereas a Polynesian adolescent who was not promiscuous would be distinctly abnormal. Some cultures enforce lifelong monogamy, others, like our own,
tolerate serial monogamy; in still other cultures, two or more women
may be joined to one man or several men to a single woman. Homosexuality has been a permitted pattern in the Greco-Roman world, in
parts of Islam, and in various primitive tribes. Large portions of the
population of Tibet, and of Christendom at some places and periods,
have practiced complete celibacy. To us marriage is first and foremost
an arrangement between two individuals. In many more societies marriage is merely one facet of a complicated set of reciprocities, economic
and otherwise, between two families or two clans.

The essence of the cultural process is selectivity. The selection is
only exceptionally conscious and rational. Cultures are like Topsy.
They just grew. Once, however, a way of handling a situation becomes

institutionalized, there is ordinarily great resistance to chance or deviation. When we speak of "our sacred beliefs," we mean of course that they are beyond criticism and that the person who suggests modification or abandonment must be punished. No person is emotionally indifferent to his culture. Certain cultural premises may become totally out of accord with a new factual situation. Leaders may recognize this and reject the old ways in theory. Yet their emotional loyalty continues in the face of reason because of the intimate conditionings of early childhood.

A culture is learned by individuals as the result of belonging to some particular group, and it constitutes that part of learned behavior which is shared with others. It is our social legacy, as contrasted with our organic heredity. It is one of the important factors which permits us to live together in an organized society, giving us ready-made solutions to our problems, helping us to predict the behavior of others, and permitting others to know what to expect of us.

Culture regulates our lives at every turn. From the moment we are born until we die there is, whether we are conscious of it or not, constant pressure upon us to follow certain types of behavior that other men have created for us. Some paths we follow willingly, others we follow because we know no other way, still others we deviate from or go back to most unwillingly. Mothers of small children know how unnaturally most of this comes to us—how little regard we have, until we are "culturalized," for the "proper" place, time, and manner for certain acts such as eating, excreting, sleeping, getting dirty, and making loud noises. But by more or less adhering to a system of related designs for carrying out all the acts of living, a group of men and women feel themselves linked together by a powerful chain of sentiments. Ruth Benedict gave an almost complete definition of the concept when she said, "Culture is that which binds men together."

It is true any culture is a set of techniques for adjusting both to the external environment and to other men. However, cultures create problems as well as solve them. If the lore of a people states that frogs are dangerous creatures, or that it is not safe to go about at night because of witches or ghosts, threats are posed which do not arise out of the inexorable facts of the external world. Cultures produce needs as well as provide a means of fulfilling them. There exists for every group culturally defined, acquired drives that may be more powerful in ordinary daily life than the biologically inborn drives. Many Americans, for example, will work harder for "success" than they will for sexual satisfaction.

Most groups elaborate certain aspects of their culture far beyond maximum utility or survival value. In other words, not all culture promotes physical survival. At times, indeed, it does exactly the opposite. Aspects of culture which once were adaptive may persist long after they have ceased to be useful. An analysis of any culture will disclose many features which cannot possibly be construed as adaptations to the total environment in which the group now finds itself.

However, it is altogether likely that these apparently useless features represent survivals, with modifications through time, of cultural forms once useful.

Any cultural practice must be functional or it will disappear before long. That is, it must somehow contribute to the survival of the society or to the adjustment of the individual. However, many cultural functions are not manifest but latent. A cowboy will walk three miles to catch a horse which he then rides one mile to the store. From the point of view of manifest function this is positively irrational. But the act has the latent function of maintaining the cowboy's prestige in the terms of his own subculture. One can instance the buttons on the sleeve of a man's coat, our absurd English spelling, the use of capital letters, and a host of other apparently nonfunctional customs. They serve mainly the latent function of assisting individuals to maintain their security by preserving continuity with the past and by making certain sectors of life familiar and predictable.

Culture is like a map. Just as a map isn't the territory but an abstract representation of a particular area, so also a culture is an abstract description of trends toward uniformity in the words, deeds, and artifacts of a human group. If a map is accurate and you can read it, you won't get lost; if you know a culture you will know your way around in the life of a society.

Many educated people have the notion that culture applies only to exotic ways of life or to societies where relative simplicity and relative homogeneity prevail. Some sophisticated missionaries, for example, will use the anthropological conception in discussing the special modes of living of South Sea Islanders, but seem amazed at the idea that it could be applied equally to inhabitants of New York City. And social workers in Boston will talk about the culture of a colorful and well-knit immigrant group but boggle at applying it to the behavior of staff members in the social-service agency itself.

In the primitive society the correspondence between the habits of individuals and the customs of the community is ordinarily greater. There is probably some truth in what an old Indian once said, "In the old days there was no law; everybody did what was right." The primitive tends to find happiness in the fulfillment of intricately involuted cultural patterns; the modern more often tends to feel the pattern as repressive to his individuality. It is also true that in a complex stratified society there are numerous exceptions to generalizations made about the culture as a whole. It is necessary to study regional, class, and occupational subcultures. Primitive cultures have greater stability than modern cultures; they change—but less rapidly.

Every culture has organization as well as content. There is nothing mystical about this statement. One may compare ordinary experience. If I know that Smith, working alone, can shovel 10 cubic yards of dirt a day, Jones 12, and Brown 14, I would be foolish to predict that the three working together would move 36. The total might well be considerably more; it might be less. A whole is different from the sum of its parts. The same principle is familiar in athletic teams. A brilliant pitcher added to a nine may mean a pennant or may mean the cellar; it depends on how he fits in.

And so it is with cultures. A mere list of the behavioral and regulatory patterns and of the implicit themes and categories would be like a map on which all mountains, lakes, and rivers were included—but not in their actual relationship to one another. Two cultures could have almost identical inventories and still be extremely different. The full significance of any single element in a culture design will be seen only when that element is viewed in the total matrix of its relationship to other elements.

Cultures vary greatly in their degree of integration. Synthesis is achieved partly through the overt statement of the dominant conceptions, assumptions, and aspirations of the group in its religious lore, secular thought, and ethical code; partly through habitual but unconscious ways of looking at the stream of events, ways of begging certain questions. To the naïve participant in the culture these modes of categorizing, of dissecting experience along these planes and not others, are as much "given" as the regular sequence of daylight and darkness or the necessity of air, water, and food for life. Had Americans not thought in terms of money and the market system during the depression they would have distributed unsalable goods rather than destroyed them.

Every group's way of life, then, is a structure—not a haphazard collection of all the different physically possible and functionally effective patterns of belief and action. A culture is an interdependent system based upon linked premises and categories whose influence is greater, rather than less, because they are seldom put in words. Some degree of internal coherence which is felt rather than rationally constructed seems to be demanded by most of the participants in any culture. As Whitehead has remarked, "Human life is driven forward by its dim apprehension of notions too general for its existing language."

In sum, the distinctive way of life that is handed down as the social heritage of a people does more than supply a set of skills for making a living and a set of blueprints for human relations. Each different way of life makes its own assumptions about the ends and purposes of human existence, about what human beings have a right to expect from each other and the gods, about what constitutes fulfillment or frustration. Some of these assumptions are made explicit in the lore of the folk; others are tacit premises which the observer must infer by finding consistent trends in word and deed.

COMMENTARY

Since culture is a given, pervasive part of man's environment, Kluckhohn once suggested that man was as likely to discover it as a fish was to discover water. He points to the ways in which culture becomes a part of the individual's psychosomatic organization, shaping his "feelings, thoughts and behavior." The implicit, assumptive, preconscious character of culture raises numerous questions for mental health professionals. It suggests that the clinician may well need to discover the cultural worlds of the patient, himself, and of the treatment system as well if he is to comprehend presenting problems and appropriate intervention approaches. Consider, for example, how the particular cultural systems of physicians, psychiatrists, social workers, or sociologists dispose them to variant perceptions of the patient. Which of these perceptions are correct? How may each be limited, distorted, or biased? To what extent are their perspectives clear and explicit? How are they competing, conflicting, or complementary?

One interesting example of this issue is found in Goffman's Asylums,[1] in which his sociological analysis challenged the prevailing view that the bizarre and exotic behavior of patients was an inherent symptom of schizophrenia. Alternatively, he suggests that much of their behavior represented reactions to the hospital as a sociocultural system. Comparable studies and concepts have been offered by social scientists and mental health professionals alike. Some of them are considered later in this volume.

If culture is deeply embedded in the patient's personality and environment—heavily implicit as well as explicit—how is it implicated in the patient's problems or adaptive strivings? Is the process of psychotherapy a process of self-discovery; of the identification of personality structure; of strengths and weaknesses? Is it a process of sociocultural discovery?

Emotions are key elements in physical and mental health. In what ways are emotional needs and reactions shaped by the particular values and beliefs of a culture? How may a culture influence the experience of sexuality, love, grief, anxiety, fear? How may a culture render emotional needs problematic?

If one allows the importance of sociocultural elements in patient problems, the issue of how one identifies, describes, and analyzes them remains a methodological concern. Simply stated, this is an issue of social diagnosis. How and how well is this being conducted by the various mental health professions or teams?

Just as the sociocultural systems in which patients live may be dysfunctional and irrational, how may this be so in the organization of treatment units? Like the self-discoveries of patients, how does a treatment team gain insight into untoward traditions, beliefs, values, and social organization? Is this achieved by comparison with other units—as in the cross-cultural method? Is it achieved by inviting the observations of outsiders; by social scientists; by community meetings or "group process" sessions? What are the values and limitations of each?

NOTE

1. Erving Goffman, *Asylums* (Garden City, N.Y.: Doubleday, Anchor Books, 1961).

CHAPTER 6

Status and Role

INTRODUCTION

In this paper Levinson examines the concepts of role in fine analytical detail, and with reference to research findings. Underlying his broadly based analysis, with its many important excursions, is a central, unifying preoccupation with the individual and the group. An important extension of our introductory remarks on status and role, it is also a paradigm illustration of what social psychology is all about. This is a notable example of the work of a critical and creative scholar who is sufficiently informed and open to point to the value and limitations of both psychodynamic and sociological approaches, and how they may contribute to each other. It should not be surprising that such an effort is necessarily a bit heavy. Yet because it treats so many important matters as simply and clearly as may be possible, we believe the reader will find a careful reading worth the effort.

Levinson notes that the view that roles are culturally defined *is an oversimplification: (1) it tends to assume that there is widespread consensus; (2) it tends to ignore that fact that role expectations in different groups vary in the degree to which they provide a blueprint for behavior; (3) it does not recognize that roles may have built-in contradictions and ambiguities; (4) it does not recognize that roles may be subject to processes of change; and (5) it does not recognize that there is a dynamic relationship between culturally defined roles and the individuals who are in a position to play them—that the person and the role are subject to mutual influence.*

The traditional concept of role requires refinement in order better to serve our efforts to describe and analyze the complex realities of social and psychological systems. Every science moves from rough to refined approximations. This demands increasingly sharp definitions of key concepts, consistency with new empirical findings, further theoretical specification, and qualification of the conditions under which empirical generalizations hold. A classic, relatively simple example is

Boyle's Law of the inverse relationship between the pressure on gases and their volume. In time this proved to hold true within a certain range of temperatures and with regard to some, but not all, gases.

Levinson shows why it is necessary to distinguish among: (1) organizationally given role demands (culturally and structurally defined roles); (2) personal role conceptions (those of any given individual); and (3) role behavior (the actual behavior of individuals in a given social position). These distinctions facilitate our understanding of the distinct properties of individuals and groups, and their interactional effects.

These distinctions are useful tools for the clinician faced, as it were, with the need for three hands: one to examine the unique constellation of factors which describe his patient; one to consider the patient's psychological processes; and one with which to grasp the dynamics of the social networks of his patient. These tasks not only require three hands, but a nervous system which permits their integration.

ROLE, PERSONALITY, AND SOCIAL STRUCTURE IN THE ORGANIZATIONAL SETTING

Daniel J. Levinson

During the past 20 years the concept of role has achieved wide currency in social psychology, sociology, and anthropology. From a sociopsychological point of view, one of its most alluring qualities is its double reference to the individual and to the collective matrix. The concept of role concerns the thoughts and actions of individuals, and, at the same time, it points up the influence upon the individual of socially patterned demands and standardizing forces. Partly for this reason, "role" has been seen by numerous writers [1] as a crucial concept for the linking of psychology, sociology, and anthropology. However, while the promise has seemed great, the fulfillment has thus far been relatively small. The concept of role remains one of the most overworked and underdeveloped in the social sciences.

My purpose here is to examine role theory primarily as it is used

Daniel J. Levinson, "Role, Personality, and Social Structure in the Organizational Setting," *Journal of Abnormal and Social Psychology* 58, 1959, pp. 170–180. Copyright 1959 by the American Psychological Association and reproduced by permission.

in the analysis of organizations (such as the hospital, business firm, prison, school). The organization provides a singularly useful arena for the development and application of role theory. It is small enough to be amenable to empirical study. Its structure is complex enough to provide a wide variety of social positions and role-standardizing forces. It offers an almost limitless opportunity to observe the individual personality *in vivo* (rather than in the psychologist's usual *vitro* of laboratory, survey questionnaire, or clinical office), selectively utilizing and modifying the demands and opportunities given in the social environment. The study of personality can, I submit, find no setting in which the reciprocal impact of psyche and situation is more clearly or more dramatically evidenced.

Organizational theory and research has traditionally been the province of sociology and related disciplines that focus most directly upon the collective unit. Chief emphasis has accordingly been given to such aspects of the organization as formal and informal structure, administrative policy, allocation of resources, level of output, and the like. Little interest has been shown in the individual member as such or in the relevance of personality for organizational functioning. The prevailing image of the organization has been that of a mechanical apparatus operating impersonally once it is set in motion by administrative edict. The prevailing conception of social role is consonant with this image: the individual member is regarded as a cog in the apparatus, what he thinks and does being determined by requirements in the organizational structure.

This paper has the following aims: (1) to examine the traditional conception of organizational structure and role and to assess its limitations from a sociopsychological point of view; (2) to examine the conception of social role that derives from this approach to social structure and that tends, by definition, to exclude consideration of personality; (3) to provide a formulation of several, analytically distinct, role concepts to be used in place of the global term "role"; and (4) to suggest a theoretical approach to the analysis of relationships among role, personality, and social structure.

Traditional Views of Bureaucratic Structure and Role

Human personality has been virtually excluded from traditional organization theory. Its absence is perhaps most clearly reflected in Weber's [2] theory of bureaucracy, which has become a major source of current thought regarding social organization and social role. I shall examine this theory briefly here, in order to point up some of its psychological limitations but without doing justice to its many virtues. In Weber's writings, the bureaucratic organization is portrayed as a monolithic edifice. Norms are clearly defined and consistently applied, the agencies of role socialization succeed in inducing acceptance of organizational requirements, and the sanctions system provides the constraints and incentives needed to maintain behavioral conformity. Every individual is given a clearly defined role and readily "fills" it. There is little room in this tightly bound universe for more complex choice, for individual creativity, or for social change. As Gouldner has said of the studies carried out in this tradition: "Indeed, the social scene described has sometimes been so completely stripped of people that the impression is unintentionally rendered that there are disembodied social forces afoot, able to realize their ambitions apart from human action." [3]

For Weber, bureaucracy as an ideal type is administered by "experts" in a spirit of impersonal rationality and is operated on a principle of discipline according to which each member performs his required duties as efficiently as possible. Rationality in decision making and obedience in performance are the pivots on which the entire system operates. In this scheme of things, emotion is regarded merely as a hindrance to efficiency, as something to be excluded from the bureaucratic process.

The antipathy to emotion and motivation in Weber's thinking is reflected as well in his formulation of three types of authority: traditional, charismatic, and rational-legal. The rational-legal administrator is the pillar of bureaucracy. He receives his legitimation impersonally, from "the system," by virtue of his *technical* competence. His personal characteristics, his conception of the organization and its component groupings, his modes of relating to other persons (except that he be fair and impartial)—these and other psychological characteristics are not taken into theoretical consideration. There is no place in Weber's ideal type for the ties of affection, the competitive strivings, the subtle forms of support or of intimidation, so commonly found in even the most "rationalized" organizations. It is only the "charismatic" leader who becomes emotionally important to his followers and who must personally validate his right to lead.

While Weber has little to say about the problem of motivation, two motives implicitly become universal instincts in his conception of "bureaucratic man." These are *conformity* (the motive for automatic acceptance of structural norms) and *status seeking* (the desire to advance oneself by the acquisition and exercise of technical competence). More complex motivations and feelings are ignored.

There has been widespread acknowledgment of both the merits and the limitations of Weber's protean thought. However, the relevance of personality for organizational structure and role definition remains a largely neglected problem in contemporary theory and research.[4] Our inadequacies are exemplified in the excellent *Reader in Bureaucracy*, edited by Merton and associates.[5] Although this book contains some of the most distinguished contributions to the field, it has almost nothing on the relation between organizational structure and personality. The editors suggest two lines of interrelation: first, that personality may be one determinant of occupational choice; and second, that a given type of structure may in time modify the personalities of its members. These are valuable hypotheses. However, they do not acknowledge the possibility that personality may have an impact on social structure. "The organization" is projected as an organism that either selects congenial personalities or makes over the recalcitrant ones to suit its own needs. This image is reflected in the editors' remark: "It would seem, therefore, that officials not initially suited to the demands of a bureaucratic position, progressively undergo modifications of personality." [6] In other words, when social structure and personality fail to mesh, it is assumed to be personality alone that gives. Structure is the prime, uncaused, cause.

The impact of organizational structure on personality is indeed a significant problem for study. There is, however, a converse to this. When a member is critical of the organizational structure, he *may* maintain his personal values and traits, and work toward structural change. The manifold impact of personality on organizational structure and role remains to be investigated. To provide a theoretical basis for this type of investigation we need, I believe, to reexamine the concept of a role.

"Social Role" as a Unitary Concept

The concept of role is related to, and must be distinguished from, the concept of social position. A position is an element of organizational autonomy, a location in social space, a category of organizational membership. A role is, so to say, an aspect of organizational physiology; it involves function, adaptation, process. It is meaningful to say that a person "occupies" a social position; but it is inappropriate to say, as many do, that one occupies a role.

There are at least three specific senses in which the term "role" has been used, explicitly or implicitly, by different writers or by the same writer on different occasions.

1. Role may be defined as the *structurally given demands* (norms, expectations, taboos, responsibilities, and the like) associated with a given social position. Role is, in this sense, something outside the given individual, a set of pressures and facilitations that channel, guide, impede, support his functioning in the organization.

2. Role may be defined as the member's *orientation* or *conception* of the part he is to play in the organization. It is, so to say, his inner definition of what someone in his social position is supposed to think and do about it. Mead [7] is probably the main source of this view of social role as an aspect of the person, and it is commonly used in analyses of occupational roles.

3. Role is commonly defined as the *actions* of the individual members—actions seen in terms of their relevance for the social structure (that is, seen in relation to the prevailing norms). In this sense, role refers to the ways in which members of a position act (with or without conscious intention) *in accord with or in violation of a given set of organizational norms*. Here, as in 2, role is defined as a characteristic of the actor rather than of his normative environment.

Many writers use a definition that embraces all of the above meanings without systematic distinction, and then shift, explicitly or implicitly, from one meaning to another. The following are but a few of many possible examples.[8]

Each of the above three meanings of "role" is to be found in the writings of Parsons: (1) "From the point of view of the actor, his role is defined by the normative expectations of the members of the group as formulated in its social traditions";[9] (2) "The role is that organized sector of an actor's orientation which constitutes and defines his participation in an interactive process";[10] and (3) "The status-role [is] the organized subsystem of acts of the actor or actors. . . ."[11]

More often, the term is used in a way that includes all three meanings at once. In this *unitary*, all-embracing conception of role, there is, by assumption, a close fit between behavior and disposition (attitude, value), between societal prescription and individual adaptation. This point of view has its primary source in the writings of Linton, whose formulations of culture, status, and role have had enormous influence. According to Linton,[12] a role "includes the attitudes, values and behavior ascribed by the society to any and all persons occupying this status." In other words, society provides for each status or position a single mold that shapes the beliefs and actions of all its occupants.

Perhaps the most extensive formulation of this approach along sociopsychological lines is given by Newcomb. Following Linton, Newcomb asserts, "Roles thus represent ways of carrying out the function for which positions exist—ways which are generally agreed upon within [the] group."[13] And, "Role is strictly a sociological concept; it purposely ignores individual, psychological facts."[14] Having made this initial commitment to the "sociological" view that individual role activity is a simple mirroring of group norms, Newcomb later attempts to find room for his "psychological" concerns with motivation, meaning, and individual differences. He does this by partially giving up the "unitary" concept of role, and introducing a distinction between "prescribed role" and "role behavior." He avers that prescribed role is a sociological concept, "referring to common factors in the behaviors required,"[15] whereas role behavior is a psychological concept that refers to the activities of a single individual. The implications of this distinction for his earlier general definition of role are left unstated.

Whatever the merits or faults of Newcomb's reformulation, it at least gives conceptual recognition to the possibility that social prescription and individual adaptation may not match. This possibility is virtually excluded in the definition of social role forwarded by Linton and used by so many social scientists. In this respect, though certainly not in all respects, Linton's view is like Weber's: both see individual behavior as predominantly determined by the collective matrix. The matrix is, in the former case, culture, and in the latter, bureaucracy.

In short, the "unitary" conception of role assumes that there is a 1:1 relationship, or at least a *high degree of congruence*, among the three role aspects noted above. In the theory of bureaucratic organization, the rationale for this assumption is somewhat as follows. The organizationally given requirements will be internalized by the members and will thus be mirrored in their role conceptions. People will know, and will want to do, what is expected of them. The agencies of role socialization will succeed except with a deviant minority—who constitute a separate problem for study. Individual action will in turn reflect the structural norms, since the appropriate role conceptions will have been internalized and since the sanctions system rewards normative behavior and punishes deviant behavior. Thus, it is assumed that structural norms, individual role conceptions, and individual role performance are three isomorphic reflections of a single entity: "the" role appropriate to a given organizational position.

It is, no doubt, reasonable to expect some degree of congruence among these aspects of a social role. Certainly, every organization contains numerous mechanisms designed to further such congruence. At the same time, it is a matter of common observation that organizations vary in the degree of their integration; structural demands are often contradictory, lines of authority may be defective, disagreements occur and reverberate at and below the surface of daily operations. To assume that what the organization requires, and what its members actually think and do, comprise a single, unified whole is severely to restrict our comprehension of organizational dynamics and change.

It is my thesis, then, that the unitary conception of social role is unrealistic and theoretically constricting. We should, I believe, eliminate the single term "role" except in the most general sense, i.e., of "role theory" as an overall frame of analysis. Let us, rather, give independent conceptual and empirical status to the above three concepts and others. Let us investigate the relationships of each concept with the others, making no assumptions about the degree of congruence among them. Further, let us investigate their relationships with various other characteristics of the organization and of its individual members. I would suggest that the role concepts be named and defined as follows.

Organizationally Given Role Demands

The role demands are external to the individual whose role is being examined. They are the situational pressures that confront him as the occupant of a given structural position. They have manifold sources: in the official charter and policies of the organization; in the traditions and ideology, explicit as well as implicit, that help to define the organization's purposes and modes of operation; in the views about this position which are held by members of the position (who influence any single member) and by members of the various positions impinging upon this one; and so on.

It is a common assumption that the structural requirements for any position are as a rule defined with a *high degree of explicitness, clarity, and consensus* among all the parties involved. To take the position of hospital nurse as an example: it is assumed that her role requirements will be understood and agreed upon by the hospital administration, the nursing authorities, the physicians, etc. Yet one of the striking research findings in all manner of hospitals is the failure of consensus regarding the proper role of nurse.[16] Similar findings have been obtained in school systems, business firms, and the like.[17]

In attempting to characterize the role requirements for a given position, one must therefore guard against the assumption that they are unified and logically coherent. There may be major differences and even contradictions between official norms, as defined by charter or by administrative authority, and the "informal" norms held by various groupings within the organization. Moreover, within a given-status group, such as the top administrators, there may be several conflicting viewpoints concerning long-range goals, current policies, and specific role requirements. In short, the structural demands themselves are often multiple and disunified. Few are the attempts to investigate the sources of such disunity, to acknowledge its frequency, or to take it into conceptual account in general structural theory.

It is important also to consider the specificity or *narrowness* with which the normative requirements are defined. Norms have an "ought" quality; they confer legitimacy and reward value upon certain modes of action, thought, and emotion, while condemning others. But there are degrees here. Normative evaluations cover a spectrum from "strongly required," through various degrees of qualitative kinds of "acceptable," to more or less stringently tabooed. Organizations differ in the width of the intermediate range on this spectrum. That is, they differ in the number and kinds of adaptation that are normatively acceptable. The wider this range—the less specific the norms—the greater is the area of personal choice for the individual. While the existence of such an intermediate range is generally acknowledged, structural analyses often proceed as though practically all norms were absolute prescriptions or proscriptions allowing few alternatives for individual action.

There are various other normative complexities to be reckoned with. A single set of role norms may be internally contradictory. In the case of the mental hospital nurse, for example, the norm of maintaining an "orderly ward" often conflicts with the norm of encouraging self-expression in patients. The individual nurse then has a range of choice, which may be narrow or wide, in balancing these conflicting requirements. There are also ambiguities in norms, and discrepancies between those held explicitly and those that are less verbalized and perhaps less conscious. These normative complexities permit, and may even induce, significant variations in individual role performance.

The degree of *coherence* among the structurally defined role requirements, the degree of *consensus* with which they are held, and the degree of *individual choice* they allow (the range of acceptable alternatives) are among the most significant properties of any organization.

In some organizations, there is very great coherence of role requirements and a minimum of individual choice. In most cases, however, the
degree of integration within roles and among sets of roles appears to
be more moderate.[18] This structural pattern is of especial interest from
a sociopsychological point of view. To the extent that the requirements
for a given position are ambiguous, contradictory, or otherwise "open,"
the individual members have greater opportunity for selection among
existing norms and for creation of new norms. In this process, personality plays an important part. I shall return to this issue shortly.

While the normative requirements (assigned tasks, rules governing authority-subordinate relationships, demands for work output, and
the like) are of great importance, there are other aspects of the organization that have an impact on the individual member. I shall mention two that are sometimes neglected.

Role facilities. In addition to the demands and obligations imposed upon the individual, we must also take into account the techniques, resources, and conditions of work—the means made available
to him for fulfilling his organizational functions. The introduction of
tranquilizing drugs in the mental hospital, or of automation in industry,
has provided tremendous leverage for change in organizational structure and role definition. The teacher-student ratio, an ecological characteristic of every school, grossly affects the probability that a given
teacher will work creatively with individual students. In other words,
technological and ecological facilities are not merely "tools" by which
norms are met; they are often a crucial basis for the maintenance or
change of an organizational form.

Role dilemmas or problematic issues. In describing the tasks
and rules governing a given organizational position, and the facilities
provided for their realization, we are, as it were, looking at that position from the viewpoint of a higher administrative authority whose
chief concern is "getting the job done." Bureaucracy is often analyzed
from this (usually implicit) viewpoint. What is equally necessary,
though less often done, is to look at the situation of the position-mem-
bers from their own point of view: the meaning it has for them, the
feelings it evokes, the ways in which it is stressful or supporting. From
this sociopsychological perspective, new dimensions of role analysis
emerge. The concept of role dilemma is an example. The usefulness
of this concept stems from the fact that every human situation has its
contradictions and its problematic features. Where such dilemmas
exist, there is no "optimal" mode of adaptation; each mode has its
advantages and its costs. Parsons,[19] in his discussion of "the situation
of the patient," explores some of the dilemmas confronting the ill
person in our society. Erikson and Pine and Levinson [20] have written
about the dilemmas of the mental hospital patient; for example, the
conflicting pressures (from without and from within) toward cure
through self-awareness and toward cure through repressive self-control.
Role dilemmas of the psychiatric resident have been studied by Sharaf
and Levinson.[21] Various studies have described the problems of the
factory foreman caught in the conflicting cross-pressures between the

workers he must supervise and the managers to whom he is responsible. The foreman's situation tends to evoke feelings of social marginality, mixed identifications, and conflicting tendencies to be a good "older brother" with subordinates and an obedient son with higher authority.

Role dilemmas have their sources both in organizational structure and in individual personality. Similarly, both structure and personality influence the varied forms of adaptation that are achieved. The point to be emphasized here is that every social structure confronts its members with adaptive dilemmas. If we are to comprehend this aspect of organizational life, we must conceive of social structure as having intrinsically *psychological* properties, as making complex psychological demands that affect, and are affected by, the personalities of its members.

Personal Role Definition

In the foregoing we have considered the patterning of the environment for an organizational position—the kind of sociopsychological world with which members of the position must deal. Let us turn now to the individual members themselves. Confronted with a complex system of requirements, facilities, and conditions of work, the individual effects his modes of adaptation. I shall use the term "personal role definition" to encompass the individual's adaptation within the organization. This may involve passive "adjustment," active furthering of current role demands, apparent conformity combined with indirect "sabotage," attempts at constructive innovation (revision of own role or of broader structural arrangements), and the like. The personal role definition may thus have varying degrees of fit with the role requirements. It may serve in various ways to maintain or to change the social structure. It may involve a high or a low degree of self-commitment and personal involvement on the part of the individual.[22]

For certain purposes, it is helpful to make a sharp distinction between two levels of adaptation: at a more *ideational* level, we may speak of a role conception; at a more *behavioral* level, there is a pattern of role performance. Each of these has an affective component. Role conception and role performance are independent though related variables; let us consider them in turn.

Individual (and modal) role conceptions. The nature of a role conception may perhaps be clarified by placing it in relation to an ideology. The boundary between the two is certainly not a sharp one. However, ideology refers most directly to an orientation regarding the entire organizational (or other) structure—its purposes, its modes of operation, the prevailing forms of individual and group relationships, and so on. A role conception offers a definition and rationale for one position within the structure. If ideology portrays and rationalizes the organizational world, then role conception delineates the specific functions, values, and manner of functioning appropriate to one position within it.

The degree of uniformity or variability in individual role conceptions within a given position will presumably vary from one organization to another. When one or more types of role conception are commonly held (consensual), we may speak of modal types. The maintenance of structural stability requires that there be at least moderate consensus and that modal role conceptions be reasonably congruent with role requirements. At the same time, the presence of incongruent modal role conceptions may, under certain conditions, provide an ideational basis for major organizational change.

Starting with the primary assumption that each member "takes over" a structurally defined role, many social scientists tend to assume that there is great uniformity in role conception among the members of a given social position. They hold, in other words, that for every position there is a *dominant, modal role conception corresponding to the structural demands,* and that there is relatively little individual deviation from the modal pattern. Although this state of affairs may at times obtain, we know that the members of a given social position often have quite diverse conceptions of their proper roles.[23] After all, individual role conceptions are formed only partially within the present organizational setting. The individual's ideas about his occupational role are influenced by childhood experiences, by his values and other personality characteristics, by formal education and apprenticeship, and the like. The ideas of various potential reference groups within and outside of the organization are available through reading, informal contacts, etc. There is reason to expect, then, that the role conceptions of individuals in a given organizational position will vary and will not always conform to official role requirements. Both the diversities and the modal patterns must be considered in organizational analysis.

Individual (and modal) role performance. This term refers to the overt behavioral aspect of role definition—to the more or less characteristic ways in which the individual acts as the occupant of a social position. Because role performance involves immediately observable behavior, its description would seem to present few systematic problems. However, the formulation of adequate variables for the analysis of role performance is in fact a major theoretical problem and one of the great stumbling blocks in empirical research.

Everyone would agree, I suppose, that role performance concerns only those aspects of the total stream of behavior that are structurally relevant. But which aspects of behavior are the important ones? And where shall the boundary be drawn between that which is structurally relevant and that which is incidental or idiosyncratic?

One's answer to these questions probably depends, above all, upon his conception of social structure. Those who conceive of social structure rather narrowly, in terms of concrete work tasks and normative requirements, are inclined to take a similarly narrow view of role. In this view role performance is simply the fulfillment of formal role norms, and anything else the person does is extraneous to role performance as such. Its proponents acknowledge that there are variations in "style" of performance but regard these as incidental. What is essential to *role* performance is the degree to which norms are met.

A more complex and inclusive conception of social structure requires correspondingly multidimensional delineation of role performance. An organization has, from this viewpoint, "latent" as well as "manifest" structure; it has a many-faceted emotional climate; it tends to "demand" varied forms of interpersonal allegiance, friendship, deference, intimidation, ingratiation, rivalry, and the like. If characteracteristics such as these are considered intrinsic properties of social structure, then they must be included in the characterization of role performance. My own preference is for the more inclusive view. I regard social structure as having psychological as well as other properties, and I regard as intrinsic to role performance the varied meanings and feelings which the actor communicates to those about him. Ultimately, we must learn to characterize organizational behavior in a way that takes into account, and helps to illuminate, its functions for the individual, for the others with whom he interacts, and for the organization.

It is commonly assumed that there is great uniformity in role performance among the members of a given position. Or, in other words, that there is *a dominant, modal pattern of role performance corresponding to the structural requirements*. The rationale here parallels that given above for role conceptions. However, where individual variations in patterns of role performance have been investigated, several modal types rather than a single dominant pattern were found.[24]

Nor is this variability surprising, except to those who have the most simplistic conception of social life. Role performance, like any form of human behavior, is the resultant of many forces. Some of these forces derive from the organizational matrix; for example, from role demands and the pressures of authority, from informal group influences, and from impending sanctions. Other determinants lie within the person, as for example his role conceptions and role-relevant personality characteristics. Except in unusual cases where all forces operate to channel behavior in the same direction, role performance will reflect the individual's attempts at choice and compromise among diverse external and internal forces.

The relative contributions of various forms of influence to individual or modal role performance can be determined only *if each set of variables is defined and measured independently of the others*. That is, indeed, one of the major reasons for emphasizing and sharpening the distinctions among role performance, role conception, and role demands. Where these distinctions are not sharply drawn, there is a tendency to study one element and to assume that the others are in close fit. For example, one may learn from the official charter and the administrative authorities how the organization is supposed to work —the formal requirements—and then assume that it in fact operates in this way. Or, conversely, one may observe various regularities in role performance and then assume that these are structurally determined, without independently assessing the structural requirements. To do this is to make structural explanations purely tautologous.

More careful distinction among these aspects of social structure and role will also, I believe, permit greater use of personality theory in organizational analysis. Let us turn briefly to this question.

Role Definition, Personality, and Social Structure

Just as social structure presents massive forces which influence the individual from without toward certain forms of adaptation, so does personality present massive forces from within which lead him to select, create, and synthesize certain forms of adaptation rather than others. Role definition may be seen from one perspective as an aspect of personality. It represents the individual's attempt to structure his social reality, to define his place within it, and to guide his search for meaning and gratification. Role definition is, in this sense, an *ego achievement*—a reflection of the person's capacity to resolve conflicting demands, to utilize existing opportunities and create new ones, to find some balance between stability and change, conformity and autonomy, the ideal and the feasible, in a complex environment.

The formation of a role-definition is, from a dynamic psychological point of view, an "external function" of the ego. Like the other external (reality-oriented) ego functions, it is influenced by the ways in which the ego carries out its "internal functions" of coping with, and attempting to synthesize, the demands of id, superego, and ego. These internal activities—the "psychodynamics" of personality—include among other things: unconscious fantasies; unconscious moral conceptions and the wishes against which they are directed; the characteristic ways in which unconscious processes are transformed or deflected in more conscious thought, feeling, and behavioral striving; conceptions of self and ways of maintaining or changing these conceptions in the face of changing pressures from within and from the external world.

In viewing role definition as an aspect of personality, I am suggesting that it is, *to varying degrees*, related to and imbedded within other aspects of personality. An individual's conception of his role in a particular organization is to be seen within a series of wider psychological contexts: his conception of his occupational role generally (occupational identity), his basic values, life-goals, and conception of self (ego identity), and so on. Thus, one's way of relating to authorities in the organization depends in part upon his relation to authority in general, and upon his fantasies, conscious as well as unconscious, about the "good" and the "bad" parental authority. His ways of dealing with the stressful aspects of organizational life are influenced by the impulses, anxieties, and modes of defense that these stresses activate in him.[25]

There are variations in the degree to which personal role definition is imbedded in, and influenced by, deeper-lying personality characteristics. The importance of individual or modal personality for role definition is a matter for empirical study and cannot be settled by casual assumption. Traditional sociological theory can be criticized for assuming that individual role definition is determined almost entirely by social structure. Similarly, dynamic personality theory will not take its rightful place as a crucial element of social psychology until it views the individual within his sociocultural environment. Lacking an adequate recognition and *conceptualization* of the individual's external reality—including the "reality" of social structure—personality researchers tend to assume that individual adaptation is primarily personality-determined and that reality is, for the most part, an amorphous blob structured by the individual to suit his inner needs.

Clearly, individual role conception and role performance do not emanate, fully formed, from the depths of personality. Nor are they simply mirror images of a mold established by social structure. Elsewhere [26] I have used the term "mirage" theory for the view, frequently held or implied in the psychoanalytic literature, that ideologies, role conceptions, and behavior are mere epiphenomena or by-products of unconscious fantasies and defenses. Similarly, the term "sponge" theory characterizes the view, commonly forwarded in the sociological literature, in which man is merely a passive mechanical absorber of the prevailing structural demands.

Our understanding of personal role definition will remain seriously impaired as long as we fail to place it, analytically, in *both intrapersonal and structural-environmental contexts*. That is to say, we must be concerned with the meaning of role definition both for the individual personality and for the social system. A given role definition is influenced by, and has an influence upon, the *psyche* as well as the *socius*. If we are adequately to understand the nature, the determinants, and the consequences of role definition, we need the double perspective of personality and social structure. The use of these two reference points is, like the use of our two eyes in seeing, necessary for the achievement of depth in our social vision.

Theory and research on organizational roles must consider relationships among at least the following sets of characteristics: structurally given role demands and opportunities, personal role definition (including conceptions and performance), and personality in its role-related aspects. Many forms of relationship may exist among them. I shall mention only a few hypothetical possibilities.

In one type case, the role requirements are so narrowly defined, and the mechanisms of social control so powerful, that only one form of role performance can be sustained for any given position. An organization of this type may be able selectively to recruit and retain only individuals who, by virtue of personality, find this system meaningful and gratifying. If a congruent modal personality is achieved, a highly integrated and stable structure may well emerge. I would hypothesize that a structurally congruent modal personality is one condition, though by no means the only one, for the stability of a rigidly integrated system. (In modern times, of course, the rapidity of technological change prevents long-term stability in any organizational structure.)

However, an organization of this kind may acquire members who are not initially receptive to the structural order, that is, who are *incongruent* in role conception or in personality. Here, several alternative developments are possible.

1. The "incongruent" members may change so that their role conceptions and personalities come better to fit the structural requirements.
2. The incongruent ones may leave the organization, by choice or by expulsion. The high turnover in most of our organizations is due less to technical incompetence than to rejection of the "conditions of life" in the organization.
3. The incongruent ones may remain, but in a state of apathetic conformity. In this case, the person meets at least the minimal requirements of role performance but his role conceptions continue relatively unchanged, he gets little satisfaction from work, and he engages in repeated "sabotage" of organizational aims. This is an uncomfortably frequent occurence in our society. In the Soviet Union as well, even after 40 years of enveloping social controls, there exist structurally incongruent forms of political ideology, occupational role definition, and personality.[27]
4. The incongruent members may gain sufficient social power to change the organizational structure. This phenomenon is well known, though not well enough understood. For example, in certain of our mental hospitals, schools, and prisons over the past 20–30 years, individuals with new ideas and personal characteristics have entered in large enough numbers, and in sufficiently strategic positions, to effect major structural changes. Similar ideological and structural transitions are evident in other types of organization, such as corporate business.

The foregoing are a few of many possible developments in a relatively monolithic structure. A somewhat looser organizational pattern is perhaps more commonly found. In this setting, structural change becomes a valued aim and innovation is seen as a legitimate function of members at various levels in the organization. To the extent that diversity and innovation are valued (rather than merely given lipservice), variations in individual role definition are tolerated or even encouraged within relatively wide limits. The role definitions that develop will reflect various degrees of synthesis and compromise between personal preference and structural demand.

In summary, I have suggested that a primary distinction be made between the structurally given role demands and the forms of role definition achieved by the individual members of an organization. Personal role definition then becomes a linking concept between personality and social structure. It can be seen as a reflection of those aspects of individual personality that are activated and sustained in a given structural-ecological environment. This view is opposed both to the "sociologizing" of individual behavior and to the "psychologizing" of organizational structure. At the same time, it is concerned with both the psychological properties of social structure and the structural properties of individual adaptation.

Finally, we should keep in mind that both personality structure and social structure inevitably have their internal contradictions. No individual is sufficiently all of a piece that he will for long find any form of adaptation, occupational or otherwise, totally satisfying. Whatever the psychic gains stemming from a particular role definition and social structure, there will also be losses: wishes that must be renounced or made unconscious, values that must be compromised, anxieties to be handled, personal goals that will at best be incompletely met. The organization has equivalent limitations. Its multiple purposes cannot all be optimally achieved. It faces recurrent dilemmas over conflicting requirements: control and freedom; centralization and decentralization of authority; security as against the risk of failure; specialization and diffusion of work function; stability and change; collective unity and diversity. Dilemmas such as these arise anew in different forms at each new step of organizational development, without permanent solution. And perpetual changes in technology, in scientific understanding, in material resources, in the demands and capacities of its members and the surrounding community, present new issues and require continuing organizational readjustment.

In short, every individual and every sociocultural form contains within itself the seeds of its own destruction—or its own reconstruction. To grasp both the sources of stability and the seeds of change in human affairs is one of the great challenges to contemporary social science.

NOTES

1. H. H. Gerth and C. W. Mills, *Character and Social Structure* (New York: Harcourt, Brace, 1953); N. Gross, W. S. Mason, and A. W. McEachern, *Explorations in Role Analysis* (New York: Wiley, 1958); E. L. Hartley and Ruth E. Hartley, *Fundamentals of Social Psychology* (New York: Knopf, 1952); R. Linton, *The Cultural Background of Personality* (New York: Appleton-Century-Crofts, 1945); G. H. Mead, *Mind, Self, and Society* (Chicago: University of Chicago Press, 1934); R. K. Merton, *Social Theory and Social Structure*, rev. ed. (New York: Free Press, 1957); T. Parsons, *The Social System* (New York: Free Press, 1951); and T. R. Sarbin, "Role Theory," in *Handbook of Social Psychology*, ed. G. Lindzey (Cambridge, Mass.: Addison-Wesley, 1954), 1:223–258.

2. M. Weber, *Essays in Sociology*, ed. H. H. Gerth and C. W. Mills (New York: Oxford University Press, 1946), and idem, *The Theory of Social and Economic Organization*, ed. T. Parsons (New York: Oxford University Press, 1947).

3. A. W. Gouldner, *Patterns of Industrial Bureaucracy* (New York: Free Press, 1954), p. 16.

4. Contemporary organization has benefited from criticisms and reformulations of Weber's theory by such writers as C. I. Barnard, *The Functions of the Executive* (Cambridge, Mass.: Harvard University Press, 1938); C. J. Friedrich, *Constitutional Government and Democracy* (Boston: Little, Brown, 1950); Gerth and Mills, *Character and Social Structure*; Gouldner, *Patterns of Industrial Bureaucracy*; Merton, *Social Theory*; and T. Parsons, Introduction to Weber, *Theory of Social and Economic Organization*. P. Selznick, *Leadership in Administration* (Evanston, Ill.:

Row, Peterson, 1957), has recently presented a conception of the administrative-managerial role that allows more room for psychological influences, but these are not explicitly conceptualized. There is growing though still inconclusive evidence from research on "culture and personality" work (A. Inkeles and D. J. Levinson, "National Character: The Study of Modal Personality and Socio-Cultural Systems," in *Handbook of Social Psychology*, ed. Lindzey, 2:977–1020) that social structures of various types both "require" and are influenced by modal personality, but this approach has received little application in research on organizations. An attempt at a distinctively sociopsychological approach, and a comprehensive view of the relevant literature, is presented by C. Argyris, *Personality and Organization* (New York: Harper, 1957).

5. R. K. Merton et al., *Reader in Bureaucracy* (New York: Free Press, 1957).

6. Ibid., p. 352.

7. Mead, *Mind, Self, and Society*.

8. An argument very similar to the one made here is presented by Gross, Mason, and McEachern, *Explorations in Role Analysis*, in a comprehensive overview and critique of role theory. They point up the assumption of high consensus regarding role demands and role conceptions in traditional role theory, and present empirical evidence contradicting this assumption. Their analysis is, however, less concerned than the present one with the converging of role theory and personality theory.

9. T. Parsons, *Essays in Sociological Theory*, rev. ed. (New York: Free Press, 1945), p. 230.

10. T. Parsons and E. A. Shils, eds., *Toward a General Theory of Action* (Cambridge, Mass.: Harvard University Press, 1951), p. 23.

11. Parsons, *Social System*, p. 26.

12. Linton, *Cultural Background*.

13. T. M. Newcomb, *Social Psychology* (New York: Dryden, 1950), p. 281.

14. Ibid., p. 329.

15. Ibid., p. 459.

16. See, for example, T. Burling, Edith Lentz, and R. N. Wilson, *The Give and Take in Hospitals* (New York: Putnam's, 1956), and C. Argyris, *Human Relations in a Hospital* (New Haven: Labor and Management Center, 1955).

17. See, for example, Gross, Mason, and McEachern, *Explorations in Role Analysis*, and A. Kornhauser, R. Dubin, and A. M. Ross, *Industrial Conflict* (New York: McGraw-Hill, 1954).

18. The reduced integration reflects in part the tremendous rate of technological change, the geographical and occupational mobility, and the diversity in personality that characterize modern society. On the other hand, diversity is opposed by the standardization of culture on a mass basis and by the growth of large-scale organization itself. Trends toward increased standardization and uniformity are highlighted in the analysis in W. F. Whyte, *The Organization Man* (New York: Simon and Schuster, 1956).

19. Parsons, *Social System*.

20. K. T. Erikson, "Patient Role and Social Uncertainty: A Dilemma of the Mentally Ill," *Psychiatry* 20 (1957):263–274; and F. Pine and D. J. Levinson, "Problematic Issues in the Role of Mental Hospital Patient," mimeographed (Center for Sociopsychological Research, Massachusetts Mental Health Center, 1958).

21. M. R. Sharaf and D. J. Levinson, "Patterns of Ideology and Role Definition Among Psychiatric Residents," in *The Patient and the Mental Hospital*, ed. M. Greenblatt, D. J. Levinson, and R. H. Williams (New York: Free Press, 1957), pp. 263–285.

22. Selznick, *Leadership in Administration*.

23. Greenblatt, Levinson, and Williamson, eds., *Patient and the Mental Hospital*; Gross, Mason, and McEachern, *Explorations in Role Analysis*; L. Reissman and J. J. Rohrer, eds., *Change and Dilemma in the Nursing Profession* (New York: Putnam's, 1957); and R. Bendix, *Work and Authority in Industry* (New York: Wiley, 1956).

24. Argyris, *Personality and Organization*, and Greenblatt, Levinson, and Williams, eds., *Patient and the Mental Hospital*.

25. Argyris, *Personality and Organization*; E. H. Erikson, *Childhood and Society* (New York: Norton, 1950); W. E. Henry, "The Business Executive: The Psychodynamics of a Social Role," *American Journal of Sociology* 54 (1949):286–291; F. H. Blum, *Toward a Democratic Work Process* (New York: Harper, 1933); and F. Pine and D. J. Levinson, "Two Patterns of Ideology, Role Conception, and Personality Among Mental Hospital Aides," in *Patient and the Mental Hospital*, ed. Greenblatt, Levinson, and Williams, pp. 209–218.

26. D. J. Levinson, "Idea Systems in the Individual and Society" (Paper presented at Boston University, Founder's Day Institute, 1954), mimeographed (Center for Sociopsychological Research, Massachusetts Mental Health Center, 1954).

27. A. Inkeles, Eugenia Hanfmann, and Helen Beier, "Modal Personality and Adjustment to the Soviet Political System," *Human Relations* 11 (1958): 3–22.

COMMENTARY

If Levinson's convictions are correct, the organizational context offers the mental health professional a uniquely revealing laboratory in which to sharpen his thinking about personality and role systems. The challenge should be compelling to the likes of psychiatric residents, nurses, social workers, and psychologists for several reasons:

1. Feasibility. *The organizational context of hospital, ward, or team is one in which the professional regularly spends numerous hours of activity.*
2. Tangibility. *With his vital self-concerns as a reference, the professional may scrutinize vividly and concretely his experiences in the organizational settings in terms of the concepts suggested. This will give them further concreteness and clarity.*
3. Relevance. *The professional's ability to comprehend "self" and "society" in the organizational setting is tied to his ability to fulfill personal goals, achieve mastery and personal growth, and comprehend and influence the role system of the setting. Understanding and influencing patient behavior is an additional incentive.*
4. Confirmability. *Professionals may "test" Levinson's formulations, although not necessarily in a strict "experimental" sense, by judging their ability to: (1) reveal, clarify, organize, and "explain" behavior; (2) predict behavior; and (3) achieve desired outcomes in deliberately conceived social strategies to meet organization goals.*
5. Mastery. *As in the learning of other ideas or information, the professional may be rewarded by the extent to which increased understanding of these formulations help him to achieve his goals more effectively and extend his personal competence.*

By illustrating these somewhat abstractly stated potentialities, we may perhaps appreciate Levinson's paper more clearly. Is it possible, for example, for a psychiatric resident to identify the "organizationally given role expectations" incumbent upon him? What consensus about the roles of the resident will he find among his peers, faculty, or co-workers? In what ways are the expectations of authorities consonant with his personal role conceptions? Are they sources of conflict, anxiety, frustration, or fulfillment? Are they appropriate to his knowledge, skill, ability, or personality traits?

In what ways may a professional's experience of conflict with faculty, supervisors, or other professionals be attributed to personality clashes, conflicting roles, or variant role expectations? Is it possible to correlate conflicting role conceptions with patient disturbances or problems in patient care? Does role standardization result in alienation or frustration due to individual differences in aptitude or career goals?

If a patient's symptomatology is expressed in terms of depression, inadequate self-esteem, or uncertain identity, how are such traits ex-

hibited by psychologists, social workers, or mental health professionals in the organizational setting? In what ways may they be attributed to personality or to organizationally given role expectations or role conceptions?

Such questions are implied by Levinson's probes and concepts. It is to be hoped that mental health professionals will be sufficiently stimulated by their suggestiveness and import to bring them to the examination of their organizational settings. As in preceding topics, there are also studies in this area, some of which are presented in Part II.

CHAPTER 7

Primary Groups

INTRODUCTION

This study of the influence of Allied propoganda exposes dramatically the role of the primary group in contributing to the maintenance of high morale, commitment, and combat effectiveness of the German soldiers during World War II. Contrary to popular opinion, the researchers discovered that commitment to a "cause" or to Nazi ideology generally characterized only a small minority of German soldiers. Apathy and ignorance about the course of the war was characteristic of the majority.

Paradoxically, the average soldier showed an intense identification with, and personal devotion to, Adolph Hitler. Apparently their identification with the Führer was not as an ideological and political symbol, but as a vicarious mechanism for achieving strength, protection, and reassurance.

The soldier's loyalty and devotion was most significantly attached to his immediate combat unit, with whom he shared a high degree of intimacy, a community of experience, and day-to-day interaction and interdependence. Reciprocally, he drew support from his group.

Recognizing the role of these factors in promoting solidarity and morale, the military leadership attempted by every possible means to keep units intact. As the war advanced, a number of factors served to break down these established groupings; desertion and defection, which had theretofore been rare even under conditions of severe casualties and setbacks, began to occur in growing numbers.

PRIMARY GROUPS IN THE GERMAN ARMY

Edward A. Shils and Morris Janowitz

This study was carried out by the intelligence unit of a Psychological Warfare Division. It analyzes the relative influence of primary and secondary group situations on the high degree of stability of the German Army in World War II. It also evaluates the impact of the Western Allies' propaganda on the German Army's fighting effectiveness.

Methods of collecting data included front-line interrogation of prisoners of war, intensive psychological interviews in rear areas, and a monthly opinion poll of random samples of prisoners of war. Captured enemy documents, statements of recaptured Allied personnel, and the reports of combat observers were also analyzed.

Although outnumbered and inferior in equipment, the German Army maintained its integrity and fighting effectiveness through a series of almost unbroken retreats over a period of several years. Disintegration through desertion was insignificant, and the active surrender of individuals or groups remained rare throughout the Western campaign.

The extraordinary tenacity of the German Army has frequently been attributed to the strong Nazi political convictions of German soldiers. It is the main hypothesis of this paper, however, that the unity of the German Army was sustained only slightly by the political convictions of its members, and that the determined resistance of the German soldier was due to the steady satisfaction of his *primary* personality needs.

The Military Primary Group

Modern social research has shown that the primary group, the chief source of affection and accordingly the major factor in personality formation in infancy and childhood, continues to be a major social and psychological support through adulthood. In the army, when isolated from civilian primary groups, the soldier depends more and more on his military group. His spontaneous loyalties are to the members of his immediate unit whom he sees daily and with whom he develops a high degree of intimacy.

A German sergeant, captured toward the end of World War II, was asked by his interrogators about the political opinions of his men. In reply, he laughed and said, "When you ask such a question, I realize well that you have no idea of what makes a soldier fight. The soldiers live in their holes and are happy if they live through the next day. If we think at all, it's about the end of the war and then home."

The combat effectiveness of the majority of soldiers depends only to a small extent on their preoccupation with the major political issues which might be affected by the outcome of the war and which are of concern to statesmen and publicists. There are, of course, soldiers to whom such motivations are important. Volunteer armies recruited on the basis of ethical or political loyalties, such as the International Brigade in the Spanish Civil War, are influenced by major political goals. In the German Army, a "hard core" of Nazis was similarly motivated.

In a conscript army, the criteria of recruitment are much less specialized, and the army is more nearly representative of the total population. Political or social values and ethical schemes do not have much impact on the determination of such soldiers to fight to the best of their ability and to hold out as long as possible. For the ordinary German soldier the decisive fact was that he was a member of a squad or section that maintained its structural integrity and coincided roughly with the *social* unit which satisfied some of his major primary needs. If he had the necessary weapons, he was likely to go on fighting as long as the group had a leadership with which he could identify and as long as he gave affection to and received affection from the other members of his squad and platoon. In other words, as long as he felt himself to be a member of his primary group and therefore bound by the expectations and demands of its other members, he was likely to be a good soldier.

Weakness of Secondary Symbols

Problems and symbols remote from immediate personal experience had relatively little influence on the behavior and attention of the German soldier. Interrogation of prisoners showed that they had little interest in the strategic aspects of the war. There was widespread ignorance and apathy about the course of the fighting. Three weeks after the fall of the city of Aachen, many prisoners who were taken in the adjoining area did not know that the city had fallen. For at least a week after the beginning of the Battle of the Bulge—an important German counter-offensive toward the end of the war—most of the troops on the northern hinge of the bulge did not know that the offensive was taking place and were not much interested when they were told of it after their capture.

Neither did expectations about the outcome of the war play a great role in the integration or disintegration of the German Army. The statistics of German soldier opinion show that pessimism about the outcome of the war was compatible with excellent combat performance. The relatively greater importance of considerations of self-preservation is shown by German prisoner recall of the contents of Allied propaganda leaflets (Table 1). During December 1944 and Jan-

TABLE 1
Allied Leaflet Propaganda Themes Remembered by German Prisoners of War

	Dec. 15–31 1944	Jan. 1–15 1945	Jan. 15–31 1945	Feb. 1–15 1945
Number of Ps/W	60	83	99	135
Themes and appeals remembered:				
a. Promise of good treatment as Ps/W and self-preservation through surrender	63%	65%	59%	76%
b. Military news	15	17	19	30
c. Strategic hopelessness of Germany's position	13	12	25	26
d. Hopelessness of a local tactical position	3	1	7	7
e. Political attacks on German leaders	7	5	4	8
f. Bombing of German cities	2	8	6	—
g. Allied Military Government	7	3	—	—
h. Appeals to civilians	5	4	2	—
	*	*	*	*

* The percentages add up to more than 100 percent since some Ps/W remembered more than one topic. Only Ps/W remembering at least one theme were included in this tabulation.

uary 1945, more than 60 percent of the sample of prisoners taken recalled references to the preservation of the individual, and the figure rose to 76 percent in February of 1945. On the other hand, the proportion of prisoners recalling references to the total strategic situation of the war and the prospect of the outcome of the war seldom amounted to more than 20 percent, while references to political subjects never amounted to more than 10 percent. The general tendency was not to think about the outcome of the war unless forced to do so by direct interrogation. Pessimism was counterbalanced by reassuring identification with a strong and benevolent *Führer*, by identification with good officers, and by the psychological support of a closely integrated primary group.

Ethical aspects of the war did not trouble the German soldier much. When pressed by Allied interrogators, the prisoners said that

Germany was forced to fight for its life. There were very few German soldiers who said that Germany had been morally wrong to attack Poland or Russia. Most of them thought that if anything was wrong about the war, it was in the realm of technical decisions. The decision to exterminate the Jews was bad not because of its immorality, but because it united the world against Germany. The declaration of war against the Soviet Union was wrong only because it created a two-front war. But these were all arguments which had to be forced from the prisoners of war; left to themselves, they seldom mentioned them.

The "hard-core" minority of fervent Nazis expressed strong political views. But National Socialism was of little interest to most of the German soldiers. "Nazism," said a soldier, "begins ten miles behind the front lines."

The soldiers did not react noticeably to attempts to Nazify the army. When the Nazi party salute was introduced in 1944, it was accepted as just one more army order, about equal in significance to an order requiring the carrying of gas masks. The *Nationalsozialistische Führungsoffizier* (Nazi indoctrination officer), known as the NSFO, was regarded apathetically or as a joke. The NSFO was rejected not for his Nazi connection but because he was an "outsider" who was not a real soldier. The highly Nazified Waffen SS divisions were never the object of ordinary soldiers' hostility, even when they were charged with atrocities. On the contrary, the Waffen SS was esteemed, not as a Nazi formation, but for its excellent fighting capacity. Wehrmacht soldiers felt safer when there was a Waffen SS unit on their flank.

In contrast to the apolitical attitude of the German infantry soldier toward most secondary symbols, an intense and personal devotion to Adolph Hitler was maintained throughout the war. There is little doubt that identification with the *Führer* was an important factor in prolonging German resistance. Despite fluctuations in expectations regarding the outcome of the war, the trust in Hitler remained strong even after the beginning of the serious reverses in France and Germany. The attachment grew in large part from the feeling of strength and protection the soldier gained from his conception of the *Führer* personality.

However, as defeat became imminent, and the danger to physical survival increased, devotion to Hitler deteriorated. The tendency to attribute virtue to the strong and immorality to the weak boomeranged, and devotion to Hitler declined. Moreover, for most of the disheveled, dirty, bewildered prisoners, Hitler was of slight importance compared with their own survival problems and the welfare of their families.

Impact of Allied Propaganda

A monthly opinion poll of German prisoners found there was no significant decline in attachment to Nazi ideology until February and

March 1945, shortly before the German surrender in May 1945. In other words, the propaganda attacks on Nazi ideology seem to have been of little avail until the smaller military units began to break up under heavy pressure. Much effort was devoted to ideological attacks on German leaders but only about 5 percent of the prisoners mentioned this topic, confirming the general failure of ideological appeals. Allied propaganda presentations of the justness of our war aims, postwar peace intentions, and United Nations unity were all ineffective.

Promises of good treatment as prisoners of war gained most attention and were best remembered. In other words, the best propaganda referred to immediate situations and concrete problems. The most effective single leaflet in communicating the promise of good treatment was the "safe conduct pass." It was usually printed on the back of leaflets which stressed self-preservation. The rank and file were attracted by its official language and legal, document-like character. Where General Eisenhower's signature did not appear on the leaflet, doubt was cast on its authenticity.

As a result of psychological warfare research, a series of leaflets was prepared which aimed at primary group organization in the German Army and omitted reference to ideological symbols. Group organization depended on the acceptance of the immediate leadership and mutual trust. Therefore, this series of leaflets tried to stimulate group discussion and to bring attention to concerns which would loosen solidarity. One leaflet declared, "Do not take our [the Allies'] word for it; ask your comrade; find out how he feels." There followed a series of questions on personal concerns, family problems, the immediate tactical situation, and supply problems. Discussion of these problems was expected to increase anxiety.

Factors Affecting Primary Group Cohesion

If the primary group was a crucial element in the German Army, it is important to know what factors strengthened or weakened primary group cohesion.

1. *The "hard core."* The stability and effectiveness of the military primary group depended in large measure on the Nazi "hard core," who approximated 10 to 15 percent of the total of enlisted men; the percentage was higher for noncommissioned officers and was very much higher among the junior officers. Most of these were young men between twenty-four and twenty-eight years of age who as adolescents were imbued with the Nazi ideology during its zenith. They were enthusiasts for the military life. The presence in the group of a few such men, zealous, energetic, and unsparing of themselves, provided models for the weaker men, and their threats served to check divisive tendencies. Although, as we have seen, political ideology was not important to most soldiers, the "hard core" provided the link between the or-

dinary soldier in his primary group and the political leadership of the German Army and state.

2. *Community of experience.* German officers saw that solidarity is fostered by the recollection of jointly experienced gratifications and, therefore, the groups who had gone through a victory together when possible were maintained as units. This principle also guided replacement policy. The entire personnel of a division would be withdrawn from the front simultaneously and refitted as a unit with replacements. New members added to the division while it was in the rear had the opportunity to assimilate themselves into the group; then the group as a whole was sent forward. This system continued until close to the end of the war and helps to explain the durability of the German Army in the face of the overwhelming numerical and material superiority of the Allied forces.

Poor morale toward the end of the war was found most frequently in hastily assembled units. These were made up of new recruits, dragooned stragglers, air force men who had been forced into the infantry (and who felt a loss of status in the change), men transferred from the navy into the infantry, older factory workers, concentration camp inmates, and older married men who had been kept in reserve throughout the war and who had remained with their families until the last moment. These reluctant infantrymen, so diverse in age composition and background, could not quickly become effective fighting units. They had no time to become used to one another and to develop the type of friendliness which is possible only when loyalties to outside groups have been renounced—or at least put into the background.

3. *Family ties.* Correspondence between soldiers and their families was generally encouraged, but the families of German soldiers were given strict instructions not to mention family hardships in their letters to the front. Even so, preoccupation with family affairs often conflicted with loyalty to the military primary group.

The pull of the civilian primary group became stronger as the coherence of the army group weakened under the pressure of Allied victories. Sometimes the strength of family ties was used to keep the men fighting in their units. For example, soldiers were warned that desertion would result in severe punishment of the deserter's family. Some men reasoned that the shortest way home was to keep the group intact and to avoid capture and a long period in an enemy prisoner of war camp. They thought those remaining in the defeated but intact army units would have only a short wait before they would be demobilized.

4. *Proximity.* Spatial proximity is important in maintaining the solidarity of military groups. In February and March of 1945, isolated remnants of platoons and companies surrendered in groups with increasing frequency. The tactical situation forced groups of three or four soldiers to take refuge in cellars, trenches, and other underground shelters. Isolation from the nucleus (officers and "hard-core" elements) of the primary group reinforced fears of destruction and helped to break down primary group relations.

Conclusion

At the beginning of World War II, many publicists and specialists in propaganda attributed much importance to psychological warfare operations. The legendary successes of Allied propaganda against the German Army at the end of World War I and the expansion of the advertising and mass communications industries in the ensuing two decades had convinced many people that human behavior could be extensively manipulated by mass communications. They emphasized that military morale was to a great extent a function of the belief in the rightness of the larger cause at issue in the war; good soldiers were, therefore, those who clearly understood the political and moral implications of what was at stake.

Studies of the German Army's morale and fighting effectiveness during the last three years of the war cast doubt on these hypotheses. Solidarity in the German Army was based only very indirectly and partially on political convictions or broad ethical beliefs. Where conditions allowed primary group life to function smoothly and where the primary group developed a high degree of cohesion, morale was maintained regardless of the political attitudes of the soldiers. When conditions fostered disintegration of the military primary group, effective propaganda ignored political issues and exploited the desire to survive.

COMMENTARY

The extreme threats of combat, and the sharing of common, interdependent survival concerns, promoted and accelerated the formation of primary groups in combat units. This study thus dramatizes the support and security functions so distinctively characteristic of primary groups. In less conspicuous ways, the forces which stimulate cohesion or disintegration are also operative in informal groups such as families and peer groups, as well as more specialized associations, such as an operating room team or psychiatric ward personnel.

Wittingly or unwittingly, many characteristics of the mental health field implicate primary group processes: the "democratization" of treatment teams; informal terms of address; "community meetings"; the therapeutic community; and so on. There is a need for a more deliberate and informed application of the literature on primary groups to the mental health field. Illustrative of relevant questions are: What factors facilitate the development of primary groups among and between staff and patients? In what ways are primary groups functional or dysfunctional to the fulfillment of individual needs and organization goals? Do primary relationships conflict with the need for authority and power in organizations? What are the indications and contraindications for the development of primary relationships between staff and patients?

There is also the need for closer examination of the patient's primary relationships and their implications for health or illness. Are the patient's disturbances associated with changing or problematic primary relationships? Does he or she need to acquire skills in the development or "management" of primary relationships? How can therapeutic groups or the therapeutic community serve to educate patients about the nature and consequences of primary group relationships? Has the impact of severe psychiatric disturbances ruptured primary relationships? How may they be repaired? Is this a therapeutic task?

CHAPTER 8

Socialization

INTRODUCTION

The late anthropologist Ruth Benedict had a deep interest in the "psychology of culture"—in the influence of culture on individuals. A gifted writer and disciplined scholar, her work combines artistic sensitivity with the scientific attempt to describe and analyze empirical facts.

The following article was originally published in the journal Psychiatry *in 1939, indicating that its major observations were early recognized as relevant to that profession. It has since become a classic in the social science literature as well.*

Socialization may be viewed in part as a process in which people are prepared to assume various roles in society. However, individuals assume different roles in society as they move through their life cycle. The question of how people are prepared to assume their changing roles thus becomes an important matter for inquiry. Benedict's major thesis is that the role expectations of children and adults in American society are sharply contrasting. At the same time, the culture fails to provide socializing experiences that would serve the progressive ability of individuals to assume their adult roles. It is in this sense that Benedict regards adult roles in American culture as marked by discontinuous cultural conditioning and as problematic for individuals.

The three types of conflicting role expectations which she examines are: (1) responsible-nonresponsible status role; (2) dominance-submission; and (3) contrasted sexual role. Using the cross-cultural, comparative method, Benedict aptly documents that many so-called primitive cultures possess less conflicting child-adult role expectations; otherwise provide for more continuous conditioning; or have special procedures which support role transitions.

CONTINUITIES AND DISCONTINUITIES IN CULTURAL CONDITIONING

Ruth Benedict

All cultures must deal in one way or another with the cycle of growth from infancy to adulthood. Nature has posed the situation dramatically: on the one hand, the newborn baby, physiologically vulnerable, unable to fend for itself, or to participate of its own initiative in the life of the group, and, on the other, the adult man or woman. Every man who rounds out his human potentialities must have been a son first and a father later and the two roles are physiologically in great contrast: he must first have been dependent upon others for his very existence and later he must provide such security for others. This discontinuity in the cycle is a fact of nature and is inescapable. Facts of nature, however, in any discussion of human problems, are ordinarily read off not at their bare minimal but surrounded by all the local accretions of behavior to which the student of human affairs has become accustomed in his own culture. For that reason it is illuminating to examine comparative material from other societies in order to get a wider perspective on our own special accretions. The anthropologist's role is not to question the facts of nature, but to insist upon the interposition of a middle term between "nature" and "human behavior"; his role is to analyze that term, to document local man-made doctorings of nature and to insist that these doctorings should not be read off in any one culture as nature itself. Although it is a fact of nature that the child becomes a man, the way in which this transition is effected varies from one society to another, and no one of these particular cultural bridges should be regarded as the "natural" path to maturity.

From a comparative point of view our culture goes to great extremes in emphasizing contrasts between the child and the adult. The child is sexless, the adult estimates his virility by his sexual activities; the child must be protected from the ugly facts of life, the adult must meet them without psychic catastrophe; the child must obey, the adult must command this obedience. These are all dogmas of our culture, dogmas which in spite of the facts of nature other cultures commonly do not share. In spite of the physiological contrast between child and adult these are cultural accretions.

It will make the point clearer if we consider one habit in our own culture in regard to which there is not this discontinuity of conditioning. With the greatest clarity of purpose and economy of training, we

Ruth Benedict, "Continuities in Cultural Conditioning," *Psychiatry*, I, 1939, pp. 161–167. Reprinted by special permission of the William Alanson White Psychiatric Foundation, Inc.

achieve our goal of conditioning everyone to eat three meals a day. The baby's training in regular food periods begins at birth and no crying of the child and no inconvenience to the mother is allowed to interfere. We gauge the child's physiological makeup and at first allow it food oftener than adults, but, because our goal is firmly set and our training consistent, before the child is two years old it has achieved the adult schedule. From the point of view of other cultures this is as startling as the fact of three-year-old babies perfectly at home in deep water is to us. Modesty is another sphere in which our child training is consistent and economical; we waste no time in clothing the baby and in contrast to many societies where the child runs naked till it is ceremonially given its skirt or its pubic sheath at adolescence, the child's training fits it precisely for adult conventions.

In neither of these aspects of behavior is there need for an individual in our culture to embark before puberty, at puberty, or at some later date upon a course of action which all his previous training has tabued. He is spared the unsureness inevitable in such a transition.

The illustration I have chosen may appear trivial, but in larger and more important aspects of behavior, our methods are obviously different. Because of the great variety of child training in different families in our society, I might illustrate continuity of conditioning from individual life histories in our culture, but even these, from a comparative point of view, stop far short of consistency and I shall therefore confine myself to describing arrangements in other cultures in which training which with us is idiosyncratic, is accepted and traditional and does not therefore involve the same possibility of conflict. I shall choose childhood rather than infant and nursing situations not because the latter do not vary strikingly in different cultures but because they are nevertheless more circumscribed by the baby's physiological needs than is its later training. Childhood situations provide an excellent field in which to illustrate the range of cultural adjustments which are possible within a universally given, but not so drastic, set of physiological facts.

The major discontinuity in the life cycle is of course that the child who is at one point a son must later be a father. These roles in our society are strongly differentiated; a good son is tractable, and does not assume adult responsibilities; a good father provides for his children and should not allow his authority to be flouted. In addition the child must be sexless so far as his family is concerned, whereas the father's sexual role is primary in the family. The individual in one role must revise his behavior from almost all points of view when he assumes the second role.

I shall select for discussion three such contrasts that occur in our culture between the individual's role as child and as father: (1) responsible-nonresponsible status role; (2) dominance-submission; and (3) contrasted sexual role. It is largely upon our cultural commitments to these three contrasts that the discontinuity in the life cycle of an individual in our culture depends.

1. Responsible-Nonresponsible Status Role

The techniques adopted by societies which achieve continuity during the life cycle in this sphere in no way differ from those we employ in our uniform conditioning to three meals a day. They are merely applied to other areas of life. We think of the child as wanting to play and the adult as having to work, but in many societies the mother takes the baby daily in her shawl or carrying net to the garden or to gather roots, and adult labor is seen even in infancy from the pleasant security of its position in close contact with its mother. When the child can run about it accompanies its parents still, doing tasks which are essential and yet suited to its powers, and its dichotomy between work and play is not different from that its parents recognize, namely the distinction between the busy day and the free evening. The tasks it is asked to perform are graded to its powers and its elders wait quietly by, not offering to do the task in the child's place. Everyone who is familiar with such societies has been struck by the contrast with our child training. Dr. Ruth Underhill tells me of sitting with a group of Papago elders in Arizona when the man of the house turned to his little three-year-old granddaughter and asked her to close the door. The door was heavy and hard to shut. The child tried, but it did not move. Several times the grandfather repeated, "Yes, close the door." No one jumped to the child's assistance. No one took the responsibility away from her. On the other hand there was no impatience, for after all the child was small. They sat gravely waiting till the child succeeded and her grandfather gravely thanked her. It was assumed that the task would not be asked of her unless she could perform it and having been asked the responsibility was hers alone just as if she were a grown woman.

The essential point of such child training is that the child is from infancy continuously conditioned to responsible social participation while at the same time the tasks that are expected of it are adapted to its capacity. The contrast with our society is very great. A child does not make any labor contribution to our industrial society except as it competes with an adult; its work is not measured against its own strength and skill but against high-geared industrial requirements. Even when we praise a child's achievement in the home we are outraged if such praise is interpreted as being of the same order as praise of adults. The child is praised because the parent feels well disposed, regardless of whether the task is well done by adult standards, and the child acquires no sensible standard by which to measure its achievement. The gravity of a Cheyenne Indian family ceremoniously making a feast out of the little boy's first snowbird is at the furthest remove from our behavior. At birth the little boy was presented with a toy bow, and from the time he could run about serviceable bows suited to his stature were specially made for him by the man of the family. Animals and birds were taught him in a graded series beginning with those most easily taken, and as he brought in his first of each species his family duly made a feast of it, accepting his contribution as gravely as the buffalo his father brought. When he finally killed a buffalo, it was only the final step of his childhood conditioning, not a new adult role with which his childhood experience had been at variance.

The Canadian Ojibwa show clearly what results can be achieved. This tribe gains its livelihood by winter trapping and the small family of father, mother, and children live during the long winter alone on their great frozen hunting grounds. The boy accompanies his father and brings in his catch to his sister as his father does to his mother; the girl prepares the meat and skins for him just as his mother does for her husband. By the time the boy is twelve, he may have set his own line of traps on a hunting territory of his own and return to his parent's house only once in several months—still bringing the meat and skins to his sister. The young child is taught consistently that it has only itself to rely upon in life, and this is as true in the dealings it will have with the supernatural as in the business of getting a livelihood. This attitude he will accept as a successful adult just as he accepted it as a child.[1]

2. Dominance-Submission

Dominance-submission is the most striking of those categories of behavior where like does not respond to like but where one type of behavior stimulates the opposite response. It is one of the most prominent ways in which behavior is patterned in our culture. When it obtains between classes, it may be nourished by continuous experience; the difficulty in its use between children and adults lies in the fact that an individual conditioned to one set of behavior in childhood must adopt the opposite as an adult. Its opposite is a pattern of approximately identical reciprocal behavior, and societies which rely upon continuous conditioning characteristically invoke this pattern. In some primitive cultures the very terminology of address between father and son, and more commonly, between grandfather and grandson or uncle and nephew, reflects this attitude. In such kinship terminologies one reciprocal expresses each of these relationships so that son and father, for instance, exchange the same term with one another, just as we exchange the same term with a cousin. The child later will exchange it with his son. "Father-son," therefore, is a continuous relationship he enjoys throughout life. The same continuity, backed up by verbal reciprocity, occurs far oftener in the grandfather-grandson relationship or that of mother's brother-sister's son. When these are "joking" relationships, as they often are, travelers report wonderingly upon the liberties and pretensions of tiny toddlers in their dealings with these family elders. In place of our dogma of respect to elders such societies employ in these cases a reciprocity as nearly identical as may be. The teasing and practical joking the grandfather visits upon his grandchild, the grandchild returns in like coin; he would be led to believe that he failed in propriety if he did not give like for like. If the sister's son has right of access without leave to his mother's brother's possessions, the mother's brother has such rights also to the child's possessions. They share reciprocal privileges and obligations which in our society can develop only between age mates.

From the point of view of our present discussion, such kinship conventions allow the child to put in practice from infancy the same forms of behavior which it will rely upon as an adult; behavior is not polarized into a general requirement of submission for the child and dominance for the adult.

It is clear from the techniques described above by which the child is conditioned to a responsible status role that these depend chiefly upon arousing in the child the desire to share responsibility in adult life. To achieve this little stress is laid upon obedience but much stress upon approval and praise. Punishment is very commonly regarded as quite outside the realm of possibility, and natives in many parts of the world have drawn the conclusion from our usual disciplinary methods that white parents do not love their children. If the child is not required to be submissive, however, many occasions for punishment melt away; a variety of situations which call for it do not occur. Many American Indian tribes are especially explicit in rejecting the ideal of a child's submissive or obedient behavior. Prince Maximilian von Wied who visited the Crow Indians over a hundred years ago describes a father's boasting about his young son's intractability when it was the father himself who was flouted; "He will be a man," his father said. He would have been baffled at the idea that his child should show behavior which would obviously make him appear a poor creature in the eyes of his fellows if he used it as an adult. Dr. George Devereaux tells me of a special case of such an attitude among the Mohave at the present time. The child's mother was white and protested to its father that he must take action when the child disobeyed and struck him. "But why?" the father said. "He is little. He cannot possibly injure me." He did not know of any dichotomy according to which an adult expects obedience and a child must accord it. If his child had been docile he would simply have judged that it would become a docile adult—an eventuality of which he would not have approved.

Child training which brings about the same result is common also in other areas of life than that of reciprocal kinship obligations between child and adult. There is a tendency in our culture to regard every situation as having in it the seeds of a dominance-submission relationship. Even where dominance-submission is patently irrelevant we read in the dichotomy, assuming that in every situation there must be one person dominating another. On the other hand some cultures, even when the situation calls for leadership, do not see it in terms of dominance-submission. To do justice to this attitude it would be necessary to describe their political and especially their economic arrangements, for such an attitude to persist must certainly be supported by economic mechanisms that are congruent with it. But it must also be supported by—or what comes to the same thing, express itself in— child training and familial situations.

3. Contrasted Sexual Role

Continuity of conditioning in training the child to assume responsibility and to behave no more submissively than adults is quite possible in terms of the child's physiological endowment if his participation is suited to his strength. Because of the late development of the child's reproductive organs continuity of conditioning in sex experience presents a difficult problem. So far as their belief that the child is anything but a sexless being is concerned, they are probably more nearly right than we are with an opposite dogma. But the great break is presented by the universally sterile unions before puberty and the presumably fertile ones after maturation. This physiological fact no amount of cultural manipulation can minimize or alter, and societies therefore which stress continuous conditioning most strongly sometimes do not expect children to be interested in sex experience until they have matured physically. This is striking among American Indian tribes like the Dakota; adults observe great privacy in sex acts and in no way stimulate children's sexual activity. There need be no discontinuity, in the sense in which I have used the term, in such a program if the child is taught nothing it does not have to unlearn later. In such cultures adults view children's experimentation as in no way wicked or dangerous but merely as innocuous play which can have no serious consequences. In some societies such play is minimal and the children manifest little interest in it. But the same attitude may be taken by adults in societies where such play is encouraged and forms a major activity among small children. This is true among most of the Melanesian cultures of Southeast New Guinea; adults go as far as to laugh off sexual affairs within the prohibited class if the children are not mature, saying that since they cannot marry there can be no harm done.

It is this physiological fact of the difference between children's sterile unions and adults' presumably fertile sex relations which must be kept in mind in order to understand the different mores which almost always govern sex expression in children and in adults in the same culture. A great many cultures with preadolescent sexual license require marital fidelity and a great many which value premarital virginity in either male or female arrange their marital life with great license. Continuity in sex experience is complicated by factors which it was unnecessary to consider in the problems previously discussed. The essential problem is not whether or not the child's sexuality is consistently exploited—for even where such exploitation is favored in the majority of cases the child must seriously modify his behavior at puberty or at marriage. Continuity in sex expression means rather that the child is taught nothing it must unlearn later. If the cultural emphasis is upon sexual pleasure the child who is continuously conditioned will be encouraged to experiment freely and pleasurably, as among the Marquesans; [2] if emphasis is upon reproduction, as among the Zuni of New Mexico, childish sex proclivities will not be exploited for the only important use which sex is thought to serve in his culture is not yet possible to him. The important contrast with our child training is that although a Zuni child is impressed with the wickedness of premature sex experimentation he does not run the risk as in our culture of associating this wickedness with sex itself rather than with sex at his age. The adult in our culture has often failed to unlearn the wickedness or the dangerousness of sex, a lesson which was impressed upon him strongly in his most formative years.

Discontinuity in Conditioning

Even from this very summary statement of continuous conditioning the economy of such mores is evident. In spite of the obvious advantages, however, there are difficulties in its way. Many primitive societies expect as different behavior from an individual as child and as adult as we do, and such discontinuity involves a presumption of strain.

Many societies of this type, however, minimize strain by the techniques they employ, and some techniques are more successful than others in ensuring the individual's functioning without conflict. It is from this point of view that age-grade societies reveal their fundamental significance. Age-graded cultures characteristically demand different behavior of the individual at different times of his life and persons of a like age-grade are grouped into a society whose activities are all oriented toward the behavior desired at that age. Individuals "graduate" publicly and with honor from one of these groups to another. Where age society members are enjoined to loyalty and mutual support, and are drawn not only from the local group but from the whole tribe as among the Arapaho, or even from other tribes as among the Wagawaga of Southeast New Guinea, such an institution has many advantages in eliminating conflicts among local groups and fostering intratribal peace. This seems to be also a factor in the tribal military solidarity of the similarly organized Masai of East Africa. The point that is of chief interest for our present discussion however is that by this means an individual who at any time takes on a new set of duties and virtues is supported not only by a solid phalanx of age mates but by the traditional prestige of the organized "secret" society into which he has now graduated. Fortified in this way, individuals in such cultures often swing between remarkable extremes of opposite behavior without apparent psychic threat. For example, the great majority exhibit prideful and nonconflicted behavior at each stage in the life cycle even when a prime of life devoted to passionate and aggressive head hunting must be followed by a later life dedicated to ritual and to mild and peaceable civic virtues.[3]

Our chief interest here, however, is in discontinuity which primarily affects the child. In many primitive societies such discontinuity has been fostered not because of economic or political necessity or because such discontinuity provides for a socially valuable division of labor, but because of some conceptual dogma. The most striking of these are the Australian and Papuan cultures where the ceremony of the "Making of Man" flourishes. In such societies it is believed that men and women have opposite and conflicting powers, and male children, who are of undefined status, must be initiated into the male role. In Central Australia the boy child is of the woman's side and women are tabu in the final adult stages of tribal ritual. The elaborate and protracted initiation ceremonies of the Arunta therefore snatch the boy from the mother, dramatize his gradual repudiation of her. In a final ceremony he is reborn as a man out of the men's ceremonial "baby pouch." The men's ceremonies are ritual statements of a masculine solidarity, carried out by fondling one another's *churingas,* the material symbol of each man's life, and by letting out over one another blood drawn from their veins. After this warm bond among men has been established through the ceremonies, the boy joins the men in the men's house and participates in tribal rites.[4] The enjoined discontinuity has been tribally bridged.

West of the Fly River in southern New Guinea there is a striking development of this Making of Man cult which involves a childhood period of passive homosexuality. Among the Keraki [5] it is thought that no boy can grow to full stature without playing the role for some years. Men slightly older take the active role, and the older man is a jealous partner. The life cycle of the Keraki Indians includes, therefore, in succession, passive homosexuality, active homosexuality, and heterosexuality. The Keraki believe that pregnancy will result from postpubertal passive homosexuality and see evidence of such practices in any fat man whom even as an old man they may kill or drive out of the tribe because of their fear. The ceremony that is of interest in connection with the present discussion takes place at the end of the period of passive homosexuality. This ceremony consists in burning out the possibility of pregnancy from the boy by pouring lye down his throat, after which he has no further protection if he gives way to the practice. There is no technique for ending active homosexuality, but this is not explicitly tabu for older men; heterosexuality and children however are highly valued. Unlike the neighboring Marindanim who share their homosexual practices, Keraki husband and wife share the same house and work together in the gardens.

I have chosen illustrations of discontinuous conditioning where it is not too much to say that the cultural institutions furnish adequate support to the individual as he progresses from role to role or interdicts the previous behavior in a summary fashion. The contrast with arrangements in our culture is very striking, and against this background of social arrangements in other cultures the adolescent period of *Sturm und Drang* with which we are so familiar becomes intelligible in terms of our discontinuous cultural institutions and dogmas rather than in terms of physiological necessity. It is even more pertinent to consider these comparative facts in relation to maladjusted persons in our culture who are said to be fixated at one or another preadult level. It is clear that if we were to look at our social arrangements as an outsider, we should infer directly from our family institutions and habits of child training that many individuals would not "put off childish things"; we should have to say that our adult activity demands traits that are interdicted in children, and that far from redoubling efforts to help children bridge this gap, adults in our culture put all the blame on the child when he fails to manifest spontaneously the new behavior or, overstepping the mark, manifests it with untoward belligerence. It is not surprising that in such a society many individuals fear to use behavior which has up to that time been under a ban and trust instead, though at great psychic cost, to attitudes that have been exercised with approval during their formative years. Insofar as we invoke a physiological scheme to account for these neurotic adjustments we are led to overlook the possibility of developing social institutions which would lessen the social cost we now pay; instead we elaborate a set of dogmas which prove inapplicable under other social conditions.

NOTES

1. Ruth Landes, *The Ojibwa Woman*, Part 1, *Youth*, Columbia University Contributions to Anthropology, vol. 31 (New York: Columbia University Press, 1938).
2. Ralph Linton, class notes on the Marquesans.
3. Henry Elkin, manuscript on the Arapaho.
4. B. Spencer and F. J. Gillen, *The Arunta*, 2 vols. (New York: Macmillan, 1927), and Geza Roheim, "Psycho-Analysis of Primitive Cultural Types," *International Journal of Psychoanalysis* 13 (1932): 1–224—in particular chap. 3, on the Aranda, The Children of the Desert.
5. Francis E. Williams, *Papuans of the Trans-Fly* (Oxford: The Clarendon Press, 1936).

ANNOTATED REFERENCES

Hiller, E. T. *Social Relations and Social Structures*. New York: Harper, 1947, pp. 331–614. Hiller, in this section of his text, analyzes the structure of society in terms of the characteristics and interrelations of social roles. This is probably the most complete description of various classes of social roles available in one volume.

Hughes, E. C. "Dilemmas and Contradictions of Status." *American Journal of Sociology*, March 1945, pp. 353–359. Contradictions between social roles sometimes grow out of peripheral elements rather than central elements. Hughes describes some of the contradictions among the roles which the individual is called upon to play in a highly mobile society and finds that frequently it is the peripheral elements which are involved.

Komarovsky, Mirra. "Cultural Contradictions and Sex Roles." *American Journal of Sociology*, November 1946, pp. 184–189. The conflict between the adult roles of the American woman are described in this article. The basic contradictions are between the pressures pushing the woman in the direction of a career and those pointing toward homemaking.

Linton, Ralph. "Age and Sex Categories." *American Sociological Review*, October 1942, pp. 589–603. Drawing on cross-cultural materials, Linton examines the range of variation among different cultures in the utilization of age and sex categories for the ascription of social position and role.

Schuetz, Alfred. "The Stranger: An Essay in Social Psychology." *American Journal of Sociology*, May 1944, pp. 499–507. Schuetz explores the problems facing the stranger in any group: the inability to predict the responses of others and a lack of knowledge as to how to conduct himself in relation to others. In order to participate in the life of the group he must be assigned a position and role and learn to act accordingly.

Znaniecki, Florian. "The Impact of War on Personality Organization." *Sociology and Social Research*, January–February 1943, pp. 171–180. Under conditions of stress changes occur in the culture of a society modifying the character of the social roles defined by the culture. Znaniecki summarizes a group of studies by his students showing the effect of war on some of the more typical social roles of our society.

COMMENTARY

A number of important socialization processes or mechanisms are well illustrated in this paper. The communication of expectations may be frank or subtle, explicit or implicit, verbal or nonverbal. In their own way, such expectations are communicated by the Papago grandfather's request to his granddaughter to close the door; the little bow given to the infant boy by the Cheyenne; and the dolls given to little American girls. Male and female names, blue and pink ribbons, are familiar examples of how early sex role expectations are communicated and differentiated.

Sanctions—rewards and punishments—are universal techniques of socialization. Although the forms and mechanism of reward and punishment have not been adequately described or analyzed, they include expressions of approval, praise, the demonstration or denial of affection, punishment, and ridicule. That "loss of face" among the Japanese can elicit suicide illustrates dramatically the power of social sanctions.

Benedict's reference to the young Ojibwa boy accompanying his father on trapping expeditions illustrates modeling mechanisms in socialization. Adults deliberately (and probably nondeliberately as well) serve as models in the socialization process. As in the games of children, modeling and role playing are also exemplified in the behavior of would-be members of the group. The themes of culture heroes and the cult of personality among American adolescents is perhaps reflective of such processes.

Certainly the ways in which a culture and social structure shape the individual's expression of responsibility, independence, assertion, and sexuality are psychiatric concerns. In what ways does contemporary American society influence their expression? What variations exist by social class, region, race, ethnicity, or religion? What role do peer groups, the family, neighborhood, school, and job play in in-

fluencing their development? Are there patterned conflicts, ambigui-
ties, inconsistences?

To what extent does Benedict's description of American culture in
the 1930s still fit today? Does it fit some subcultural groups better
than others? Do these discontinuities create "storm and stress" among
American adolescents, as Benedict contends? Such questions deserve
the clinician's continuing attention.

While Benedict describes and analyzes some specific observations,
her paper also illustrates one general concern of sociopsychiatric in-
quiry: the identification of social sources of psychiatric disturbance.
As an illustrative exercise, assuming that Benedict's characterization
was accurate, what kinds of psychiatric, interpersonal, and situational
disturbances might American adolescents be expected to manifest?
What kinds of intervention might be attempted?

While there have always been competing schools of thought in
the mental health field, debates about "models" of psychiatric dis-
turbance are perhaps more lively today then ever before. It is always
instructive to attempt to discern the merits of different formulations.
For example, does Benedict's contention about adolescent turmoil com-
pete with, conflict with, or complement biological or psychoanalytic
formulations?

Through socialization the individual learns the norms, values, be-
liefs, and goals characteristic of the group. To the extent that he is
socialized, he learns his appropriate role functions. Yet individuals
are unique and reactive. What conflicts may occur for an individual
in the socialization process?

CHAPTER 9

Social Stratification

INTRODUCTION

Belief in social and economic mobility—in its importance and possibility—is a major theme in American society. In this paper Rosen examines some of the factors which might be expected to lead to different rates of upward mobility among the social classes. Specifically, he focuses on the roles of achievement motivation *and* value orientations.

On the basis of data gathered from high school students, Rosen found that middle-class students show significantly higher levels of achievement motivation than lower-class students. However, Rosen argues that this "drive to excel" is not a sufficient cause of upward mobility, since it can be expressed in ways that are not necessarily conducive to that end. For example, it could be expressed in religious piety, hobbies, or excellence in welding. "Whether the individual will elect to strive for success in situations which facilitate mobility in our society," Rosen proposes, "will in part be determined by his values." Values serve to define both the ends and means of action.

Measuring certain value orientations theoretically consistent with successful mobility strivings, the author demonstrates that they are characteristic of the upper and middle classes, but not the lower social classes. He also observes that these value orientations are associated with the desire to get an education beyond high school, but achievement motivation is not!

This is an elegant illustration of the refined use of scientific theory and method, the more impressive because it addresses itself to important, complex ideas and phenomena. Using measures of his theoretical variables, and statistical techniques to assess their association, the investigator proceeds to test hypotheses and discern the functions of the variables.

Rosen's treatment of social mobility also demonstrates a "double concern": understanding the sociocultural system (the class structure) and *the individual (psychocultural aspects of the class structure). This dual concern is at the center of social psychology and social psychiatry as well.*

THE ACHIEVEMENT SYNDROME:
A PSYCHOCULTURAL DIMENSION
OF SOCIAL STRATIFICATION

Bernard C. Rosen

The empirical generalization that upward mobility is greater among members of the middle class than those of the lower strata has been explained in several alternative ways.[1] It has been suggested, for example, that social strata possess different physical characteristics which affect mobility, that as a result of certain selective processes persons in the upper and middle strata are, on the average, more intelligent, healthier, and more attractive than those in the lower strata.[2] More frequently, differential mobility is described as a function of the relative opportunities available to individuals in the social structure. This structural dimension of stratification is explicit in the "life chances" hypothesis in which it is argued that money, specialized training, and prestigeful contacts—factors which affect access to high position—are relatively inaccessible to individuals in the lower social strata.[3] Such explanations are relevant and consistent with one another. They lack exhaustiveness, however, since neither explanation takes into account the possibility that there may be psychological and cultural factors which affect social mobility by influencing the individual's willingness to develop and exploit his talent, intelligence, and opportunities.

It is the thesis of this paper that class differential rates of vertical mobility may be explicated also in terms of a psychocultural dimension of stratification, that is, as a function of differences in the motives and values of social classes.[4] More specifically, this study examines empirically the notion (long current in sociology, but for which there is as yet insufficient empirical verification) that social classes in

Bernard Rosen, "The Achievement Syndrome: A Psychocultural Dimension of Social Stratification," *American Sociological Review* 21, April 1946, pp. 203–211.

American society are characterized by a dissimilar concern with achievement, particularly as it is expressed in the striving for status through social mobility.[5] It is hypothesized that social classes possess to a disparate extent two components of this achievement orientation. The first is a psychological factor involving a personality characteristic called *achievement motivation* (or, in Murray's terminology, *need achievement*) which provides an internal impetus to excel. The second is a cultural factor consisting of certain *value orientations* which define and implement achievement-motivated behavior. Both of these factors are related to achievement; their incidence, we suggest, is greater among persons of the middle class than those in the lower class.

The task of this paper is threefold: (1) to make a preliminary attempt at determining whether social strata are dissimilar with respect to these two factors by examining their incidence among a group of randomly selected adolescents stratified by social position; (2) to indicate the significance of these factors for differential occupational achievement; and (3) to suggest some class-related origins of achievement motivation and values.

Research Procedure

The universe from which the study sample was drawn is the entire male population of sophomores in two large public high schools in the New Haven area. This group was stratified by the social position of the main wage-earner in the family (in most cases the father) through data secured by questionnaire and according to a scheme developed by Hollingshead.[6] His Index of Social Position utilizes three factors: (1) occupation; (2) education; and (3) ecological area of residence. Each factor is scaled and assigned a weight determined by a standard regression equation. The combined scores group themselves in five clusters (social strata) and to each of these a numerical index is assigned. The highest status group is labeled Class I; the others follow in numerical order, Class V being the lowest. Respondents were drawn randomly from each stratum: five subjects from Class I (the entire Class I sophomore population in the two schools), twenty-five from Class II, and thirty each from Classes III, IV, and V. In all there are 120 subjects, all of them white, ages fourteen through sixteen; the modal age is fifteen.

It was hypothesized that social strata are dissimilar with respect to two factors related to achievement: that is, achievement motivation and achievement value orientation. By achievement motivation we mean an anticipation of an increase in affect aroused by cues in situations involving standards of excellence. The behavior of people highly motivated for achievement is persistent striving activity, aimed at attaining a high goal in some area involving competition with a standard of excellence. In relation to these standards of excellence the achievement-oriented person directs his efforts toward obtaining the pleasure of success and avoiding the pain of failure. Value orientations are defined (following the manner described in Williams' *American Society*) as meaningful and affectively charged modes of organizing behavior, as principles that guide human conduct. They establish the criteria which influence the individual's preferences and goals; they act as spectacles through which the individual sees himself and his environment. Two techniques were employed to measure these factors. A projective test (a technique which does not rely upon the person's self-knowledge) was used to measure the adolescent's achievement motivation; the direct questionnaire was used to measure his values.

The personality correlate of achievement called "achievement motivation" has been investigated by McClelland and his associates.[7] Using a Thematic Apperception Test-type measure, they have developed a projective test whose scoring system is designed to detect and measure the degree to which a person thinks about and is emotionally involved in competitive task behavior that is evaluated against a standard of excellence. As is customary in the TAT testing procedure, the subject is presented with a set of fairly ambiguous pictures and asked to tell a story about each of them. His imaginative responses are then scored for evidences of achievement motivation. Two criteria must be satisfied before a story can be scored as containing achievement imagery. First, the events and people in the stories must show some evaluation of individual performance in relation to and competition with a standard of excellence, e.g.: "The boy has done a *good* job in the exam." Second, some affect, either positive or negative, must be connected with the evaluated performance, e.g.: "He is *unhappy* because he lost the essay contest." It is the assumption of the test that the more the individual shows indications of evaluated performance connected with affect in unstructured situations, the greater the degree to which achievement motivation is part of his personality.

This projective test was administered to the subjects in the following standardized way. Subjects were assembled during the school day in small groups (twenty to thirty persons) in a school room equipped with a screen and a slide projector. The test administrator explained to the students that they were going to see a series of pictures and that their task was to write a story about each picture. In his instructions to the subjects the administrator made no effort to manipulate the motive of the students. Since all testing was done in the school, it was expected that each boy would bring to the test his normal achievement motivation level induced by the cues of the school. The same administrator was used throughout the tests.[8]

Following the test, the subjects were asked to fill out a structured questionnaire, part of which contained items (the content of which is described in a later section of this paper) designed to index their value orientations. These items took the form of statements with which the subjects were asked to agree or disagree, and are centered around certain kinds of values that we felt are related to scholastic and vocational achievement.

Research Findings

Social Stratification and the Achievement Motive. The findings of this study support the hypothesis that social strata differ from one another in the degree to which the achievement motive is characteristic of their members. Furthermore, the data indicate that members of the middle class tend to have considerably higher need achievement scores than individuals in the lower social strata. Plotted on a graph, the mean achievement scores of the social classes fall along a regression curve: the highest mean score in Class II (the group most likely to be described as middle class when the trichotomy of upper, middle, and lower class is used), a somewhat lower score in Class I, and progressively lower scores in an almost linear fashion in Classes III, IV, and V. Reading in numerical order from Class I to V, the mean score for each class is 8.40, 8.68, 4.97, 3.40, and 1.87. The mean score for Class II is more than four times as great as the score for Class V.[9]

A test of the statistical significance of this association between social position and achievement motivation is shown in Table 1. In or-

TABLE 1
Achievement Motivation by Social Class

Achievement	Social Class			
Motivation Score	I and II	III	IV	V
Low	17%	57%	70%	77%
High	83	43	30	23
Number	(30)	(30)	(30)	(30)

x^2: 26.6
$P < .001$.

der to simplify presentation, subjects whose scores fall below the approximate median for the entire sample are categorized as having low achievement motivation;[10] Classes I and II are collapsed into one group because of the scarcity of cases in Class I.[11] The data indicate a clear relationship between social position and motivation score. For example, 83 percent of the subjects in Classes I and II have high motivation scores, as compared with 23 percent in Class V, a difference that is statistically significant at the .001 level.

Social Stratification and Value Orientation. In itself the achievement motive is not a sufficient cause of upward mobility. Obviously the lack of innate capacity and/or structural opportunities may frustrate the achievement drive, but in addition there are cultural factors which are related to mobility. Among these factors are certain values which affect mobility in that they provide a definition of goals, focus the attention of the individual on achievement, and prepare him to translate motive into action. For example, before the achievement motive can be translated into the kinds of action that are conducive to culturally defined achievement (and hence operate as a factor in social mobility), there must be some definition of the kinds of situations in which achievement is expected and of the goals to which one should or may aspire.

Achievement-oriented situations and goals are not defined by the achievement motive; it may provide the impetus to excel, but it does not delineate the areas in which such excellence should or may take place. Achievement motivation can be expressed through a wide range of behavior, some of which may not be conducive to social mobility in our society. The achievement motive can be, and perhaps frequently is, expressed through nonvocational behavior, for example lay religious activity of an individual whose drive to excel finds release though piety or mastery of sacred literature; or it may find an outlet in nonprofessional "hobby-type" behavior. Even when expressed through vocational activity, the achievement motive may be canalized into culturally defined deviant occupations (e.g., the criminal), or into low-status vocations (e.g., the individual whose achievement drive is expressed and satisfied through his desire to be the *best* welder among his peers). Whether the individual will elect to strive for success in situations which facilitate mobility in our society will, in part, be determined by his values.

Furthermore, before the achievement motive can be expressed in culturally defined success behavior, there needs to be more than a desire to achieve success; there must also be some awareness of and willingness to undertake the steps necessary for achievement. Such steps involve, among other things, a preparedness to plan, to work, and to make sacrifices. Whether the individual will understand their importance and accept them will, in part, be affected by his values. It must follow, therefore, that differential interclass rates of mobility cannot be entirely explained as a function of differences in achievement motivation; social classes must also be shown to differ in their possession of these implementary values necessary to achievement.

The notion that social classes possess dissimilar values as part of their distinctive subcultures has been suggested by a number of investigators, for example, the Kluckhohns, who have delineated a wide range of differences in the value systems of social strata in American society.[12] In Florence Kluckhohn's schema [13] these values are part of a configuration of value orientations which grow out of man's effort to solve five basic problems that are everywhere immanent in the human situation. While all five of Kluckhohn's orientations are relevant to the problem of achievement, three were selected as especially pertinent for examination in this study: (1) what is the accepted approach to the problem of mastering one's physical and social environment; (2) what is the significant time dimension; and (3) what is the dominant modality of relationship of the individual to his kin. We were interested in determining whether social classes are dissimilar in their possession of these orientations. A brief description of their content (modified somewhat from the way in which they appear in the Kluckhohn schema), and examples of the items used to index each of them, are as follows: [14]

1. *Activistic-passivistic orientation* concerns the extent to which a society or sub-group encourages the individual to believe in the possibility of his manipulating the physical and social environment to his advantage. In an activistic society the individual is encouraged to believe that it is both possible and necessary for him to improve his status, whereas a passivistic orientation promotes the acceptance of the notion that individual efforts to achieve mobility are relatively futile.

 Item 1. "All I want out of life in the way of a career is a secure, not too difficult job, with enough pay to afford a nice car and eventually a home of my own."

 Item 2. "When a man is born the success he is going to have is already in the cards, so he might just as well accept it and not fight against it."

2. *Present-future orientation* concerns a society's attitude toward time and its impact upon behavior. A present-oriented society stresses the merit of living in the present with an emphasis upon immediate gratifications; a future-oriented society urges the individual to believe that planning and present sacrifices are worthwhile, or morally obligatory, in order to insure future gains.

 Item 3. "Planning only makes a person unhappy since your plans hardly ever work out anyway."

 Item 4. "Nowadays with world conditions the way they are the wise person lives for today and lets tomorrow take care of itself."

3. *Familistic-individualistic orientation* concerns the relationship of the individual to his kin. One aspect of this orientation is the importance given to the maintenance of physical proximity to the family of orientation. In a familistically oriented society the individual is not urged, or perhaps not permitted, to acquire independence of family ties. An individualistically oriented society does not expect the individual to maintain the kinds of affective ties which will impede his mobility.

 Item 5. "Nothing in life is worth the sacrifice of moving away from your parents."

Responses which indicate an activistic, future-oriented, individualistic point of view (the answer "disagree" to these items) are considered those which reflect values most likely to facilitate achievement and social mobility. These items were used to form a value index, and a score was derived for each subject by giving a point for each achievement-oriented response.[15]

An analysis of the data supports the hypothesis that the middle class is characterized by a larger proportion of persons with achievement-oriented values than are the lower social strata. The plotting of mean value scores for each class reveals an almost linear relationship between social position and values: the higher the class the higher the value score. Thus the mean scores for the five social strata are in descending order, with Class I first and Class V last, 4.6, 4.1, 3.8, 3.0, and 2.5. This relationship is shown to be statistically significant in Table 2 in which social position is cross-tabulated with value score. To simplify presentation value scores are dichotomized: respondents whose score falls above the approximate median for the entire sample

TABLE 2
Value Orientations by Social Class

Value	Social Class			
Score	I and II	III	IV	V
Low	23%	30%	67%	83%
High	77	70	33	17
Number	(30)	(30)	(30)	(30)

χ^2: 28.9
P < .001.

are designated as having a high score. The data reveal that of those adolescents in Class I or II, 77 percent score high on the value scale, as compared with 17 percent of the adolescents in Class V. For the entire table, the probability of this level of association occurring by chance is less than one out of a thousand.

Achievement Correlates of Achievement Motivation and Values. Achievement motivation and value orientation were found to be related to different kinds of behavior that affect social mobility. We have stated that the achievement motive expresses itself in concern with performance evaluated against a standard of excellence. In the school situation this performance may be canalized within the framework of scholastic achievement. That this is probably frequently the case can be seen in Table 3 in which motivation scores are cross-tabulated with average

TABLE 3
Average School Grade by Achievement Motivation

Average	Achievement Motivation Score		Value Orientation Score	
School Grade	High	Low	High	Low
"B" or above	69%	35%	54%	46%
"C" or below	31	65	46	54
Number	(54)	(66)	(59)	(61)

χ^2: 13.5. χ^2: .833.
P < .001.   P > .30.

school grades. The data show that subjects with high motivation scores are proportionately more likely to achieve grades of "B" or better than are adolescents with low motivation scores: 69 percent of the former as against 35 percent of the latter. Value scores, however, proved not to be related to academic achievement, although they are associated with a kind of behavior that is, if not in itself an act of achievement, at least a factor in social mobility in our society. It was found that the individual's value score, but *not* his motivation score, is related to educational aspiration. Thus the data in Table 4 indicate that subjects with high value scores are proportionately more likely to want to go to college than are those with low scores: 61 percent of the former as

TABLE 4
School Aspiration by Value Orientation

School	Value Orientation Score		Achievement Motivation Score	
Aspiration	High	Low	High	Low
Aspires to go to college	61%	33%	51%	46%
Does not aspire to go to college	39	67	49	54
Number	(59)	(61)	(54)	(66)

x^2: 13.3.　　　　　　　　　　　　　　　　　　x^2: 1.2.
P < .001.　　　　　　　　　　　　　　　　　　P > .20.

compared with 33 percent of the latter. The relationships between motivation and grades and between values and aspiration level are statistically significant at the .001 level.

Since high need achievement and value scores tend to occur more frequently among members of the upper and middle than in the lower strata, it is not surprising to find that social strata are different in their academic achievement and educational aspiration levels. This is particularly marked in the case of educational aspiration level, which was found to be considerably higher for adolescents in the upper and middle strata than for those in the lower strata. Thus when subjects were asked, "If you could arrange things to suit yourself, how far would you go in school?" 93 percent of respondents in the combined category of strata I, II, and III aspired to continue their education beyond high school, either in college or in a technical school; whereas of

TABLE 5
Value Score by Aspiration Level and Social Class

	Social Class			
	I–II–III		IV–V	
Aspiration Level	Under-Aspirers	Other-Aspirers	Over-Aspirers	Other-Aspirers
Value Score				
Low	57%	23%	65%	79%
High	43	77	35	21
Number	7	53*	17	43†

* Includes those individuals whose aspiration level represents the modal choice for their status group.
† Includes those subjects whose aspiration level is below or at the modal choice for their group.

the combined strata IV-V only 47 percent aspired to go beyond high school.[16]

The hypothesis that this differential in education aspiration is, in part at least, a function of value orientation differences is supported by the data shown in Table 5, in which under- and overaspirers are examined. Underaspirers are those respondents in strata I, II, or III whose educational aspiration level is lower than the modality for their group (i.e., those who do not aspire to go beyond high school); overaspirers are those adolescents in strata IV-V whose aspiration level is higher than the norm for their group (i.e., those who aspire to go beyond high school). The data in Table 5 in which over- and underaspirers are compared with one another, and with other members of their class, in terms of their value scores show a clear relationship between over-under-aspiration level and value orientations. Thus fewer underaspirers have high value scores than do other members of their strata —43 percent of the former as compared with 77 percent of the latter, whereas overaspirers are more likely to have high value scores than are other members of their class—35 percent as compared with 21 percent. Furthermore, the class differences in value scores shown in Table 2 virtually disappear when aspiration level is held constant: an earlier difference of more than 40 percent between categories I-II-III and IV-V is reduced to 8 percent when over- and underaspirers are compared with one another, whereas it is increased when the "other" categories are compared.

The relationship between academic achievement (as measured by average grades) and social class appears to reflect to a considerable extent strata differentials in achievement motivation. Class differences in academic achievement which appear significant on first inspection (e.g., 17 percent of the subjects in the combined category of Classes I-II-III have average grades of "A"; only 3 percent of those in Classes IV-V have grades this high; also, 54 percent of the former have average grades of "B" or higher, as compared with 42 percent of the lower status category) are markedly altered when need achievement score is introduced as a test variable. As can be seen in Table 6, the earlier relationship between class and grades is virtually erased for those

TABLE 6
School Grades by Achievement Motivation and Social Class

Achievement Motivation Score	Social Class			
	I–II–III		IV–V	
	High	Low	High	Low
Average School Grades				
"B" or above	66%	32%	75%	36%
"C" or below	34	68	25	64
Number	38	22	16	44

with low achievement motivation and slightly reversed for those with high motivation. However, although the differences *between* strata are reduced to a statistically insignificant level, *within* strata differences between individuals with high and low motivation scores remain, thus pointing up the relationship between motivation and academic achievement.

Achievement motivation and achievement-oriented values are not, of course, the only factors related to academic success and educational aspiration. The fact that *all* the cells in the contingency tables described here contain some cases clearly indicates that other variables are at work. Among these variables may be such factors as sibling rivalry, the operation of ego-defense mechanisms, or motives other than need achievement, for example, the need for power. Furthermore, social classes may be dissimilar in ways other than in their motives or values, and these differences can have significance for achievement. Classes are said to be different in manners, richness of cultural-esthetic experiences, and possibly with respect to intelligence, to a general sense of well-being, power, and past history of successful endeavor. All of these factors may contribute to differential class rates of mobility by affecting academic and vocational success and aspiration level. The task of this paper, however, has been to focus upon the factors of achievement motivation and values, although probably in the empirical situation many of the above factors are operative and interactive at the same time.

Whatever the importance present and future studies may show the other factors listed above to have for achievement, the fact remains that this study reveals a significant relationship between achievement motivation and grades, and between values and educational aspiration. This fact is of more than academic interest. There is a nexus, though it is of course not a perfect one, between educational and vocational achievement in our society. Furthermore, the college degree is becoming an increasingly important prerequisite for movement into prestigeful and lucrative jobs, hence an aspiration level which precludes college training may seriously affect an individual's opportunity for social mobility. Since we have shown that achievement-oriented motives and values are more characteristic of the middle than the lower strata, it is reasonable to suggest that these variables are, in part at least, factors which tend to create differential class rates of social mobility.

Class-Related Origins of Achievement Motivation and Values. The achievement motive and values examined here, while related, represent genuinely different components of the achievement syndrome, not only in their correlates but also in their origins. Value orientations, because they tend to be on a conceptual level, are probably acquired in that stage of the child's cultural training when verbal communication of a fairly complex nature is possible. Achievement motivation, on the other hand, probably has its origins in certain kinds of parent-child interaction that occur early in the child's life and are likely to be emotional and unverbalized. Analytically, then, the learning of achievement-oriented values can be independent of the acquisition of the achievement motive, though empirically they often occur together.

Several empirical studies have shown that achievement motivation is most likely to be high when the child is urged to obtain, and rewarded for achieving, independence and mastery, accompanied by few restrictions after mastery has been acquired.[17] Winterbottom's study,[18] for example, indicates that mothers of children with high achievement motivation differ from mothers of children who have low motivation in that they: (1) make more demands (particularly for evidences of independence, maturity, and achievement) at early ages; and (2) give more intense and frequent rewards for fulfilled demands.

These are the patterns which are believed to be especially characteristic of middle-class families, although it must be emphasized that the data to substantiate this conclusion are still tentative and often conflicting and that child-rearing practices, like other aspects of American culture, are in constant flux.[19] From babyhood on much of the middle-class child's affect is likely to be associated with achievement-related behavior structured for him by the training practices and values of his parents. In the preschool period the tendency for middle-class parents to make early demands upon their children is reflected in such practices as early toilet training and the intense concern with cleanliness. As the child grows he is frequently urged and encouraged to demonstrate his developing maturity (e.g., early walking, talking, and self-care). Signs of precocity are signals for intense parental pride and often lavish rewards. It is precisely this atmosphere which provides, if Winterbottom is correct, a most fertile environment for the growth of the achievement motive.

When the child starts his formal schooling, the achievement-oriented demands and values of his parents tend to be focused on the school situation. From the beginning of his school career the middle-class child is more likely than his lower-class counterpart to have standards of excellence in scholastic behavior set for him by his parents. In fact, the relatively higher position which scholastic attainment has in the middle-class than in the lower-class value system means that more frequently for the middle- than for the lower-class child parental demands and expectations, as well as rewards and punishments, will center around school performance.

Associated with the stress on scholastic achievement are other achievement-oriented values that are more characteristic of the middle than the lower class. While it is probably true that the notion that success is desirable and possible is widespread in our society, the implementary values—those which encouraged behavior that facilitates achievement—have long been more associated with the culture of the middle than of the lower class. Middle-class children are more likely to be taught not only to believe in success, but also to be willing to take those steps that make achievement possible: in short, to embrace the achievement value system which states that given the willingness to work hard, plan, and make the proper sacrifices, an individual should be able to manipulate his environment so as to ensure eventual success.

NOTES

1. Cf. N. Rogoff, *Recent Trends in Occupational Mobility* (New York: Free Press, 1953); K. B. Mayer, *Class and Society* (Garden City, N.Y.: Doubleday, 1955); and R. Albrecht, "Social Class in Old Age," *Social Forces* 29 (May 1951): 400–405.

2. Cf. P. Sorokin, *Social Mobility* (New York: Harper, 1927). For the relationship of intelligence to social mobility, see C. A. Anderson et al., "Intelligence and Occupational Mobility," *Journal of Political Economy* 60 (June 1952): 218–239.

3. Factors of this sort have been abundantly studied. See H. Pfautz, "The Current Literature on Social Stratification: Critique and Bibliography," *American Journal of Sociology* 58 (January 1953), esp. pp. 401–404.

4. A review of recent investigations of some psychological dimensions of social stratification can be found in Pfautz, "Current Literature." While a number of personality correlates of social class have been delineated, there have been no studies of the relationship of class to the achievement motive as such, though C. W. Mills' notion of the "competitive personality" comes closest to approximating the personality characteristic examined in this study. See his *White Collar* (New York: Oxford University Press, 1953). Of the many studies of the cultural correlates of social class, two which have particular relevance for the problem examined in this paper are H. Hyman, "The Value System of Different Classes: A Social Psychological Contribution to the Analysis of Stratification," in ed. R. Bendix and S. Lipset, *Class, Status, and Power* (New York: Free Press, 1953), pp. 425–442, and T. Parsons, "A Revised Analytical Approach to the Theory of Social Stratification," ibid., pp. 92–128.

5. A. Green, in his introductory text, *Sociology* (New York: McGraw-Hill, 1952), regards the middle class' high level of achievement drive, as expressed through status striving, as its single most pronounced characteristics. However, the data to support this conclusion are largely of an anecdotal or highly qualitative nature. See C. W. Mills, *White Collar*, and A. Davis, B. Gardner, and M. Gardner, *Deep South* (Chicago: University of Chicago Press, 1941).

6. For a fuller exposition of this scheme see A. Hollingshead and F. C. Redlich, "Social Stratification and Psychiatric Disorders," *American Sociological Review* 18 (April 1953): 163–169.

7. D. McClelland et al., *The Achievement Motive* (New York: Appleton-Century-Crofts, 1953).

8. Experiments have shown that motivation scores vary with the conditions under which the test is given. The kinds of instructions preceding the test are known to affect the test scores. These instructions are basically of three kinds: *achievement-oriented* instructions which produce cues aimed at increasing the score; *relaxed* instructions which tend to deemphasize the arousal of the motive; and *neutral* instruction that are aimed at obtaining a measure of the normal level of motivation a subject brings to a situation. Instructions used in this study were of a neutral type. The impact of the school situation upon the scores is unknown, but we believe that in effect this factor was controlled since all subjects were tested in the same situation. Further information on the various methods for administering this test, and their significance for the test results, can be found in ibid., chap. 3. The test protocols were scored by two judges. The Pearson product moment correlation between the two scorings was plus .89, an estimate of scoring reliability similar to those reported in earlier studies with this measure.

9. In a study of personality and value differences between upper-class Harvard freshmen (private school graduates) and middle-class freshmen (public school graduates), C. McArthur, "Personality Differences Between Middle and Upper Classes," *Journal of Abnormal and Social Psychology* 50 (March 1955): 247–254, found that the need achievement level of the middle class was significantly higher than that of the upper class. The difference between the two groups in the writer's study was in the same direction noted by McArthur, but was not statistically significant. However, since sampling methods, TAT pictures, and scoring procedures used in the two studies are different, the data are not comparable.

10. Four pictures were used in this study. The approximate median score for the entire sample was + 4. Sixty-six subjects have a score of + 4 or less; fifty-four subjects a score of + 5 or more. Scores ranged from − 4 to + 15. It should be under-

stood that the terms "high" and "low" used in this study do not refer to absolute standards but to relative ranks for individuals in this sample. As yet there are not sufficient data to permit the setting up of norms for broad cross-sections of the population for either achievement motivation or value orientation.

11. Analysis of the data in which persons in Classes I and II are examined together in one cell or part reveals that the conclusions noted above are not affected when the cells are collapsed.

12. C. Kluckhohn and F. Kluckhohn, "American Culture: Generalized Orientations and Class Patterns," in *Conflicts of Power in Modern Culture*, ed. L. Bryson et al. (New York: Harper, 1947), pp. 106–128. See also M. Gordon, "*Kitty Foyle* and the Concept of Class as Culture," *American Journal of Sociology* 53 (November 1947): 210–217. Other investigators are cited in Pfautz, *Current Literature*, pp. 403–404.

13. F. Kluckhohn, "Dominant and Substitute Profiles of Cultural Orientations: Their Significance for the Analysis of Social Stratification," *Social Forces* 28 (May 1950): 376–393.

14. In all, fourteen items were used to index certain of the adolescent's values and perceptions. The nine additional items are as follows:

1. Even though parents often seem too strict, when a person gets older he will realize it was beneficial.
2. If my parents told me to stop seeing a friend of my own sex, I'd see that friend anyway.
3. Parents seem to believe that you can't take the opinion of a teenager seriously.
4. Parents would be greatly upset if their son ended up doing factory work.
5. It's silly for a teenager to put money in a car when the money could be used to get started in a business or for an education.
6. The best kind of job is one where you are part of an organization all working together, even if you don't get individual credit.
7. Education and learning are more important in determining a person's happiness than money and what it will buy.
8. When the time comes for a boy to take a job, he should stay near his parents even if it means giving up a good job.
9. Even when teenagers get married their main loyalty still belongs to their mother and father.

15. The writer is indebted to an earlier, somewhat different scale (based in part on work done by the writer as a member of the "Cultural Factors in Talent Development" project), put together by Fred L. Strodtbeck.

16. Class differentials in educational aspiration level have been noted by a number of investigators. See, for example, J. A. Kahl, "Educational and Occupational Aspirations of 'Common Man' Boys," *Harvard Educational Review* 23 (Summer 1953): 186–203.

17. McClelland, *Achievement Motive*, chap. 9.

18. M. Winterbottom, "The Relationship of Childhood Training in Independence to Achievement Motivation" (Ph.D. Diss., University of Michigan, 1953).

19. The uncertain character of data relating to class differences in child rearing is pointed up in the article, R. J. Havighurst and A. Davis, "A Comparison of the Chicago and Harvard Studies of Social Class Differences in Child Rearing," *American Sociological Review* 20 (August 1955): 435–442. See also M. C. Erickson, "Social Status and Child-rearing Practices," in *Readings in Social Psychology*, ed. T. Newcomb and E. Hartley (New York: Holt, 1947), and A. Davis, *Social-class Influences Upon Learning* (Cambridge, Mass.: Harvard University Press, 1951).

COMMENTARY

As in the area of socialization, a number of questions arise regarding the influence of the stratification system on psychiatric disturbances. With reference to Rosen's paper, the following questions may be instructively entertained: In what ways is this a study of personality development? What levels or types of achievement motivation and value orientations may be regarded as normal, healthy, or problematic? What sources of developmental or situational stress would one expect an individual with high achievement motivation to experience? Studies indicate that the most severe psychiatric disturbances in the United States are concentrated in the lowest social classes. How might this fact be related to the culture complex of achievement and social mobility?

Rosen documents variations in achievement motivation and value orientations within each social class. What conflicts or stresses are experienced by individuals whose motives and values differ from group norms? For example, what happens to the middle-class boy who wants to be an automobile mechanic, or the lower-class chap who wants to be a doctor? What factors other than his family culture influence his achievement motivation and value orientation?

In what ways is the culture of a society a framework for self-fulfillment and an obstacle to it? It may be argued that in any society the individual has strivings for acceptance, self-esteem, and mastery. Moreover, he will have a unique endowment and developmental history which influence his capabilities and wishes. What will be the "fit" between "self" and "society"?

CHAPTER 10

The Family in Society

INTRODUCTION

*All education is piecemeal. We learn bits of concepts and informa-
tion, and no sooner come to appreciate their value than we realize
their incompleteness, imperfection, and lack of cohesion. Perhaps that
is what drives researchers and scholars—this gratification with new
knowledge, dissatisfaction with inadequacies, and the ever beckoning
challenge to revise, extend, and integrate. In a small way this is the
challenge that invites review of the next selection.*

*We have explored a number of sociological concepts: culture,
status and role, primary groups, socialization, and stratification. In
Campisi's study of the Italian family in the United States, each of
these concepts may be brought together—not only further to illustrate
and clarify each of them, but to show their interrelations in the social
system (which has a certain integrity). The paper also leads us into
new concerns: the family as a special type of human group; the relationships of family to society; sociocultural conflicts; disorganization
and change.*

*Campisi examines changes in the cultural characteristics of the
Italian family associated with its immigration from the Old World to
America. He succinctly provides an abundantly detailed description
of three family types: the Old World, southern peasant family; the
first-generation Italian American family; and the second-generation
Italian American family.*

*The paper illustrates concretely the numerous facets of group
life and individual existence which are defined and regulated by culture. The meaning of sexuality; the relationships between men and
women; the respective rights and obligations of parents and children;
the ethical, social, and supernatural function of religion—these are
among the profoundly consequential views and behavior patterns
shaped decisively by culture. Significant variations in such patterns*

are sharply exposed by Campisi's brief but cogent and comprehensive review.

The Old World family, not unlike the late, agriculturally based rural American family, was a unit of economic cooperation and consumption. It was a rather comprehensive group which served multiple functions for its members: economic, affectional, recreational, educational, religious, and so on. The family was thus a dominant institution, both in the lives of its members and in the functioning of community and society.

The Old World family was a close-knit primary group bound by tradition, resistant to change, and concentrating authority in the status of the father. The transformation of the culture and structure of the Old World family after its relocation in America stems from several sources, including its detachment from a larger cultural and social system of which it was a part to a world in which it was a minority, alien culture; the fact that it had been based on an agricultural economy in small-village settings rather than one which was urban-industrial; and its extensive contact with a different culture which was its new medium of survival and which imposed economic, political, and social pressures for "Americanization."

These pressures lead to acculturation—*the acquisition of culture (in this case American culture). Campisi describes and analyzes the movement of the first- and second-generation Italian American family away from the Old World form and toward that of the contemporary urban American family in terms of three stages: (1) initial contact; (2) conflict; and (3) accommodation.*

ETHNIC FAMILY PATTERNS:
THE ITALIAN FAMILY IN THE UNITED STATES

Paul J. Campisi

The changes in the Italian family in America can be visualized in terms of a continuum which ranges from an unacculturated Old World type to a highly acculturated and urbanized American type of family. This transformation can be understood by an analysis of three types

Paul J. Campisi, "Ethnic Family Patterns: The Italian Family in the United States," *The American Journal of Sociology* 53, 1948, pp. 443–449. Reprinted with permission of the author and The University of Chicago Press.

of families which have characterized Italian family living in America: the Old World peasant Italian family which existed at the time of the mass migration from Italy (1890–1910) and which can be placed at the unacculturated end of the continuum; the first-generation Italian family in America, which at the beginning of contact with American culture was much like the first but which changed and continues to change increasingly so that it occupies a position somewhere between the two extremes; and, finally, the second-generation Italian family which represents a cross-fertilization of the first-generation Italian family and the American contemporary urban family, with the trend being in the direction of the American type. Consequently, the position this family assumes is near the American-urban end of the continuum.

Since there are significant differences between the northern Italian and southern Italian families and since there are even greater differences among peasant, middle-class, and upper-class families, it seems expedient to single out one type of family for discussion and analysis, namely, the southern Italian peasant family. During the period of mass migration from Italy the bulk of the immigrants were from southern Italy (including Sicily).[1] These immigrants came mostly from small-village backgrounds as peasant farmers, peasant workers, or simple artisans, and as such they brought with them a southern Italian folk-peasant culture. It is this type of background which the majority of Italian families in America have today.[2]

This paper cannot possibly present an adequate analysis of all the important changes observed in the Italian family. Therefore, a simple tabular form (see Table I) is used to display the most important details.

The Southern Italian Peasant Family in America

At the time of the great population movement from Italy to America, beginning at the end of the nineteenth century, the southern Italian peasant family was a folk societal family. One of the chief characteristics of the folk society is that its culture is highly integrated, the separate parts forming a strongly geared and functionally meaningful whole.[3] This intimate interconnection between the various parts of a folk culture indicates that it would be artificial and fruitless to attempt to isolate, even for the sake of study and analysis, any one part, such as the family, and to proceed to discuss that as a discrete and distinct entity. All the characteristics of the Old World Italian peasant family are intimately tied in with such institutions and practices as religion, the planting and gathering of food, the celebrations of feasts and holidays, the education of the children, the treatment of the sick, the protection of the person, and with all other aspects of small-village folk culture. In the final analysis Old World peasant-family life meant small-village life, and the two were inseparable aspects of a coercive folk-peasant culture. This fact sharply distinguishes the Old World

TABLE 1

Differences Between the Southern Italian Peasant Family in Italy and the First- and Second-Generation Italian Family in America

	Southern Italian Peasant Family in Italy	First-Generation Southern Italian Family in America	Second-Generation Southern Italian Family in America
A. General characteristics:			
1.	Patriarchal	Fictitiously patriarchal	Tends to be democratic
2.	Folk-peasant	Quasi-urban	Urban and modern
3.	Well integrated	Disorganized and in conflict	Variable, depending on the particular family situation
4.	Stationary	Mobile	High degree of mobility
5.	Active community life	Inactive in the American community but somewhat active in the Italian neighborhood	Inactive in the Italian neighborhood, but increasingly active in American community
6.	Emphasis on the sacred	Emphasis on the sacred is weakened	Emphasis on the secular
7.	Home and land owned by family	In the small city the home may be owned, but in a large city the home is usually a flat or an apartment	Ownership of home is an ideal, but many are satisfied with flat
8.	Strong family and community culture	Family culture in conflict	Weakened family culture reflecting vague American situation
9.	Sharing of common goals	No sharing of common goals	No sharing of common goals
10.	Children live for the parents	Children live for themselves	Parents live for the children
11.	Children are an economic asset	Children are an economic asset for few working years only and may be an economic liability	Children are an economic liability
12.	Many family celebrations of special feasts, holidays, etc.	Few family celebrations of feasts and holidays	Christmas only family affair, with Thanksgiving being variable
13.	Culture is transmitted only by the family	Italian culture is transmitted only by family, but American culture is transmitted by American institutions other than the family	American culture is transmitted by the family and by other American institutions
14.	Strong in-group solidarity	Weakened in-group solidarity	Little in-group solidarity
15.	Many functions: economic, recreational, religious, social, affectional, and protective	Functions include semirecreational, social, and affectional	Functions reduced to affectional in the main
B. Size:			
1.	Large-family system	Believe in a large-family system but cannot achieve it because of migration	Small-family system

Southern Italian Peasant Family in Italy	First-Generation Southern Italian Family in America	Second-Generation Southern Italian Family in America
2. Many children (10 is not unusual)	Fair number of children (10 is unusual)	Few children (10 is rare)
3. Extended kinship to godparents	Extended kinship, but godparent relationship is weakened	No extended kinship to godparents

C. *Roles and statuses:*

Southern Italian Peasant Family in Italy	First-Generation Southern Italian Family in America	Second-Generation Southern Italian Family in America
1. Father has highest status	Father loses high status, or it is fictitiously maintained	Father shares high status with mother and children; slight patriarchal survival
2. Primogeniture: eldest son has high status	Rule of primogeniture is variable; success more important than position	No primogeniture; all children tend to have equal status
3. Mother center of domestic life only and must not work for wages	Mother center of domestic life but may work for wages and belong to some clubs	Mother acknowledges domestic duties but reserves time for much social life and may work for wages
4. Father can punish children severely	Father has learned that American law forbids this	Father has learned it is poor psychology to do so
5. Family regards itself as having high status and role in the community	Family does not have high status and role in the American community but may have it in the Italian colony	Family struggles for high status and role in the American community and tends to reject high status and role in the Italian community
6. Women are educated for marriage only	Women receive some formal education as well as family education for marriage	Emphasis is on general education with reference to personality development rather than to future marriage
7. The individual is subordinate to the family	Rights of the individual increasingly recognized	The family is subordinate to the individual
8. Daughter-in-law is subservient to the husband's family	Daughter-in-law is in conflict with husband's family	Daughter-in-law is more or less independent of husband's family
9. Son is expected to work hard and contribute to family income	Son is expected to work hard and contribute to family income, but this is a seldom-realized goal	Son expected to do well in school and need not contribute to family income

D. *Interpersonal relations:*

Southern Italian Peasant Family in Italy	First-Generation Southern Italian Family in America	Second-Generation Southern Italian Family in America
1. Husband and wife must not show affection in the family or in public	Husband and wife are not demonstrative in public or in the family but tolerate it in their married children	Husband and wife may be demonstrative in the family and in public
2. Boys are superior to girls	Boys are regarded as superior to girls	Boys tend to be regarded as superior to girls, but girls have high status also
3. Father is consciously feared, respected, and imitated	Father is not consciously feared or imitated but is respected	Father is not consciously feared. He may be imitated and may be admired

TABLE 1—Continued

Southern Italian Peasant Family in Italy	First-Generation Southern Italian Family in America	Second-Generation Southern Italian Family in America
4. Great love for mother	Great love for mother but much ambivalence from cultural tensions	Love for mother is shared with father
5. Baby indulgently treated by all	Baby indulgently treated by all	Baby indulgently treated by all with increasing concern regarding sanitation, discipline, and sibling rivalry
E. Marriage:		
1. Marriage in early teens	Marriage in late teens or early twenties	Marriage in early or middle twenties
2. Selection of mate by parents	Selection of mate by individual with parental consent	Selection of mate by individual regardless of parental consent
3. Must marry someone from the same village	This is an ideal, but marriage with someone from the same region (i.e., province) is tolerated; very reluctant permission granted to marry outside nationality; no permission for marriage outside religion	Increasing number of marriages outside nationality and outside religion
4. Dowry rights	No dowry	No dowry
5. Marriage always involves a religious ceremony	Marriage almost always involves both a religious and a secular ceremony	Marriage usually involves both, but there is an increasing number of marriages without benefit of religious ceremony
F. Birth and child care:		
1. Many magical and superstitious beliefs in connection with pregnancy	Many survivals of old beliefs and superstitions	Few magical and superstitious notions in connection with pregnancy
2. Delivery takes place in a special confinement room in the home; midwife assists	Delivery takes place generally in a hospital; may take place in home; family doctor displaces midwife	Delivery takes place almost always in a hospital; specialist, obstetrician, or general practitioner assists
3. Child illnesses are treated by folk remedies; local physician only in emergencies or crises	Child illnesses are treated partially by folk remedies but mostly by the family doctor	Child illnesses are treated by a pediatrician; much use of latest developments in medicine (vaccines, etc.)
4. Child is breast-fed either by the mother or by a wet nurse; weaning takes place at about end of second or third year by camouflaging the breasts	Child is breast-fed if possible; if not, it is bottle-fed; some practice with variations regarding weaning	Child is bottle-fed as soon as possible; breast-feeding is rare; no weaning problems
5. No birth control	Some birth control	Birth control is the rule

Southern Italian Peasant Family in Italy	First-Generation Southern Italian Family in America	Second-Generation Southern Italian Family in America
G. *Sex attitudes:*		
1. Child is allowed to go naked about the house up to the age of 5 or 6; after this there is rigid enforcement of the rule of modesty	Variable, depending on the individual family's situation	This is variable, depending on the individual family; development of modesty is much earlier than in Old World peasant family
2. Sex matters are not discussed in family	Sex matters are not discussed in family	Sex matters increasingly discussed in family but not as freely as in "old" American family
3. Adultery is severely punished by the man's taking matters into his own hands	Adultery results in divorce or separation	Adultery may result in divorce or separation
4. Chastity rule rigidly enforced by chaperonage; lack of it grounds for immediate separation at wedding night	Attempts to chaperon fail, but chastity is an expectation; lack of it is grounds for separation, but there are few cases of this kind in America	No chaperonage; chastity is expected, but lack of it may be reluctantly tolerated
5. No premarital kissing and petting are allowed	No premarital kissing and petting are allowed openly	Premarital kissing and petting are allowed openly
6. Boys and girls attend separate schools	Schools are coeducational	Schools are coeducational
H. *Divorce and separation:*		
1. No divorce allowed	No divorce allowed, but some do divorce	Religion forbids it, but it is practiced
2. Desertion is rare	Desertion is rare	Desertion is rare
I. *Psychological aspects:*		
1. Fosters security in the individual	Fosters conflict in the individual	Fosters security with some conflict lags
2. The family provides a specific way of life; hence, there is little personal disorganization	Family is in conflict, hence cannot provide a specific way of life; yields marginal American-Italian way of life	Family reflects confused American situation, does not give individual a specific way of life, but marginality is weakened
3. Recreation is within family	Recreation is both within and outside the family	Recreation is in the main outside the family; this is variable, depending on individual family situation

peasant family from the first- and second-generation families in America.

The First-Generation Southern Italian Peasant Family in America

By the first-generation Italian family is simply meant that organization of parents and offspring wherein both parents are of foreign birth and wherein an attempt is made to perpetuate an Italian way of life in the transplanted household. This is a family in transition, still struggling against great odds to keep alive those customs and traditions which were sacred in the Old World culture. As a result of many internal and external pressures which have cut it off from its Old World foundations, the first-generation family is marked by considerable confusion, conflict, and disorganization. The uncertain and precarious position of the first-generation Italian family today is further aggravated by the loss of that strong family and community culture which had been such an indispensable part of the Old World peasant family. It is this loss in the first-generation family which pushes it away from the unacculturated end of the continuum to a position somewhere in the middle.[4]

The Second-Generation Southern Italian Peasant Family in America

This refers to that organization of parents and offspring wherein both the parents are native American-born but have foreign-born parents who attempted to transmit to them an Italian way of life in the original first-generation family in America.

Among the significant characteristics of this type of family is the orientation which the American-born parents make to the American culture. This adjustment tends to take three forms. One is that of complete abandonment of the Old World way of life. The individual changes his Italian name, moves away from the Italian neighborhood and in some cases from the community, and has little to do with his foreign-born parents and relatives.[5] The ideal is to become acculturated in as short a time as possible. This type of second-generation Italian generally passes for an American family and is rare. A second form of second-generation Italian family is a marginal one. In this type there is a seriously felt need to become Americanized and hence to shape the structure and functions of the family in accordance with the contemporary urban American type of family. The parental way of life is not wholly repudiated, although there is some degree of rejection. This family is likely to move out of the Italian neighborhood and to communicate less and less with first-generation Italians, but the bond with the first-generation family is not broken completely. Intimate communication is maintained with the parental household, and the relationships with the parents as well as with immigrant relatives are affectionate and understanding. A third form which the second-generation family takes is of orientation inward toward an Italian way of life. This type of family generally prefers to remain in the Italian neighborhood, close to the parental home. Its interaction with the non-Italian world is at a minimum, and its interests are tied up with those of the Italian community. Of the three, the second type is the most representative second-generation Italian family in America. This is the family depicted in Table 1.

Table 1 reveals the movement of the first- and second-generation Italian families away from the Old World peasant pattern and toward the contemporary American family type. In this persistent and continuous process of acculturation there are three stages: (1) the initial-contact stage; (2) the conflict stage; and (3) the accommodation stage.

The Initial-Contact Stage

In the first decade of Italian living in America the structure of the Old World family is still fairly well intact, but pressures from within and outside the family are beginning to crack, albeit imperceptibly, the Old World peasant pattern. Producing this incipient distortion are the following: the very act of physical separation from the parental family and village culture; the necessity to work and operate with a somewhat strange and foreign body of household tools, equipment, gadgets, furniture, cooking utensils, and other physical objects, in addition to making an adjustment to a different physical environment, including climate, urban ecological conditions, and tenement living arrangements; the birth of children and the increasing contact with American medical practices regarding child care; the necessity to work for wages at unfamiliar tasks, a new experience for the peasant farmer; the attendance of Italian children in American parochial and public schools; the informal interaction of the children with the settlement house, the church associations, the neighborhood clubs, the neighborhood gang, and other organizations; the continuing residence in America and increasing period of isolation from the Old World; the acceptance of work by the housewife outside the home for wages; the increasing recognition by both parents and children that the Italian way of life in the American community means low status, social and economic discrimination, and prejudice; and the increasing pressure by American legal, educational, political, and economic institutions for the Americanization of the foreigner.

Nonetheless, the first-generation Italian family in this phase is a highly integrated one, as in the Old World. The demands of the American community are not seriously felt in the insulated Italian colony, and the children are too young seriously to articulate their newly acquired needs and wishes. The Italian family is stabilized by the strong drive to return to Italy.

The Conflict Stage

In this period the first-generation family experiences its most profound changes and is finally wrenched from its Old World foundation. It is now chiefly characterized by the conflict between two ways of life, the one American and the other Italian, and by the incompatibility of parents and children. This phase begins roughly during the second decade of living in America—specifically, when the children unhesitatingly express their acquired American expectations and attempt to transmit them in the family situation, and when the parents in turn attempt to reinforce the pattern of the Old World peasant family. Conflicting definitions of various family situations threaten to destroy whatever stability the family had maintained through the first period. This is the period of great frustration and of misunderstanding between parents and children. In this undeclared state of war between two ways of life it is the parents who have the most to lose, for their complete acceptance of the American way of living means the destruction of the Old World ideal.

The first-generation Italian family is also constantly made to feel the force of external pressures coming from outside the Italian colony. It is inevitable that the family structure should crumble under the incessant hammering. Not able to draw upon a complete culture and social system to support its position, the family pattern, already weakened, now begins to change radically: the father loses his importance, the daughters acquire unheard-of independence; in short, the children press down upon the first-generation family an American way of life.

Accommodation Stage

This period begins with the realization by parents and children that the continuation of hostility, misunderstanding, and contraventive behavior can result only in complete deterioration of the family. The ambivalent attitude of the children toward the parents, of great affection, on the one hand, and hostility, on the other, now tends to be replaced by a more tolerant disposition. This stage begins when the offspring reach adulthood and marry and establish households of their own, for by this time the control by the parents is greatly lessened.

Among the many factors which operate to bring about a new stability in the family are the realization on the part of the parents that life in America is to be permanent; the adult age of the offspring; the almost complete dependence of the parents on the offspring, including use of the children as informants, interpreters, guides, and translators of the American world; recognition on the part of the parents that social and economic success can come to the offspring only as they become more and more like "old Americans"; the conscious and unconscious acculturation of the parents themselves with a consequent minimizing of many potential conflicts; the long period of isolation from the Old World which makes the small-village culture and peasant family seem less real; the decision by the parents to sacrifice certain aspects of the Old World family for the sake of retaining the affection of the children; the acknowledgment by the children that the first-generation family is a truncated one and that complete repudiation of the parents would leave them completely isolated; the success of the first-generation family in instilling in the offspring respect and affection for the parents; and the gradual understanding by the children that successful interaction with the American world is possible by accepting marginal roles and that complete denial of the Old World family is unnecessary.

The accommodation between parents and offspring permits the second-generation Italians to orientate themselves increasingly toward an American way of life. The second-generation household, therefore, tends to pattern itself after the contemporary urban American family. Considerable intermarriage, the advanced age of the parents, the loosening of ties with the Italian neighborhood, and the development of intimate relationships with non-Italians make the transition of the second-generation family comparatively easy.

NOTES

1. During the decade of 1900–1910, of the 2,045,877 Italians who came to America, the majority were from southern Italy.

2. The observations in this paper are based on the literature in the field, on my own specific research in America on the acculturation of Italians, and, finally, on personal impressions and conclusions as a participant observer. A visit to southern Italy and Sicily three years ago gave me an opportunity to come in contact with the Old World peasant-type family. While this type of family has changed considerably from the time of the mass migration to America, enough structural and functional family lags exist to make the reconstruction of it in this paper reasonably valid.

3. See Robert Redfield, "The Folk Society," *American Journal of Sociology* 52 (1947): 293–308.

4. For an excellent analysis of the importance of a strong family and community culture see Margaret Park Redfield, "The American Family: Consensus and Freedom," *American Journal of Sociology* 52 (1946): 175–183.

5. See Carlo Sforza, *The Real Italians* (New York: Columbia University Press, 1942), for an interesting account of Italian-Americans who change their names.

COMMENTARY

The social, cultural, and psychological dynamics described and analyzed by Campisi were not unique to the experience of Italian-Americans. In many respects they characterized the experience of Irish Catholics, European Jews, Swedes, Germans, and others during the great period of American immigration. While examining a specific ethnic-historical experience, the study reflects many generalizable principles of culture change, including the fact that cultures are adapted to particular environments; the resistance of core values and beliefs to change; the fact that cultures serve to organize the lives of individuals in meaningful terms; and the fact that cultures are organized wholes whose total functioning may be threatened by the introduction of even a single alien cultural trait.

That the social dynamics of immigration are fundamental to social change in general is colorfully illustrated by Tevye's agonizing struggle with the decline of tradition in the musical play Fiddler on the Roof, *and contemporary Japan's widespread appreciation of that ostensibly parochial drama. Moreover, many of the stresses and strains of the present gap between "American-Americans" and their "next-generation" children implicate the same principles of social change.*

One area of social-psychiatric interest in this rich human document concerns the ways in which individuals located in various parts of the family structure were subjected to patterned stresses. For example, what problems of self-esteem are attached to the changing status and role of the first-generation Italian American father? How might such problems be manifested? What stresses are associated with the position of mother or son?

As mentioned earlier in this book, an eighteen-year-old girl who had recently immigrated to the United States was assigned to a first-year psychiatric resident. She shows symptoms of anxiety and depression. She talks at length about her father, a construction worker, and complains she doesn't know what to do with her life. She reports that she is very close to her father, but they have constant arguments about what hours she must come in at night and whom she may date. In what ways are a clinician's understanding of and approach to this patient informed by Campisi's study? How may the various key concepts considered be applied here? Is it possible to act in a value-free role as a therapist in this situation?

Speaking generally, and with some oversimplification, psychoanalytic formulations tend to emphasize personality processes, while sociological formulations emphasize interpersonal relationships. Is either focus adequate for clinical roles? How do they complement or compete with each other?

If sources of stress and conflict and issues of growth and adaptation are attached to the social positions of the Italian Americans de-

scribed, do such matters bear routine examination in the lives of patients seeking psychiatric help? Are changing forms of psychiatric disturbance associated with economic, political, or religious changes in the United States? Can an individual's disturbances be comprehended apart from the family's sociocultural characteristics and its adaptation to the community? If so, how? If not, why not?

PART II

THE TREATMENT SETTING AS A SOCIAL SYSTEM

CHAPTER 11

The Treatment Setting As a Social System

Alan M. Kraft

Scientific medicine has tended to understand illness by a study of the disease process as it takes place inside the patient. Psychiatry has adopted this perspective, particularly in its examination of the hereditary and neurophysiological aspects of psychic disorders. It has been possible in this way to objectify the patient and his disorder and in this sense to isolate the individual from his environment, at least for the purposes of study. This methodology, especially suited to biological pathology, enables the investigator to narrow his examination and to disregard a great many concurrent and intercurrent events. This approach to the study of disordered feelings, thoughts, and behavior is suited to the laboratory, where events can be controlled and data isolated, but it becomes more complex in clinical practice. The person who over an extended time feels sad in the absence of any reason he can easily describe may be called clinically depressed. The neurophysiology and neurochemistry of this condition may be studied by isolating and examining the blood, cerebral electrical activity, cerebrospinal fluid, galvanic skin response, and other such elements of biological activity. These observations will illuminate one complex dimension of clinical depression, a dimension which is valid and important, yet is only one among several.

The Biological-Psychological-Social Triad

The biological dimensions may be added to by the examination of other aspects of the individual—those having to do with his psychological and social being. The process of examining and understanding these kinds of data differs from examining and understanding biological data.

Psychological processes are not so easily objectified. Many data are by definition "subjective," personal, and idiosyncratic, unavavailable for outside verification. The person's feelings of sadness, his thoughts of hopelessness and futility, cannot be verified independently; they must be accepted or rejected as reported. More "objective" observations may be made; for example, the person who feels sad may move about slowly, may be unsmiling and tearful, and may be uninvolved with people who are with him. He may speak in subdued tones, and his verbalizations may be characterized as dealing with morbid subject matter. To complicate matters further, the person may respond in different ways to different examiners, or in different ways to the same examiner, who might be sympathetic at one time and aggressive and provocative at another. Objective study becomes more difficult because the very act of examination changes the process being observed.

The study of social forces is at least as complex. Social forces are concerned with patterned group behavior, and also with beliefs and attitudes. It is possible for a relatively uninvolved observer to examine interactional patterns in a social group, or to investigate beliefs and attitudes, without running the same high order of risk of altering the process which he observes. But he does run the risk of becoming personally involved as an actor and believer in this process (see Chapter 12). Furthermore, research into social forces requires an examination of social processes as they happen. These processes are highly complex, and it is not a simple matter to isolate parts of them. The sad and depressed man will feel and behave differently, and will have a different impact upon others in his environment, if he is an office worker who sits weeping and morose at his desk, or if he is on a ward exhibiting the same behavior. The responses of others to him, and his responses to them, will be quite different in those two very different social situations. Similarly, the same individual in a hospital will respond selectively to different kinds of social settings. On one ward there may be little social interaction, with patients left more or less to their own devices; he would react quite differently on a ward in which a newly admitted patient was approached very quickly by other patients and the staff and *expected* to interact.

Each of the dimensions—biological, psychological, and social—is valid and does not negate the validity of another observation. The same clinically depressed individual may have a disturbance of catacholamine metabolism, suicidal thoughts, and unfriendly social behavior. Furthermore, it may be possible to alter the experience of the person who is feeling sad by biological (psychopharmacologic), psychological (psychotherapeutic interpretation or support), and/or social (group or family) intervention. A treatment plan might include all three kinds of intervention.

One intervention is no better or more valid than the other, except perhaps as measured by its effectiveness. There is evidence that interventions of all three types are effective in producing change. Some interventions are more powerful than others, but few would argue that clinical practice should depend upon only one kind of intervention to the exclusion of others.

When we explore social forces as they affect thought, feeling, and behavior, we must bear in mind that for heuristic purposes we are addressing ourselves to but one of the triad of forces. In practice it is seldom possible to isolate social forces from biological and psychological forces. The clinician is skillful and effective to the extent that his understanding and knowledge enable him to intervene usefully in all three dimensions.

The Hospital as a Social System

The psychiatric hospital has occupied a central role in the training of psychiatrists. There has been a temptation to view psychiatric hospitalization as though it were simply another kind of medical event analogous to hospitalization for pneumonia or gall bladder surgery. While there are many similarities between psychiatric and medical or surgical hospitalization, there are some very important differences. During hospitalization for medical or surgical treatment the patient as a person is a passive recipient of the interventions. It matters little, within broad limits, how the patient feels or thinks about his fellow patients or the staff, or how he understands his illness, so long as he is treated voluntarily. The staff have technical skills which require the patient's cooperation, but only infrequently, and only for special procedures is the patient's active participation required. Furthermore, hospitalization for medical and surgical care tends to be briefer than psychiatric hospitalization.

In contrast, psychiatric hospitalization introduces the patient into a ward or unit where his person, emotional responses, and behavior are foci for attention and response. The unit is made up of staff and patients whose interrelationships constitute a social system. Each individual becomes a member of that small society by virtue of working or living there, whether or not he wishes to be so (see Chapters 4, 5, and 8).

What is a social system? A social system is a group of individuals (varying in size from a dyad to an entire society) in which there is interaction and interdependence between the individuals. There are exchanges between the individuals and between the social system and its environment.[1]

Individuals in interaction behave as they do for many reasons. Some motivations are unique to the individual, based upon his idiosyncratic experience and history. He may be attracted or repelled by another person because of previous personal experience with someone of whom he is reminded. Or he may have special interests in certain activities, such as a hobby or type of work, based upon his past individual experience. Other motivations are based not so much on personal history as on social role. For example, the role of doctor calls forth certain kinds of expected behavior relatively independent of individual differences. Doctors characteristically are accorded respect by patients and staff and act with dignity and a certain reserve in a medical setting. Some behaviors are usually considered "inappropriate" for doctors; for example, doctors may be discreetly sexually assertive with nurses but not with patients. Patients' behavior is also determined in part by role expectation and the expectations of the setting relatively independent of idiosyncratic differences. Medical patients are expected to be passive, uncomplaining, cooperative, and unquestioning. Virtually every medical or surgical ward nurse staff categorizes its patients as "good" or "bad" according to whether their behavior complies with the staff's role definition.

A social system develops regulatory mechanisms (such as role definitions) which control exchanges between individuals and between the social system and its environment (see Chapter 6). Interactions among individuals in social systems may result in significant changes in the individuals and in the system itself, so that both the individual and the system constantly face the possibility of change and adaptation to change.

The concept of the social system is especially useful for the psychiatrist and behavioral scientist because it stresses the contextual view of group and individual behavior. By studying the human interrelationships in a treatment setting it is possible to observe these forces as they influence, constrain, or offer opportunities for change of behavior. In such a setting it is also possible to observe the ways in which an individual's behavior is responsive to his social environment. The small psychiatric unit is especially suited to learning about social forces which influence behavior because of its relatively small size and relative insulation from the myriad forces which affect other small systems, such as a classroom. As the ward becomes more open and its boundaries more permeable, it also becomes a more complex system—and therefore more difficult to study.

Examination of the social system of a psychiatric unit opens possibilities of studying the mutuality of influences, such as the influence of patients on staff; how the behavior of one group affects the other; the spoken and covert "rules" that govern their behavior; the sharing of power in the social organization; and the overt and covert belief systems regarding such issues as mental illness, treatment, recovery, and responsibility for one's behavior.

Total Institutions

For the above reasons the mental hospital has become one of the more frequently studied social institutions. The work of Goffman, *Asylums*,[2] is an important example which deserves study. Though it is not feasible to include this work in this volume, some of the important concepts will be discussed. A sociologist, Goffman examined a large mental hospital with the goal of understanding the complex social forces at work in such an institution, and to learn about the social world of the patient. He chose a mental hospital as an example of a "total institution," which he defines as "a place of residence and work where a large number of like situated individuals, cut off from the wider society for an appreciable period of time together, lead to an enclosed, formally administered round of life." [3] Prisons, mental hospitals, and military academies are total institutions. Ordinarily people live, work, and recreate in different places with different people. In a total institution these activities occur in one place with one group.

He discovered that life in such institutions has created specific role behaviors not only for patients, but for staff and employees. The belief systems and role expectations of such institutions call for individuals to behave in ways independent of their unique characteristics as individuals. The social system creates pressures in which patients are expected to behave in certain ways and forbidden to behave in other ways. They are permitted access to specified spaces and prohibited from others. Patients adapt in response to the constraints and expectations of the total institution. As the total institution becomes more encompassing in the control of the person's behavior, individuals and groups within the institution develop patterns of behavior aimed at maintenance to some degree of personal integrity. These behaviors are outside the "legitimate" prescribed institutional behaviors and are described by Goffman as comprising the "underlife" of the institution.

One of the central points that Goffman develops is that institutions provide structure and substance to an individual's stability and sense of self. However, when the strength of the institutional forces becomes overwhelming, there is a threat to the individual's sense of autonomy, which leads him to resist the pressures to conform. There is a dynamic reciprocal balancing between senses of belonging and of individuality. In the institution he describes, the individuals are able to maintain some sense of individuality by finding ways within the system to escape from being totally enveloped. Goffman's point is that this conflict is an issue for all people and all institutions, not just in total institutions, though he uses these for illustration.

This issue of the struggle by an individual for his sense of self and sense of belonging transcends institutional life. It is a nuclear problem of adolescence, of young adulthood, and in marriage. Though less clear than the forces in a total institution, the social systems in which we live require resolution of the same conflicting issues. Goffman's descriptions raise serious questions about the therapeutic effects of such institutions. Also called into question is the behavioral description of hospitalized mental patients which credits patients' peculiarities entirely to idiosyncratic individual illness. In contrast, Goffman's view is that these are descriptions not of people who "are" chronic schizophrenic, but rather of troubled people in a particular social system whose behavior is partially the product of response to their internal disturbance, but also a response to influences of their social environment. The long-term hospitalized individual with a diagnosis of schizophrenia behaves differently from the individual with the same diagnosis who has lived in some kind of open community setting.[4]

The role expectations of individuals who live and work in a mental hospital are determined in part by the needs of the outside community, in part by the needs of the hospital staff and administration, but also, importantly, by the needs of the patients. Public mental hospital patients are frequently dependent, ambivalent toward authority, and plagued by doubts about their own worth. Thus the observed behavior is not simply a result of social forces or an internal process, but a product of the complex interaction of social, psychological, and biological forces. The characteristics of the patient group affect the social system, and vice versa.[5]

The University Hospital Unit

One has only to compare the mental hospital with another kind of institution, such as a psychiatric unit in a university hospital setting, to observe expectations and behaviors by patients which differ from those in the larger public institutions. In either setting the behavior of patients and staff is powerfully influenced by the social system, drawing our attention to the potentials of social forces for therapeutic purposes (see Chapter 13). If an institution can be dehumanizing in its effect on individuals, may it be restructured so as to be helpful and growth enhancing? The "moral treatment" facilities of the early to mid-nineteenth century were institutions whose social organization was structured to influence patients to behave in more socially acceptable ways. Though the concepts may be new, the practice is not.

Thus our attention is drawn to the social organization of the hospital (or any other treatment setting) so that it may be structured to be as beneficial as possible to the patients. This led Greenblatt to write a paper [6] in which he pointed out that in order to make sophisticated use of the social system for this purpose, the clinician should understand the dynamics of such organizations and of group behavior.

Task and Socioemotional Activities

Mental health organizations share many characteristics with other kinds of service organizations. Of course, they possess unique characteristics as well. Such institutions share a characteristic of many working organizations insofar as their personnel frequently are assigned tasks requiring that they work in small groups in order to achieve their purposes. The product of the system is a service rather than material goods, a fact which makes it more difficult to evaluate its work. Groups of individuals in psychiatric treatment centers typically collaborate on wards, units, and clinical teams. In the course of their joint efforts such teams inevitably are involved in two simultaneously operating processes.

The discussions and activities of the individuals and the team are directed toward accomplishment of the accepted task. As they participate together each contributes his thinking, skills, and knowledge toward the specific task, whether it be group therapy, diagnostic evaluation, treatment planning, food service, interteam coordination, budgetary process, a research project, or a teaching program. As this collaboration is under way, a varying proportion of the time is spent in working directly on accomplishment of the task. An observer examining interactions among members of the group would note that some, but not all, discussions and activities were directly related to achievement of the prescribed task. These activities might be called *task directed* or *instrumental*. The observer would also hear and see another kind of interaction which, while not task directed, seems to be integral to all group process and necessary in order to accomplish the task. This second kind of activity includes such behavior as apparently humorous distractions, flirtations, angry disagreements, leadership struggles, cliquish groupings, and interdisciplinary squabbles. It becomes apparent that as people work together, personal and interpersonal tensions are a usual part of the interaction. These intragroup tensions and needs must be dealt with if the task is to be accomplished; they are a necessary part of group behavior, and may be referred to as the *socioemotional* or *maintenance* work of the group.

The task-directed activities meet the external requirements for work performance. The socioemotional activities provide for the expression and management of personal and interpersonal stresses. Though often covert, casual, informal and unnoticed, the socioemotional processes are necessary if the group is to accomplish its task. Both kinds of activities are necessary and legitimate. The maintenance activities should enhance the motive power for the task-directed activities. In most groups and organizations the socioemotional activities go unrecognized, and there is no deliberate attempt to make them more effective. But every group must provide or allow for mechanisms for the denial, dissipation, or resolution of socioemotional tensions, as well as providing means of enhancing esteem and giving encouragement.

Mental health staffs are usually more aware than most groups of the socioemotional process, and they have frequently evolved mechanisms for dealing directly rather than covertly with it. It may be that mental health workers are unique in that their instrumental task is the provision of socioemotional services to their patients, so that they are more in touch with their own maintenance processes. Some work groups have evolved a method by which they set aside special times to examine the intragroup process. In this way there is an attempt to make sophisticated use of their knowledge of the maintenance needs. Ordinarily, however, task-directed and socioemotional-directed activities alternate throughout the group process and are not easily separated.

Therapeutic Community

Persons who seek and receive help in a psychiatric unit have had interpersonal problems and have experienced difficulties in the socioemotional functions of the family, friendship, work, and other relationships. One of the ways in which the social system of the treatment setting may be helpful to such individuals is in assisting them to improve their abilities (or reduce their problems) in interpersonal socioemotional relationships. The social system does this by making a wide variety of relationships available and by examining the processes of the relationships as they take place (see Chapter 14). Such learning about interpersonal relationships hopefully may then be transferred to relationships outside the treatment setting. In such a therapeutic milieu the instrumental task of the staff is to provide the patients with socioemotional supports and opportunities to learn.

Too frequently socioemotional needs and activities remain covert because they are considered illegitimate and detracting from, rather than enhancing, task performance. An examination of most social systems reveals that overt and covert socioemotional processes help shape the system. The quality of interpersonal relationships in the social system determines not only which people talk to each other but also where, how, when, and about what. It also shapes work output by influencing the process of communication and individual commitment to the task.

Leadership, Managership, Power, and Authority

Authority has become a concept which carries a burden of ill feeling that beclouds its meaning. In its nontechnical meaning authority has come to designate established order. Pejorative attitudes are often related to the *users* of authority. Authority may be exercised effectively and for good purposes or ineffectively and for evil purposes. Authority in the technical, sociologic sense is the right to influence people to behave in specified ways within an organization. Authority flows from positions in an organization. It is the organization's legitimate way of ordering its tasks, assigning work, and delivering its goods or services. Authority is seldom absolute. The individual is influenced in his behavior by internal, social, and interpersonal pressures as well as by authority. An individual may refuse to accept the authority as legitimate; even if he accepts its legitimacy, he may simply refuse to comply with its directives. In so doing he will have to accept the organizational sanctions which follow. For example, the chief of a service may direct a professional to take charge of a patient's treatment. If the person in question refuses to do so he faces sanctions within the limits of his organizational life. Personal morale and values influence one's response to authority. A legitimate directive may be resisted because of personal values. For example, nurses assigned to work on abortion cases have frequently refused to do so when this work was morally repugnant to them.

Individuals in a social system may have influence on others even without authority. The charismatic individual may be very persuasive and have a profound effect on the way individuals and a group behave even though he has no authority to direct their behavior. Or an individual may be able, because of special knowledge, to influence behavior without having the authority to order it. A consultant has this kind of influence if his ideas are translated into action by a team when he is not in a position of authority over the team.

The term "power" generally refers to the ability to influence others. Authority is but one kind of power. The most direct kind of power is coercive power in which one individual or group forces its will upon another. Though this kind of power is generally associated with military, legal, and criminal processes, there are current examples of its exercise in mental health organizations. For example, on a locked ward coercive power is used with the justification that it is "for the patient's own good." Coercive power may be latent, but it is very much a part of a therapeutic relationship between clinician and patient if the clinician has the power to incarcerate, seclude, or send a patient away.

The individual or group of individuals who have authority in an organization are *managers*. The "director" or "chief" is the manager of the enterprise. He has responsibility to some individual or group for the performance of certain work and is accountable to his supraordinate for the resources he receives and the work to be done. The manager is responsible for the planning and implementing of the activities of the unit.

Leadership differs from managership. Leadership is a function of group life in which a person speaks for the sentiments, goals, ideals, concepts, or wishes of a group. Leaders influence behavior. They may or may not be the managers of the group. Leadership typically shifts on various issues. One individual may be the socioemotional leader while another is the accepted leader in specific tasks. Leadership may be shared among several members of the group. From time to time members of a group may develop sentiments of anger, resentment, and hostility toward their manager. The leadership which may express these sentiments speaks without authority but with potential influence in its confrontation with managership. Since this kind of conflict is frequent and the sentiments are virtually universal, the success of any social system in achieving its instrumental purposes depends on the skills and motivations of leadership and managership in conflict resolution. For example, in a community mental health center the issue of differing status and remunerative compensation of various disciplines may give rise to conflict between managers and various groups of staff. This issue is not unique and is almost always present in a multidisciplinary staff. The outcome of the process by which the conflict is dealt with will be influenced heavily by the skills of the managers as well as the leaders of the various groups who may have grievances. Skillful negotiation tempered by the wish to achieve a workable resolution is required on both sides.

Decision Making

Social systems must incorporate a decision-making procedure, for even if the process is not explicit, decisions will be made nonetheless. Legitimate decisions are those made by methods and people designated by legitimate authority. Illegitimate decision making takes place outside this structure, with decisions made by people without legitimate authority.

The methods by which decisions are made vary along a continuum of sharing of authority. At one end of the continuum one person makes all the decisions; at the other end the authority to make a decision is delegated to the whole social system and the decision arrived at by vote or discussion ending in consensus. A social system seldom makes all its decisions in the same way or at either extreme. Usually the decision-making process is differentiated so that the power is shared to varying degrees for separate kinds of issues. For example, a decision regarding the admission policies of a unit may be made at the highest executive level, while a decision about a choice of recreational activity may be shared among patients and staff. In either case it should be recognized that the authority to make decisions within an organization rests with management and is shared when delegated.

In this sense it is useful to distinguish between *democracy* and *democratization.* A democracy is a political system in which the authority to rule is delegated by the people to elected officials. Democratization is a process by which managers in a social system share their authority for decision making. The difference is that in democracy the authority at its origin lies with the public, who entrust it to their elected and appointed officials. In contrast, in a mental health organization the authority of the manager almost always derives from a supraordinate body, and not from employees and patients. Power is shared by managers with staff and patients by delegation of decision-making authority.

Managers should share authority for several reasons. There is the possibility that the decision-making process arrives at better decisions when it is delegated to a knowledgeable group, rather than being retained by the manager. People who have had a hand in making decisions usually have a greater stake in assuring success, and thus the process of sharing power increases commitment. Sharing power for decision making enhances information flow in an organization because more people are involved significantly in the working of the institution, and they want to know more. Psychiatric treatment is a process in which patients may wish to place themselves in a totally dependent position, and it may be useful therapeutically to share power in the treatment setting with patients so that they may learn and gain in self-esteem by making decisions and exercising authority. Finally, we are in an era of consumerism during which staff, patients, and community groups are increasingly interested in and involved with decision making. Managers are influenced by social pressures of the larger society to share their authority. Sharing of power is useful insofar as it helps achieve the goals of an organization, and it is best evaluated in these terms rather than by an ideological belief that power *should* be shared. Sharing decision making is a means to an end, though it sometimes may be viewed as an end in itself.

Socialization

Socialization is the process whereby an individual is brought into and finds his place in a social system (see Chapters 4 and 8). If the individual is resistive to the process the system may be coercive in forcing him to take his place. An example of this is imprisonment. More often the process is reciprocal—the individual wishes to find his place and the system wants him.

In a psychiatric unit socialization is a process without end because new people are always entering the social system. Patients, staff, and students come and go, and each must be socialized.

A new patient learns the formal and informal rules for his behavior. In other words, he learns the role of patient, what he may or may not do, how he is to behave in structured and informal situations, how long the treatment usually lasts, what kinds of subject matter he is expected to discuss and not to discuss, and what responsibilities he will be expected to assume. Of course each patient responds to his role expectations in a different way. However, if one visits different psychiatric units one soon comes to see distinctive patterns of units which do not vary so much in response of the individual patients but rather are characteristic of the social system itself.

Similarly, new staff members learn their place or role in the system. For example, the psychiatric resident is not only involved in the process of socialization into the unit on which he works, he is also being socialized into the profession of psychiatry. He learns the values, skills, knowledge, behaviors, and life styles that characterize psychiatrists.

Socialization may come to have a pejorative implication in this society. Among twentieth-century middle-class Americans it is highly valued to be self-actualized, self-motivated, and nonconforming although law abiding. Yet the pressures for socialization are present and strong, and in a social system they are inevitable. In order for a social system to work, certain values must be shared if the people are to survive. As a result there is a constant tension between the individual and the group.

This is an issue not just for patients but for everyone. A person might prefer to think he makes all his conscious choices autonomously, yet he should also be aware that he is not entirely autonomous; he is part of a larger scene, a larger system which pulls and tugs and influences him profoundly. He is not free to do whatever he wishes. Moreover, the social system not only demands things of him, it provides him with relationships, goods, and services he wants and needs. Most human behavior is not a response to coercion. People in groups exchange and trade—they give and they get.

NOTES

1. Walter Buckley, "Society as a Complex Adaptive System," in *Modern Systems Research for Behavioral Scientists,* ed. Walter Buckley (Chicago: Aldine, 1968), pp. 490–513.
2. Erving Goffman, *Asylums* (Garden City, N.Y.: Doubleday, Anchor Books, 1961).
3. Ibid., p. xiii (Introduction).
4. Ernest Gruenberg and Jack Zusman, "The Natural History of Schizophrenia," in *International Psychiatric Clinics,* ed. Lawrence C. Kolb, Frank J. Kallmann, Philip Polatin (Boston: Little Brown, 1964), 1:699–710 (4). See also Ernest Gruenberg, "The Social Breakdown Syndrome and Its Prevention," in *American Handbook of Psychiatry,* ed. Silvano Arieti, vol. 2, 2d ed. (New York: Basic Books, 1974), pp. 697–711.
5. Howard B. Kaplan, Ina Boyd, and Samuel E. Bloom, "Patient Culture and the Evaluation of Self," in *Deviance: The Interactionist Perspective,* ed. Earl Rubington and Martin S. Weinberg (Toronto: Collier-Macmillan, 1973), pp. 355–367.
6. Milton Greenblatt, "The Psychiatrist as Social System Clinician," in *The Patient and the Mental Hospital,* ed. Greenblatt et al. (New York: Free Press, 1957), pp. 317–323.

CHAPTER 12

The Experience of Patienthood

INTRODUCTION

Historically the psychiatric hospital has been considered a place in which troubled people have been isolated from the community, protected from noxious stimuli, and housed while receiving medical and psychological treatment. Until recent years little study had been made specifically of the social setting of the psychiatric hospital as it affects the patient's thoughts, feelings, and behavior. For example, during the time of moral treatment the daily life of the inmate was regulated in order to build desired mental attitudes and discipline, but interaction between patients was not considered a major element of the corrective experience.

In the early twentieth century, attention was focused upon the therapeutic effects of the doctor-patient relationship. However, this, too, overlooked the informal but influential social network of patients and staff who worked and lived together on the ward. In the post–World War II period Stanton and Schwartz [1] opened the way for a new era in the study of the mental hospital as a social system with their now classical studies of the informal relationship among the staff and between the staff and patients. Their studies demonstrated that often unrecognized but powerful influences were exerted on patients by the informal, unplanned, often covert social relationships on the unit. Their studies led to the examination of the treatment unit as a social system.

The following paper was one of the first to examine carefully the psychological and social influences within the psychiatric unit. It brings our attention to the experience of a person admitted to a psychiatric ward, and particularly to the experience of becoming one of the group of other patients. The authors describe how the thoughts, feelings, and behavior of the patient are shaped by the social interactions with other patients, and how in turn these interactions are influenced by the expressed and unexpressed values, beliefs, and expectations of both patients and staff. It is a study of patienthood as experienced by a social

*scientist who was admitted to a psychiatric unit without the knowl-
edge of the staff and other patients that he was not a bona fide patient.*

NOTE

1. A. Stanton and M. Schwartz, *The Mental Hospital* (New York: Basic Books,
1954).

SOCIAL STRUCTURE AND INTERACTION
PROCESSES ON A PSYCHIATRIC WARD

William Caudill, Frederick C. Redlich,
Helen R. Gilmore, and Eugene B. Brody

The individual who enters a mental hospital finds himself placed in a
number of new social situations, all of which influence his behavior
and treatment. The patient's relationship to his therapist, both in its
administrative and therapeutic aspects, has received the most study.
This holds true where the course of treatment is through insight psychotherapy [1] and also where it involves a structuring of the patient's
social milieu by prescribing how hospital personnel shall react to him.[2]
More recently, the influence on the patient of the overall social structure of the hospital has been investigated,[3] as well as the structure of
certain types of wards [4] and the social processes at work in the split
social field existing between patients and staff.[5]

For information on a third social influence, the interpersonal relationships of patients with each other, we must, however, rely largely on
patients' autobiographical accounts of their experiences.[6] Despite the
importance of this area of life in the mental hospital, it has, beyond an
occasional astute reference,[7] received little systematic attention, and
no methods have been developed for pursuing such a problem. The

---

William Caudill, Ph.D., Frederick C. Redlich, M.D., Helen R. Gilmore, M.D., and
Eugene B. Brody, M.D., "Social Structure and Interaction Processes on a Psychiatric
Ward," *American Journal of Orthopsychiatry* 22, April 1952, pp. 314–334. This article
is abridged with permission of author and publisher. Copyright © the American
Orthopsychiatric Association, Inc. Reproduced by permission.

problem becomes a particularly crucial one when thought of in terms of the effect on each other of those less disturbed neurotic and psychotic patients who remain intact, and utilize many of their social personality characteristics and interaction techniques.

Because it is so important a variable, we wished to make a study of this area of social influence in the lives of patients despite the recognition of the many difficulties which would be encountered in obtaining adequate data. Although we are fully aware of the importance of unconscious determinants of interpersonal behavior, the present study has concerned itself primarily with a definition of the social reality in which the patients find themselves. Before field work was begun, an outline was made of the most pertinent problems to be explored:

1. The interpersonal relations on the ward between patients and patients, patients and nurses, and patients and physicians.
2. The social-psychological processes involved in becoming a patient after admission, and ceasing to be a patient as the time of discharge approached.
3. The value and belief systems of the patient group, and the general attitudes to life in the hospital centering around both administration and therapy.
4. The difficulties experienced by the patients as a group in communicating with the various levels of the staff hierarchy, and the reflection of these difficulties in the operation of the control and decision-making functions invested in the staff.

Two methods were used in gathering data: Initially, in order to determine some of the social and therapeutic problems of life in a mental hospital as seen through the eyes of the patients, we decided to have an observer undergo the experience of being a patient. Known only to two senior members of the staff, he was admitted to the less disturbed ward of the hospital and, upon being assigned to one of the psychiatric residents for therapy, he followed a course of treatment for two months.[8] Secondly, after a turnover in the patient population, the same observer acted as an assistant in the activities program for several months. This paper will present material only from the first set of observations, but the major points emphasized here were found to hold true for both of the patient populations.

Neither of the methods used was completely satisfactory. In the first, the observer, by living on the ward, was in a position to experience the full round of life and to interact with the patients as people. Coupled with these advantages there were, however, disadvantages. While to our knowledge no discernible harm was done to the therapeutic progress of any of the patients, it was recognized that this might have occurred. We were also mindful of other ethical considerations, of the personal strain on the observer in undergoing psychotherapy, and of the fact that the observer's identification with the patients would inevitably result in some degree of subjectivity in the data. A partial check on such biasing was provided by having the observer include in his daily record many of his own emotional reactions to the events of hospital life. As the observer had going-out privileges after his first week of treatment, he left the hospital each afternoon for a few hours and used this time to work up his material. Despite its disadvantages, the first method provided a rich body of data concerning many problems, hitherto only incompletely recognized, which were faced by the patients as a social group in their life on the ward. The second method, while allowing the observer to be known, had the disadvantages of restricting his participation to specific ward activities which were essentially isolated from the flow of day-to-day life. It might be feasible to work out an alternative procedure whereby a known observer could live on the ward on a twenty-four-hour-a-day basis.[9]

The observations were carried out in a small private mental hospital connected with a psychiatric training center. Treatment of the patients was primarily through dynamically oriented psychotherapy. Each patient was assigned to a psychiatric resident who was under the supervision of a physician-in-charge. The resident assumed direct responsibility for most of the management and for the therapeutic care of his patients. Apart from routine contacts on rounds, a patient usually saw his therapist for one hour a day, five days a week. The remainder of a patient's schedule was worked out very sketchily, as only a limited recreational and activities program was available.

The hospital was divided into three wards. Two of these were locked wards located on the second floor where the more severely disturbed psychotic patients were treated. The third was a less disturbed ward on the first floor which accommodated both male and female patients, most of whom were diagnosed as suffering from various types of severe psychoneuroses. This paper will be concerned only with the patients on this last ward, in which each sex occupied a separate wing containing eight private rooms, a four-bed dormitory, and a living room. Men and women intermingled in the two living rooms except at mealtime.

As the average stay in the hospital was over two months, the patient population was quite stable during the period in which the observations were made. All told, there were twelve male and fifteen female patients on the ward, most of whom were between twenty and thirty-five years of age. The majority came from upper-middle-class homes, although there were a few from upper-lower-, lower-middle-, and upper-class backgrounds. Three were Jewish; two were Catholic; the rest were Protestant. There was one Negro patient.

Observations

From the moment the observer left his room on his first day in the hospital and joined the patient group at the evening meal, he felt pressure upon him to act in certain ways.[10] As he took his food tray from the cart, he was told by several patients that they had been unable to eat during their first meal at the hospital. As a consequence, he only toyed with his food. During the meal he mentioned that he should write some letters, and was told, "You can't be very sick if you are going to write letters." He feebly parried this by saying that he probably would not get an answer anyway. After the supper trays had been removed by a nurse, and the therapists had made their evening rounds, the group asked him if he played bridge, and was overjoyed to find that he did. After several rubbers, it seemed expected of him that he would retire to his room, and he did so. At ten o'clock he heard a nurse ask the group to go to their rooms, but two of the patients later returned to the living room and he overheard them discussing their problems for several hours until he fell asleep.

Although he would have been unable to categorize them so neatly at the time, there had been, even in his first day's experience, pressures exerted on the observer by the other patients for adherence to certain attitudes in four areas of life—toward the self, toward other patients, toward therapy and the therapist, and toward nurses and other hospital personnel.

Pressures for Attitudes Toward the Self. On the second day, following a conference with his therapist, the observer expressed resentment over not having going-out privileges to visit the library and work on his book—his compulsive concern over his inability to finish this task being one of the factors leading to his hospitalization. Immediately two patients, Mr. Hill and Mrs. Lewis,[11] who were later to become his closest friends, told him he was being "defensive"; since his doctor did not wish him to do such work, it was probably better "to lay off of it." Mr. Hill went on to say that one of his troubles when he first came to the hospital was thinking of things that he had to do or thought he had to do. He said that now he did not bother about anything. Mrs. Lewis said that at first she had treated the hospital as a sort of hotel and had spent her therapeutic hours "charming" her doctor, but it had been pointed out to her by others that this was a mental hospital and that she should actively work with her doctor if she expected to get well.

The observer later saw such pressure applied time and again to other patients, and he came to realize that the group attempted to push its members toward a middle ground where they would not, as in his case and that of Mrs. Lewis, attempt to deny the reality of the hospital. On the other hand, pressure was also brought to bear on those patients who went to other extremes by engaging in too much immature acting-out behavior, who regressed too far, or who denied the emotional basis of their illness. For example, one day shortly after his arrival, the following incident, thereafter to be repeated almost exactly each day, occurred:

> Dr. Johnson came by on evening rounds and Mr. Davis made a great fuss, taking him down the hall and swearing violently at him. After Dr. Johnson had left, Mr. Davis stormed back to the table saying that Dr. Johnson told him that by such actions he was trying to destroy all the patients on the ward. But, Mr. Davis continued, all that he wanted out of life was to be a pants presser; he did not want any of that intellectual stuff. Mr. Brown and Mr. Hill told Mr. Davis that he only created these scenes when his doctor showed up; he did not need to do this as he was all right and quiet at all other times. Mr. Davis admitted this.

The patients felt certain that their doctors had as one of their major aims the requiring of patients to give up their "defenses." As the patients interpreted most of their ordinary social activities as defenses, the problem was phrased by Mr. Hill when he said that his doctor kept telling him he had to give up all his defenses but that he could not see this, as what would he have left?

Pressures for Attitudes Toward Other Patients. During his first few days in the hospital the observer was frequently told, "You cannot really refuse anything people ask of you around here," and he saw this belief put into action in many small ways. He was also told many stories of recent dramatic incidents, such as that of a recent suicide and what a swell person the patient had been; and he was introduced to what might be called the folklore of the group concerning stories of bizarre and rather humorous behavior on the part of previous patients, such as that of the patient who had been brought in nude upon a stretcher screaming that she expected a telephone call from a producer in Hollywood, and who later did receive the call. Late one night a patient upstairs created a violent and noisy commotion which awakened a number of patients who congregated in the hall. The observer was told, in the warmest terms, of this patient's personal sexual problems and, at the same time, of what a nice person he really was. It was to be noted that such incidents and stories were often treated humorously, but they were almost never treated negatively. The gossip and backbiting that might be expected to develop in a closely confined group were far overshadowed by an emphasis on the positive qualities of a person and a suspension of the direct expression of judgment in other areas.

The patients felt that many of the ordinary conventions and social gestures of the outer world were made temporarily meaningless by hospital life. On one occasion the observer, who had been asked if he cared to go downtown, said he would like to do so if his friend did not mind waiting until he changed his clothes. The friend laughingly chided him to the effect that he had forgotten where he was, that in the hospital one had all the time in the world. On the other hand, small courtesies and expressions of approval that would be carried out almost unconsciously in the outer world often became conscious problems. If one overheard, and enjoyed, a patient playing the piano, should one applaud the performance, or would such approval call forth a neurotic response? Would others overreact and feel hurt if several patients wished to go to a movie alone and did not freely extend the invitation to the entire group? Such problems as these formed part of the belief that one was not free to release oneself fully in the hospital, and that it was very difficult for an individual to satisfy his need to be alone at times.

Although acquaintances among the patients would be made on the basis of similar backgrounds and interests, and much time was spent in gossiping about the social characteristics of others, these activities lacked the invidious overtones they would have carried in the outer world. Along with this went a muting of outer-world distinctions on the basis of race, ethnic group, or social class—it was as if the patients had agreed that such categories had little meaning in a hospital. Such an orientation of one's behavior was made easier by the commonly held belief that since none of the group expected to see the others again, it was not necessary to relate one's outside status to life on the ward.

While there was a suspension of the direct expression of judgment, and a much greater tolerance of wide ranges of behavior than would have been true in social situations on the outside, there were limits to such behavior even in the patient group. For example:

> One evening a number of the patients had brought in several kinds of cheese, rye bread, and Coca Cola, which they were sharing with the group. Mr. Davis, whose behavior was characterized by aggressive, adolescent outbursts of ranting toward his therapist, immediately began to grab large amounts of the food in a very ill-mannered way. The three women to whom the food belonged became angry and gave Mr. Davis a severe tongue-lashing, calling him "an ill-bred, emotionally immature kid," etc. However, one of the women shortly brought the group together again by saying, "Well, what the hell, we are all in the same boat in this place, so don't worry about it, it's all right." Unity was reestablished, the food was shared, and the group then proceeded to get a great deal of enjoyment out of playing a crossword-puzzle game introduced by Mr. Davis.

Beyond the simple supporting of others, it quickly became apparent that a type of therapy—characterized by sympathetic listening and the making of suggestions—would be carried out among close acquaintances. For example:

> Mr. Davis and Mr. Wright were close friends. When Mr. Wright went out with his wife one night, Mr. Davis sat up until 1 A.M. waiting for him in order to see how he would be feeling. On the other hand, the next day Mr. Davis was stirring up a great storm over trying to get out of the ward because he had received some letters from his wife that made him want to leave. Mr. Wright took Mr. Davis to his room, talked to him, got him a glass of milk, and calmed him down. Such scenes were repeated daily between these two patients; after one particularly bad period, Mr. Davis jokingly said that Mr. Wright was going to send him a bill for consultation services since Mr. Wright had sat up and talked with him all night.

Pressures for Attitudes Toward Therapy and Therapists. When, on the morning of his second day, the observer attributed his sick stomach to the colorless, liquid sedative that he had been given the night before, the patients told him that this had been paraldehyde, that it was given to alcoholics, and was one of the most powerful sedatives used in the hospital. This led to a discussion of the nature of each other's problems which concluded with the agreement that every case was different and that one could not generalize. Partly because of this attitude, there was a strong feeling that a patient should keep his actual relations with his therapist, and what went on during his conference hours, separate from his life on the ward. However, while the patients often adopted the pose that "the conferences weren't helping very much," they would privately discuss their progress with their closer friends, and felt they had to hold to the belief that one's doctor was competent in his therapeutic capacity; one must cooperate with him in order to make any progress and should not question his authority.

The patients believed that therapy was "somehow psychoanalytical," that one had "to go back into childhood," and that therapy went on "twenty-four hours a day." One evening a group of eleven patients were discussing the lack of activities in the hospital, and they came to the conclusion that it was part of a conscious plan by the staff to increase the intensity of "twenty-four-hour-a-day" therapy. The matter was summed up when one patient said he thought that therapy in the hospital was better than having a psychoanalysis on the outside, because in the latter case your hour of therapy was sandwiched between many other activities, whereas in the hospital you could work on your problems all the time.

Not infrequently, many patients despaired of the seemingly endless one-way talk involved in psychotherapy. They felt that they were repeating the same story over and over again until it lost all emotional feeling and became rote. They felt that their doctors never told them anything in their conferences. They were concerned about the end goal of therapy, feeling that this was kept concealed and that they never seemed to be moving toward whatever it was. Somewhat fatalistically, they felt that the doctors took "a long-range view" and did not think of the financial expense involved. While they had to believe that psychotherapy was helpful, they were disturbed because few patients seemed to get better, or to leave the hospital as "cured." Since the patients all shared in such frustrations and doubts, the group was tolerant of occasional aggressive outbursts about one's doctor in his therapeutic capacity, and sanctioned criticism and caricature of the staff's behavior, as this manifested itself in attending to administrative duties, making rounds, or in unexpected meetings outside of the hospital.

The patients generally agreed that while they all shared some similar experiences in their conferences, there were also great differences depending on the individual patient and doctor. The characterizations made by the patients of the doctors' personalities seemed to be a blend of projection by the patient of his problems onto the doctor, and a very astute, intuitive grasp of the doctor's own emotional or social problems.

Pressures for Attitudes Toward Nurses and Other Hospital Personnel.   As the observer was playing bridge on his second day, a nurse came by and said to one of the players, "I bet you are beating them at this game, I'll bet." After she had left, Mr. Davis commented that she had "treated us like seven-year-olds." Shortly, another nurse did essentially the same thing. At another time, the staff, without consulting the patients, decided to give them a Valentine party. Many of the patients did not wish to go, but did so anyway as they felt that they should not hurt the feelings of the student nurses who had organized the party. The games introduced by the nurses were on a very childish level; many of the patients felt silly playing them and were glad when the party was over and they could go back to activities of their own choosing.

The patients knew that the nurses, particularly the students, sat around in the living rooms "in order to get material for their reports," and hence the patients felt that the nurses were fair game for occasional kidding. For example:

> A nurse was listening to a conversation between Mrs. Lewis and Mr. Brown. So Mrs. Lewis joked with Mr. Brown by saying, "You didn't come in and say good night to me last night." Then she turned to the nurse and said, "You know, Mr. Brown is in and out of my room all night long." Mr. Brown smiled and said, "Yes, of course, that's true."

While the patients ignored the fact that the nurses overheard many of their conversations, there was a definite feeling in the group that one should not inform on another patient in answer to a direct request for information from the nurse:

> During the night, Mr. Sullivan had had an anxiety attack and had been taken care of by Mr. Brown, who wrapped him in a blanket and rubbed his temples until he went to sleep. When Mr. Sullivan awakened again, another patient read to him for several hours. The night nurse, of course, must have observed this behavior. Nevertheless, when a student nurse asked at breakfast the next morning how late Mr. Sullivan had been up, none of the group of male patients would answer her.

Life on the Ward. One of the observer's strongest impressions during his first day on the ward was the feeling of boredom and ennui existing among the patients, several of whom told him that "tomorrow would be just another day with nothing to do but sit around, or play bridge and ping-pong." Actually, as there were few organized activities or secondary types of therapy available, the patients, for the most part, utilized each other to develop a social life. Bridge was played interminably, endless numbers of crossword puzzles were worked cooperatively, while the daily cryptogram in the newspaper was copied out and the patients avidly competed for the solution.

The staff tended to look upon the games and activities of the patients as "fads," in the sense of a passing fashion or fancy. They were much more than this, as they provided simple settings for realistic role taking and helped to bind the group together. The considerable quantity of food the patients brought in from the outside to share with others served much the same function. Snacks, such as salami, cheese, pumpernickel, popcorn, and Coca-Cola, lent a zest lacking in the crackers and chocolate milk provided by the hospital twice a day as "nourishment." Despite the frequent tacit disapproval of the nurses, the consumption of these snacks was usually made into a social rite which complemented the evening-at-home atmosphere the patients created in the living rooms. The social stimulus value of these evening gatherings was heightened by the interaction of small friendship groups which were supported by the patients because they increased the potential for social participation and conversation in the group. Such activities provided reassurance for the patients that they could still, in some measure, interact on an adult level, and also represented a partly conscious resistance to those aspects of the hospital routine which were unduly "infantilizing."

Given the situation in the hospital, the patient group, if it wished a social life, had no choice but to turn inward and, so far as possible, to develop the potentialities of its members. This is what happened, and the resulting social structure is best seen in terms of the implementation of the values of the patient group through the role and clique system that operated in the life on the ward.

Value and Role Systems

As the sorts of pressures that have been discussed were felt by the observer, he came gradually to realize that the attitudes held by the patients were formed into a pattern of values, some of which were verbalized, while others might be inferred from the consistency of behavior. This *value system* might, in summary form, be stated as follows:

1. Toward oneself: (a) A patient should not deny the reality of being in the hospital for therapeutic purposes, (b) should give up his "defenses," and (c) should try to bring himself to a middle ground where he neither engaged in extreme regressive behavior nor attempted to carry on life as if the hospital did not exist.
2. Toward other patients: (a) A patient should suspend judgment and attempt to see all sides of a person, (b) sustain and support others, and (c) if requested, try actively to help them with their problems by doing a sort of therapy with them.
3. Toward therapy and the therapist: (a) A patient should try to believe in the ability and competence of his doctor, (b) cooperate in working with him, and (c) feel that treatment on a "twenty-four-hour-a-day" basis in the hospital was better than therapy received in the outer world.
4. Toward nurses and other personnel: (a) A patient should try to be thoughtful and pleasant, and (b) cooperate by abiding by the rules of the hospital up to the point where either the demands of the nurses became unreasonable, or the rules conflicted with a more important value toward other patients.

This value system of the patient group was translated into action by ascribing to each new member what may be called the *role of a patient*. This role required that one act in accordance with the complex of values and behavior patterns expected of every patient as described above. In addition, each individual played a *personal role* rooted in his background outside the hospital; that is, he presented himself as a certain kind of person to the patient group. The individual patient, then, had the task of integrating his personal role with the role of a patient; or, at least, seeing to it that the values and behavior characteristic of his personal role did not directly conflict with those of the patient role.

If a patient would accept and play the ascribed role of a patient, especially as it entailed mutual tolerance and responsibility for others, then the group would, in turn, support the patient in his personal role. Particularly this was true if the personal role of the patient served some positive function in the group. For example, Mr. Brown's imitations of the doctors, nurses, and other patients were a real source of catharsis for the group; and Mr. Davis's immature explosions toward the staff provided vicarious satisfaction for others,[12] while his expertness at bridge and at solving cryptograms was a source of recreation.

The integration of one's personal role with that of the patient role often required that an individual make a conscious effort to channel his personal abilities and resources into the helping of others. For example, Mrs. Lewis was a fashionably dressed woman who purposely went out of her way to help Miss Wood with her clothes; Miss Wood, in her turn, had considerable competence in massage and provided this service for a number of the women patients. The group went so far as to try to establish a function for a patient's personal role if one did not seem self-evident, and through this process the observer's library work and interest in music were drawn into the orbit of the group by having him obtain books and record albums for others.

It was possible to set up a continuum on the basis of the degree of success achieved by the patients in the integration of their personal roles with the role of a patient. The nature of such an integration had a great deal to do with the place occupied by a patient in the total structure of the group.

One extreme was represented by Mr. Hill, whose personal role coincided almost completely with what was expected of him in the role of a patient. He was a passive, nonthreatening person who was very sensitive to group approval and pressure; he had good social techniques and skills for relating to others, and a nice dry sense of humor which he utilized a great deal but never in such a way as to hurt other patients. He was always willing to sustain any activity of the group and was receptive when others came to him for support or therapy. On the other hand, he frequently sought out other patients to ask their advice. While it would be difficult to speak of "leadership" among the patients because, owing to the nature of their situation in the hospital, there were few goals toward which the group as a whole might have been led, Mr. Hill represented the most highly pivotal person on the ward, with whom all of the patients acknowledged some ties.

The other extreme was represented by Miss Ford, whose personal role conflicted in almost all respects with what was expected of her in the role of a patient. Since she felt a need to belong to the patient group, this conflict of roles was a source of anxiety for her. She said that she thought of the hospital as "just like college" and treated her doctor as a professor who would hand her the answers to her problems. She stated that she wanted nothing to do with anyone else's troubles, and hence she made little effort to support other patients. She openly expressed anti-Semitism, was aggressive and hostile to the Negro patient, and was snobbish and class-conscious. Indeed, while she continually tried to participate socially, most of her conversation was derogatory of others. As a consequence, she incurred the hostility of the group and was rejected and isolated because, although she wished to belong to the patient group, she would not carry out its values and responsibilities. Hers was a very different type of isolation from the occasional self-imposed withdrawal of Mrs. Gray, which was respected by the patients, or from the complete isolation imposed on himself by Mr. Reed.

Though physically present on the ward, Mr. Reed never entered the social field of the patients, who held an entirely neutral attitude toward him and scarcely recognized his existence.

Most of the patients interacting in the group fell somewhere between the extremes sketched above. Their personal roles did not completely coincide with the role of a patient, but they did accept the society's values and in turn received support. It cannot be said that the place occupied by a patient in the group structure was entirely what might have been expected from his previous psychodynamic history. Mr. Hill was much more highly rewarded for his type of behavior in the patient group than he would have been in the outer world, where he would have been marked as too passive a person. On the other hand, Miss Ford would probably not have been so rigidly censored for her nonsupportive and often hostile behavior by the outer world. This does not mean that she would have exhibited less anxiety, or found life easier, on the outside as the hospital still served as a refuge. It is indicated, however, that the nature of a patient's social integration into the group will affect his therapeutic progress, and both Mr. Hill and Miss Ford, for opposite reasons, experienced more than ordinary difficulty in ultimately leaving the protection of the hospital environment—the former because of his overdependence on the group, the latter because she received too little support.

A further aspect of the social structure of the patient group lay in its encouragement of various types of cliques, one of which was the boy-and-girl team. For example, Mr. Brown and Miss Gaynor spent a great deal of their time together and often joked about the amusing incidents that happened in town when clerks would mistake them for man and wife; they formed a unit in the "evenings at home" held by the group in the living rooms, where Mr. Brown would work on his cloth animals and Miss Gaynor would knit. Once, when Mr. Brown and Miss Gaynor gave a popcorn party for the group, Mrs. Gray jokingly said that all they needed were "His" and "Her" aprons. Such romantic attachments were approved so long as they remained flirtatious and casual because they served to increase social interaction, which was one of the main sociological functions of the clique. If, however, such attachments went beyond this point, they were frowned upon because any behavior which might lead to serious social consequences was felt as threatening by the group. In general, if a clique, for whatever reasons, became so interested in itself that it drew away from the group, this was felt as a social loss and pressure was applied to bring it again into the wider social field.

A second function of the clique, examples of which have already been given, was to act as a mutual therapy group; a third was to provide opportunities to let off steam and thus act as a safety valve since it was not always easy for a patient to maintain a constant attitude of tolerance and support toward all other patients; while a fourth function became operative when a patient felt disturbed and wished to draw away from the group, but did not want to isolate himself completely.

Another type of clique, restricted to a predominantly social function, was formed, especially among the women, on the basis of similarity in background outside the hospital. There was a clique of young adolescent girls; a second composed of those women who like to sew, cook, and follow other domestic pursuits; while a third consisted of those women with interests in literature, music, art, and fashion.

In general, the women remained separated in small cliques, whereas the men formed a single, loosely integrated group that functioned with little discord. Many patients remarked on the fact that the women's side seemed to be in a state of constant minor turmoil in contrast to the relative peace reigning among the men.

From the patients' point of view, the purpose of the group structure just described was, first of all, to develop among themselves the opportunities for social activities otherwise lacking in the hospital environment by maximizing the number of interpersonal relationships and roles available to an individual, while at the same time trying to keep any serious social consequences of these relationships at a minimum; and, secondly, to provide the members of the group with as supportive and ego-sustaining a milieu as was possible without coming into conflict with the staff or the routine of the hospital. Nevertheless, conflicts did arise because the staff, both doctors and nurses, seemed unacquainted with many aspects of life in the patient group, and dealt with each individual as a separate entity in administrative details as well as in therapeutic matters. In part, this was due to the fact that there was no channel provided by which the patients, as a group, could voice their desires to the staff. If a group of patients wished to make a request, this could be done only by each patient's taking the matter up, as an individual, with his therapist.

The lack of a channel of communication, and an insufficient separation between administration and therapy, increased the mutual isolation of patients and staff. Both patients and staff structured their actions in accordance with a set of values and beliefs, but because the values and beliefs of each group were only incompletely known or understood by the other, the two groups viewed one another in terms of stereotypes which impeded an accurate evaluation of social reality. Such a situation, when coupled with alternating periods of permissive and restrictive administrative control, probably helps to account for the mood swings in the patient group. One week a general air of depression would prevail, at other times the ward had the atmosphere of a hotel, while again a feeling of rebellion would come over the entire group.

Discussion

This paper has emphasized the point that psychoneurotic patients on a less disturbed ward of a mental hospital should not be thought of as an aggregate of individuals, but as a group which tries to meet many of its problems by developing a shared set of values and beliefs translated into action through a system of social roles and cliques. Some of the problems faced by the patient group in ordering the interaction of its members would seem to have been due directly to the factor of emotional illness. Since all of the members were emotionally disturbed, they had all experienced a high level of anxiety during their life in the outer world over the inability to play certain required social roles without introducing extraneous behavior stemming from neurotic conflicts. The particular patient group reported on here recognized this problem and provided for it by its values of suspension of judgment and support. In so doing, the patients were acting in ways very similar to those noted by Rowland [13] for the patients on the less disturbed wards of another mental hospital where interaction was characterized by "small, closed friendship groups," having "a maximum of insight and sympathetic interpenetration," with a "rigid control of affect in terms of group standards."

The patient group also sensed that because of hospitalization, an individual was not only relieved from playing roles in those areas of life where he experienced particular difficulty, but was also cut off from playing those roles in other areas of life which furnished him with some measure of self-esteem. Since few substitutes for these latter roles, in the form of short-range realistic goals and activities, were provided in the hospital, the patient group attempted to meet this problem by increasing opportunities for role taking through utilizing the personal attributes of the patients.

Many other problems of the patient group arose, however, because the patients and staff lived, as Rowland [14] has expressed it, "in two entirely separate social worlds, yet . . . in the closest proximity." While the staff exercised control over the patients, they did not give recognition to the patient world as a social group, but rather, they interpreted the behavior of the patients almost solely in individual dynamic-historical terms. The patient group, thus lacking an adequate channel of communication to the staff, protected itself by turning inward, and by developing a social structure which was insulated as much as possible from friction with the hospital routine. Nevertheless, such friction did occur, and the subsequent frustration led to behavior on the part of the patients which, although it overtly resembled neurotic behavior arising from personal emotional conflicts, was, in fact, to a considerable extent due to factors in the immediate situation. Such phenomena are similar to the "increased agitation and dissociative behavior" observed by Stanton and Schwartz [15] when two staff members with power over a patient disagree as to how the case should be handled. Stanton and Schwartz conclude:

> If our hypothesis is correct that the patient's dissociation is a reflection of, and a mode of participation in, a social field which itself is seriously split, it accounts for the sudden cessation of excitement following any resolution of this split. . . . In other words, the phenomena are not completely "autistic" in the sense that they are not derived entirely from

the patient's past history or from an unconscious which is isolated from reality.

Some aspects of the above situation seem almost inevitable in the nature of the hierarchical hospital structure. It is necessary to exercise some degree of control over patients; they will be cut off from the positive as well as the negative aspects of their outside life by hospitalization, and some frustration due to close living will occur in any institutional setting which must, by its nature, restrict the personal liberty of its members. If this is true, then some of the behavior of the patients is due to the nature of the situation rather than to their condition of emotional illness, and such behavior should be shared by groups living in other settings which have some *structural* similarities in common with mental hospitals. Sullivan asks this question in his discussion in the Stanton and Schwartz [16] material when he says: "Is this a pattern which is a function of the particular larger group setting, or is it one that has relatively wide validity? . . . Is it to be seen in essential rudiments among the complements of a naval vessel, among the population of a penitentiary, in any hospital which has a relatively chronic patient population, [or] on the wards of most mental hospitals only . . . ?"

A review of the work done on behavior in such settings would seem, at least tentatively, to answer this question in the affirmative. A group of less disturbed patients in a mental hospital would seem to represent one point of a continuum of types of groups all of which share some structural characteristics—e.g., membership in these groups is transitional, positive goals for the members other than their successful removal from the group are mostly lacking, and control is largely authoritarian. Despite other great differences, such as voluntary or involuntary entrance and helping or punishing aims, these characteristics tend to be shared by groups in mental hospitals,[17] tuberculosis sanitariums,[18] orphanages,[19] displaced persons camps,[20] wartime posts relatively free from danger,[21] and under various conditions of imprisonment.[22] In general, the accounts of behavior in these types of settings all stress the phenomena, so many of which are noted in hospitalized mental patients, of apathy and depersonalization, regression, denial of reality, attempts to maintain threatened self-esteem, increased wish-level and fantasy, and the formation of stereotypes concerning those who control the authority and power.

For example, the previously emotionally mature, female political prisoners observed by Jacobson [23] exhibited, as did many of the patients discussed in this paper, initial feelings of depersonalization and denial of reality; a seeming regression to adolescence with its heightened affect lability; an increased, but unstable, sensitivity to aesthetic and intellectual stimulation; and a strong upsurgence of oral cravings. Also, Jacobson's prisoners and the patients showed, as a sort of group reaction formation, increased morality and superego severity, great concern over the welfare of other members, and a constant effort to control irritability.

Such similarities in behavior as are sketched above for the various types of settings would seem to be in line with the experimental results and theoretical conceptualizations of Lewin, Lippit, White and others [24] as to the direct effect on behavior of differences in social climate.

Beyond this the patient group seemed to develop certain types of behavior shared with all human groups whether they be, as Homans [25] has pointed out, a bank wiring room in an industrial plant, a street-corner society, or a Polynesian community. Since social life is never wholly utilitarian, the patients were acting like any human group when they tended to overelaborate their interaction beyond the point required by the purely practical problems of the environment in which they found themselves. This tendency, noted by Linton [26] and detailed by Homans,[27] accounts, in part, for the fact that the bank wiring employees restricted their output in accordance with their own norms and helped each other on piecework even though this was forbidden by management; similarly, the patients supported the activities of others even if this meant going against a rule of the hospital.

Research stemming from the observations discussed here might lead to an investigation of the following problems:

1. Further studies of the value systems of patient groups, and of the roles by which these values are implemented.
2. An exploration of the somewhat separate value systems of the various communication- and mobility-block strata of the hospital staff hierarchy.
3. A detailed analysis of interaction processes between the groups making up the hierarchy in light of the differences in values that might be found to exist.
4. Related to the foregoing problems, a study of what happens to reports on patient behavior, in terms of distortions, omissions, and additions, as these reports are channeled upward through the hospital strata to the point where decisions are made, and then down again.

A review would also seem to be indicated of the important question of whether neurotic patients who are still able to function in some areas of life should be admitted to a hospital beyond the need for diagnostic studies. It is quite possible that a great many neurotic patients now admitted to our hospitals would fare better in ambulatory treatment than in a hospital setting. At the same time, many neurotic patients must temporarily be removed from the anxiety-provoking setting of the home in order to facilitate therapeutic progress. This dilemma raises many theoretical and practical problems, and would seem to call for research on other types of environmental settings that might be more conducive to the successful psychotherapeutic treatment of such patients.

There are many questions of ward management to which this study has drawn attention. Our main emphasis, however, has been on a theoretical investigation of basic problems of social structure and interaction processes. Much further study is needed before well-founded, practical applications can be made.

NOTES

1. Frieda Fromm-Reichmann, *Principles of Intensive Psychotherapy* (Chicago: University of Chicago Press, 1950). "Problems of Therapeutic Management in a Psychoanalytic Hospital," *Psychoanalytic Quarterly* 16, no. 4 (1947): 325–356.

2. E. C. Adams, "Problems in Attitude Therapy in a Mental Hospital," *American Journal of Psychiatry* 105 (1948): 456–461; W. C. Menninger, "Psychoanalytic Principles Applied to the Treatment of Hospitalized Patients," *Bulletin of the Menninger Clinic* 1 (1937): 35–43; H. S. Sullivan, "Socio-Psychiatric Research: Its Implications for the Schizophrenia Problem and for Mental Hygiene," *American Journal of Psychiatry* 87 (1931): 977–991.

3. J. B. Bateman and H. W. Dunham, "The State Mental Hospital as a Special Community Experience," *American Journal of Psychiatry* 105 (1948): 445–448; H. Rowland, "Friendship Patterns in a State Mental Hospital," *Psychiatry* 2 (1939): 363–373; H. Rowland, "Interaction Processes in a State Mental Hospital," *Psychiatry* 1 (1938): 323–337.

4. G. Devereux, "The Social Structure of a Schizophrenic Ward and Its Therapeutic Fitness," *Journal of Clinical Psychopathology* 6 (1944): 231–265.

5. R. W. Hyde and H. C. Solomon, "Patient Government: A New Form of Group Therapy," *Digest of Neurology and Psychiatry* 18 (1950): 207–218; Morris S. Schwartz and A. H. Stanton, "A Social Psychological Study of Incontinence," *Psychiatry* 13 (1950): 399–416.

A. H. Stanton and Morris S. Schwartz, "The Management of a Type of Institutional Participation in Mental Illness," *Psychiatry* 12 (1949): 13–26.

A. H. Stanton and Morris S. Schwartz, "Medical Opinion and the Social Context in the Mental Hospital," *Psychiatry* 12 (1949a): 243–249.

A. H. Stanton and Morris S. Schwartz, "Observations on Dissociation as Social Participation," *Psychiatry* 12 (1949b): 339–354.

S. A. Szurek, "Dynamics of Staff Interaction in Hospital Psychiatric Treatment of Children," *American Journal of Orthopsychiatry* 17 (1947): 652–664.

6. C. W. Beers, *A Mind That Found Itself,* 5th ed. (New York: Longmans, 1921.)

A. Boison, *The Exploration of the Inner World* (New York: Willett Clark, 1939).

J. Hillyer, *Reluctantly Told* (New York: Macmillan, 1926).

J. A. Kindwall and E. F. Kinder "Postscript on a Benign Psychosis," *Psychiatry* 3 (1940): 527–534.

M. King, *The Recovery of Myself* (New Haven: Yale University Press, 1931).

F. Peters, *The World Next Door* (New York: Farrar, Straus, 1949).

7. Noble, 1941.

8. Upon admission to the hospital, the observer told his therapist that he had recently been compulsively trying to finish the writing of a scholarly book, but felt that he was not getting ahead; worry over his work drove him to alcoholic episodes ending in fights; he was withdrawn and depressed, and had quarreled with his wife who had then separated from him. Beyond these fictions, the observer gave a somewhat distorted version of his own life in which he consciously attempted to suppress his own solutions to certain problems and to add a pattern of neurotic defenses.

9. The methodological aspects of the study will be reported later in detail.

10. The observer also, of course, felt pressure upon him in his first contacts with nurses, his therapist, and other members of the staff. These are not discussed here, however, because the major focus of this paper is upon the relationships developed by patients with each other.

11. All names appearing here are pseudonyms.

12. In psychoanalytic terms, much of what would be considered primitive instinctual "antisocial" behavior in the outer world became "social" behavior in the hospital because of the wider range of tolerance and suspension of judgment among the patients. Seen in this way, a mental hospital ward is not only, in the traditional sense, a place where the patient should be free, if need be, to regress with some degree of comfort, but it is also a place where primitive instinctual forces are themselves enmeshed and utilized in the subculture and role system of the patient group. Thus, psychotherapy carried out in the hospital must not only contend with such forces due to regression, but also with such forces supported by a social system.

13. H. Rowland, "Interaction Processes in a State Mental Hospital," *Psychiatry* 1 (1938): 323–373.

14. H. Rowland, "Friendship Patterns in a State Mental Hospital," *Psychiatry* 2 (1939): 363–373.

15. A. H. Stanton and M. S. Schwartz, "Observations on Dissociation as Social Participation," *Psychiatry* 12 (1949b): 339–354.

16. A. H. Stanton and M. S. Schwartz, "The Management of a Type of Institutional Participation in Mental Illness," *Psychiatry* 12 (1949): 13–26.

17. T. Dembo and E. Haufmann, "The Patient's Psychological Situation Upon Admission to a Mental Hospital," *American Journal of Psychology* 47 (1935): 381–408.

18. T. Mann, *The Magic Mountain* (New York: Knopf, 1930); G. S. Todd and E. Wittkower, "The Psychological Aspects of Sanitarium Management," 254 (January 10, 1948): 49–53.

19. W. Goldfarb, "The Effects of Early Institutional Care on Adolescent Personality," *Journal of Experimental Education* 12 (1943): 106–129.

20. D. P. Boder, *I Did Not Interview the Dead* (Urbana, Illinois: Univ. of Illinois Press, 1949); P. Friedman, "Some Aspects of Concentration Camp Psychology," *American Journal of Psychiatry* 105 (1949): 601–605.

21. R. R. Greenson, "Psychology of Apathy," *Psychoanalytic Quarterly* 18 (1949): 290–302; T. Heggen, *Mister Roberts* (Boston: Houghton Mifflin, 1946).

22. B. Bettelheim, "Individual and Mass Behavior in Extreme Situations," *Journal of Abnormal Social Psychology* 38 (1943): 417–452.

23. H. O. Bluhm, "How Did They Survive? Mechanisms of Defense in Nazi Concentration Camps," *American Journal of Psychotherapy* 2 (1948): 3–32; N. S. Hayner and E. Ash, "The Prisoner Community as a Social Group," *American Sociological Review* 4 (1939): 362–369; E. Jacobson, "Observations on the Psychological Effect of Imprisonment on Female Political Prisoners," *Searchlights on Delinquency*, ed. K. R. Eissler (New York: International Universities Press, 1949), pp. 341–368.

24. T. M. French, "An Analysis of the Goal Concept Based Upon Study of Reactions to Frustration," *Psychoanalytic Review* 28 (1941): 61–71; K. Lewin, "Psychoanalysis and Topological Psychology," *Bulletin of the Menninger Clinic* 1 (1937): 202–211; R. Lippitt and R. K. White, "An Experimental Study of Leadership and Group Life," *Readings in Social Psychology*, ed. T. M. Newcomb and E. L. Hartley (New York: Holt, 1947), pp. 496–511; R. Lippit, "Field Theory and Experiment in Social Psychology: Autocratic and Democratic Group Atmospheres," *American Journal of Sociology* 45 (1939): 26–49.

25. G. C. Homans, *The Human Group* (New York: Harcourt, 1950).

26. R. Linton, *The Study of Man* (New York: Appleton, 1936).

27. G. C. Homans, *The Human Group* (New York: Harcourt, 1950).

COMMENTARY

One of the major points developed in this paper is that patients on a ward should not be thought of as merely an aggregate of individuals. Patients and staff on a ward are an entity which, like other social systems, resolves its problems by developing a set of values and beliefs translated into action through a system of social roles and small subgroups of individuals.

The paper also makes the point that psychiatric hospitalization is a process far more complex than simply removal of a disturbed individual into a treatment facility where he receives some kind of intervention called "therapy" and is then discharged. The findings of these authors demonstrate that the setting is a complicated social organization. Doctors, nurses, aides, janitors, clerks, administrators, and patients have overt and covert roles in the organization, and all are bound together by organizational and societal imperatives. While individual differences are permitted, they must be within prescribed ranges, and deviance from a prescribed role within the mental hospital may be dealt with as harshly as is deviance outside the hospital.

This paper serves to remind us that when a person is hospitalized, or for that matter introduced into a small social system, he is subject to the very strong influence of that system. Unless one examines the nature of the social environment, it is possible to overlook a host of forces which are acting on the person. Not only are medications and psychotherapy influencing the patient, but so are the values of the unit and the social role relationships, demands, and opportunities. The social environment of a hospital unit may be useful to individuals, and presumably it may also create problems. This raises questions about what considerations should be given the influence of a specific ward's social system on specific individuals. Some patients may find opportunities for learning in a social system which would offer few benefits for another person. In view of the importance of the social network within the ward, Maxwell Jones and others [1] have stressed the influence of a community meeting of all patients and staff to discuss their relationships and the events on the ward.

The paper suggests possible answers to such questions as: Why do individuals who happen to live on a ward in a hospital form social groups? Why don't they ignore each other and develop relationships only with the staff? In what ways does the staff on a psychiatric ward influence patient-patient relationships? In what ways is it possible to change patient-patient relationships by the administrative rules of the ward? By the behavior of the staff with each other? Under what conditions might social organization and/or patient-patient relationships be useful, i.e., therapeutic? Harmful? [2]

The authors point out that psychotherapists tend to look at social behavior for its psychodynamics (or ego defense) mechanisms and frequently overlook the adaptive social function of behavior. On reflection, this observation may be related to our own clinical experiences.

The paper challenges the reader to think about what application can be made in planning for a treatment unit with specific regard to its social system. How would a unit for acutely disturbed patients differ from one for patients who have been hospitalized for a long time or for a day-treatment program?

This paper focuses on interpersonal and social forces as they act on the individual, and suggests that social forces act in complementarity with intrapsychic forces. It underscores the necessity for the clinician to understand both intrapsychic and social dynamics. Social dynamics include a variety of elements, such as the concepts of interpersonal conflict and gratifications; the variety of roles the individual is assigned and accepts; conflicts between and about these roles; the individual's cultural beliefs, values, and expectations, and those of his important others, and the conflict between these; his social class; the influence upon him of his peers, friends, and relatives; the ways in which he is socialized or feels or is seen to be deviant;

and the importance in his life of primary groups. The challenge to the clinician is an integration of the two perspectives of both social and intrapsychic dynamics.

NOTES

1. Maxwell Jones, "Training in Social Psychiatry at Ward Level," *American Journal of Psychiatry* 118 (1962): 705.
2. Alan M. Kraft, "The Therapeutic Community," *American Handbook of Psychiatry,* ed. Silvano Arieti, vol. 3 (New York: Basic Books, 1966).

CHAPTER 13

Instrumental and Maintenance Functions

INTRODUCTION

For every organization it is possible to identify one or a group of end products or services for which the organization exists. Factories manufacture goods; farms produce food or raw material; schools provide educational services. These end products or services are called the instrumental functions of an organization. Usually, though not always, they are easy to identify. These functions generally have meaning and value in the external world of the organization.

Organizations require nurturance from their environments in the form of resources, and these resources are paid for by the production of goods or services.

Individuals also require nurturance if they are to perform work. Investigations regarding motivation [1] indicate that people are motivated in complex ways. For example, while everyone has certain minimal requirements for sustenance, when these are provided they do not satisfy or motivate the worker. The threat of removal of these minimal resources may induce the person to continue at work, but the threat does not increase his interest in the work or his commitment to it.

What motivates people to perform to their maximal abilities? Possible answers include achievement, recognition, self-actualization, responsibility, advancement, and personal growth.

Organizations require an output of services or goods in order to survive. The organization's ability to produce depends on the effectiveness of its staff. In order to produce, the organization must provide inducements, supports, and sustenance to motivate its staff. These are *called the* maintenance *functions of the organization. They are aimed at meeting the emotional, social, and economic needs of the members.*

Hospitals are complex social organizations. Their instrumental functions are usually apparent. Their maintenance functions, though invariably of crucial importance to their success, are less apparent. The following reading is a concise consideration of the relationship between maintenance and instrumental functions in a mental hospital.

NOTE

1. C. Argyris, *Integrating the Individual and the Organization* (New York: Wiley, 1964); F. Herzberg, G. Mausner, and A. Snyderman, *The Motivation to Work* (New York: Wiley, 1959); Abraham Maslow, *Eupsychian Management* (Homewood, Ill.: Richard D. Irwin, 1965).

THE MAJOR AIMS AND ORGANIZATIONAL CHARACTERISTICS OF MENTAL HOSPITALS

Harvey L. Smith and Daniel J. Levinson

Mental hospitals, like all other organizations for work, are established to fill a set of recognized social needs. That is to say, the justification for their existence lies in their serving a variety of instrumental functions for patients and for society at large. To implement these goals each hospital develops certain structures and modes of operation that comprise its maintenance organization. One of the major problems confronting any hospital is whether its form of working structure is best suited for the goals intended. For example, mental hospitals may differ in their treatment goals. One may attempt to resolve the patient's crisis and return him speedily to the community. Another may aim at fundamental changes in the patient's long-established modes of adaptation. Others seek chiefly to provide care for "incurables." Many hospitals have multiple goals of patient care, staff training, and research. These different goals pose distinctive tasks for hospital structures; they may need to be met with quite different forms of maintenance organization.

Harvey L. Smith and Daniel J. Levinson, "The Major Aims and Organizational Characteristics of Mental Hospitals," in *The Patient and the Mental Hospital*, edited by Milton Greenblatt, M.D., Daniel J. Levinson, Ph.D., and Richard H. Williams, M.D. New York: The Free Press, 1957, pp. 3–8. Reprinted with permission of Macmillan Publishing Co., Inc. Copyright © The Free Press, a Corporation, 1957.

It is crucial for an understanding of problems of hospital life to recognize that every maintenance organization develops its own set of derived needs. Traditions arise to channel action; problems of prestige appear; failures rankle; promotions please, or inspire jealousy; informal rules become powerful; feuds with forgotten origins constantly inflame; incumbents need their wage and job security; roles and personalities may become incompatible or conflictful. Dealing with these problems and needs may come to absorb the major energies of the organization. Basic conflicts often arise between the short-run needs of the maintenance structure and the primary instrumental goals. It must therefore be asked: What is the relevance of the maintenance organization for instrumental goal-implementation? To what extent are the hospital's energies centered in the derived needs of the maintenance organization?

All human organizations for work are self-serving in many important respects. This is as true of organizations devoted to the healing arts as it is of frankly financial organizations. In all working organizations we find a complex blending of instrumental and of maintenance functions. In the former we see the goal-directed, purposive functions of the organization—the general needs it was established to serve. In the latter set of functions we see that an organization exists to persist. It is at the same time a mobilization of people to serve the common good, and to meet the social, economic, and emotional needs of its component workers. This blending of related but often conflicting functions provides mental hospitals with many problems shared with other working institutions. In addition, their unique sets of functions provide them with problems of a more specific nature. We shall attempt here to indicate some of the organizational problems that mental hospitals share with other complex organizations, and some that are their unique creation.

The social milieu provided by the hospital may aid or hinder its patients' recovery from illness. Social structural stressors, stemming from faulty communication, for example, are shown to be intimately involved in the course of illness. For the mental hospital, the problems of maintenance organization and the modes of dealing with them can hardly be dissociated from the instrumental tasks of therapy.

Problems of Status and Authority

One of the primary organizational problems faced by hospitals, a problem shared with universities, is the task of administering professional persons. For one thing, each profession is built around some hard core of inviolate skills and knowledge. In a certain sense, each professional faces members of another profession as a layman. He does not really share their intrinsic competence. Accordingly he must be most wary of exerting certain controls over members of other professions. Seen more narrowly, even members of different specialties must avoid infringing upon each other's competence. In fact, any physician finds difficulty giving "orders" concerning professional matters to another physician. Doctors, like university professors, are sensitive in this regard. The case may be even more difficult when the orders come from an administrator. Thus the organizational structure of a hospital is permeated with nodes of resistance to (or indifference to) authority.

The very nature of professional authority is involved in this problem. The form of such authority is best described in Max Weber's term "charismatic." This is not the usurpation by or emanation of power from an individual, but the attribution of powers to him by a group of followers. This is power by social definition. In these terms our culture endows the physician with power; he is defined as an authoritative figure. In Weber's formulation, an important characteristic of the charismatic form of authority is that it is defiant of administrative regulation and partially immune from it.

The presence of administrative and professional persons in hospitals entails additional problems in that they represent two different forms of status. Chester Barnard has noted the concurrent, and often conflicting, presence of "scalar" and "functional" status systems within complex organizations. Scalar status is the familiar hierarchical arrangement of positions found in clearest form in bureaucratic organizations. Power, the chain command, flows downward through the hierarchy. The administrative organization in hospitals is clearly a system of scalar statuses. Functional status, on the contrary, does not depend upon one's rank in a system, but inheres in the nature of the work one performs. High functional status is an intrinsic attribute of highly skilled work and is accordingly an attribute of professional persons. Thus, the "lowliest" (in scalar terms) physician in the hospital is fairly secure in a position of high functional status, relative to other workers. Orders also flow from occupants of high functional positions. These orders need not necessarily accord with those operative within the scalar system. Hence the coordination of activities in hospitals, always a complex problem, may become a source of conflict among hospital personnel. The implications for the carrying out of therapeutic activities are manifold.

Underlying the frequent conflicts of directives within hospitals is a basic duality of values. This is linked closely to the central institutional problem of effectively integrating the hospital's instrumental and maintenance functions. Personnel in the hospital may be oriented primarily toward one of these main functions to the exclusion of the other. For some, service to the patient is the overriding institutional goal. They are impatient with, or stoutly ignore, administrative contingencies that appear to limit service to patients or that deflect their occupational goals. Others are chiefly concerned, and are hired to be so concerned, with the institution's survival contingencies. They are attuned to the master economic problem—the allocation of scarce means to seemingly unlimited wants. Their administrative decisions, geared to the hospital's economy, delimit its service goals and impinge upon professional wants. It is small wonder, therefore, that hospitals seem to have a built-in sense of outrage. They are a form of organization which must constantly strive to minimize tensions.

Problems of Communication

Another problem of coordination faced by hospitals is that the skills and needs of each occupational group involved may remain little known to the others. Characteristically, promotions are within occupational groups and not to other occupational groups. This contrasts with the situation in many industries, where people may "work up" through a series of jobs, thus learning the skills and values of various occupations. This may involve "earned" promotions or a planned training system. It provides that at least some executives will have intimate knowledge of the work, and perhaps even the workers, which they may direct. The hospital does not offer such paths of mobility. Few physicians have ever been aides, nor will the nurse become a physician. Each occupational level therefore tends to operate as a somewhat closed system. Its skills, values, and attitudes are acquired within the occupation or profession and may be little known outside it.

For the effective coordination of an enterprise as complex as a hospital there must be meaningful communication among the many levels and occupational groupings within it. For such communication to take place with minimal distortion (if at all), the conceptions and expectations that each group has of the others must be mutually congruent, and, within limits, accurate. Research on relations among the professions has shown that this is not the case in hospitals. The conceptions that members of any given occupation hold of the skills, tasks, and attitudes of other occupational groupings do not appear to be congruent, nor do they appear to be accurate. Clearly, if the physician does not know what a nurse will do, and if he expects her to be doing something quite different from what she will actually do, therapeutic plans may fail to be communicated at all, or may be drastically altered in transmission. Similarly, the nurse may wait for the physician to apply an unequivocal diagnostic label to a patient before implementing the nursing plan; if the physician does not intend to do so—if, indeed, he cannot do so—the patient's needs may again go unmet.

Relationships Between and Within Occupational Groupings

The presence in the hospital of many component occupational groups and levels of training poses special problems. A university hospital, or one affiliated with a teaching institution, may embody several simultaneous but not necessarily compatible goals, notably service, research, and teaching. These goals are not intrinsically incompatible. However, personnel of the hospital may come to acknowledge—in fact, they may be hired specifically to perform—only one of these many sets of functions. For them the proper execution of their job is the means of running the hospital and achieving those of its goals to which they are a party. Competing goals and alternate functions may be seen as a hindrance. The researcher may be intolerant of service demands; the teacher may want quick turnover of varied cases; the administrator may press the needs for bed occupancy regardless of variety. In many hospitals these problems are never really "solved": A sort of chronic imbalance exists, shifting now this way, now that, as contingent pressures vary. Again, this may lead to a milieu rife with strains.

Relations among the professions lead to another form of strain within hospitals. It has been noted that mobility in the hospital is peculiarly patterned; personnel are not usually promoted into other occupational groups. Yet the different groups are not completely insulated from each other and one group may seek occupational mobility at the expense of another. This is effected through competition for certain functions and may be achieved by dropping tasks which lack prestige or by taking on tasks which have high prestige, or by both means. Thus the nurse relinquishes certain of her less satisfying tasks to the aide. This enhances the nurse's self-image as well as that of the aide, who sees herself performing nursing duties. Similarly the nurse may enhance her position by performing duties, e.g., anesthetic administration or venipuncture, which formerly were more clearly the duty of the physician. There is always, therefore, an unstable margin of competition for specific functions between occupational groups. In psychiatric contexts, where the allocation of duties and functions to the professional groups has not yet achieved clarification, there may be continuing conflict along these ill-defined borders. The recurring skirmishes can threaten to become war when the conflicting claims and sanctions of competing professional associations and colleague groups are injected into the hospital situation.

Ambiguities of role and status differentiation present other important problems. This is perhaps particularly true of mental hospitals where the overlapping of skills among the professions is more extensive and where the designation of duties to specific professions is less precise than in the general hospital. The problem is aggravated when professions with approximate status, coequals in the "outside" world, find themselves subordinated to psychiatrists in the hospital world. Psychologists, for example, are distressed, in moving from classroom to hospital, to find that their status as fully fledged academician becomes transmuted into that of paramedical or ancillary (which of course means subordinate) medical professional. The independent academician becomes a dependent professional. Since the psychologist feels that his skills are in no way less complex or important in dealing with psychiatric patients, a chronic situation of interprofessional status unease may exist within many hospitals. Pressures from outside colleagues and from professional associations often operate to reinforce or renew problematic relationships within the hospital.

Problems of relationship may occur as well within a single professional group. Among psychiatrists, for example, many incompatible points of view are held concerning diagnosis and therapy. The professional label of "psychiatrist" covers a range of orientations including the neurological, the psychoanalytic, and the social psychiatric. The profession as a whole may handle such a range of difference quite amicably through the proliferation of sections within the master association. The small staffs of hospitals cannot be so sectioned off and differences of orientation are often brought into face-to-face conflict. Differences of orientation, real though they may be, are often not real in their consequences. Psychiatrists of quite different theoretical orientations may arrive at similar diagnoses and formulate identical therapeutic plans. But other personnel on the ward may be unaware that the different languages used are finally in agreement or close accord. They may conclude that broad disagreements persist among psychiatric staff and may accordingly have grave difficulty in relating their activities to the master plan of therapy.

The Individuation-Standardization Dilemma

Psychiatric therapy, geared to the life histories and behavioral needs of specific patients, probably requires greater individuation or prescriptions for care for its patients than do the therapies of other specialties. Whereas many surgical and medical procedures are applicable to all patients, routinization comes less easily in the mental hospital or on the psychiatric ward. This makes the task of maintaining orderly routines a difficult one in psychiatric contexts. Problems of "individuation" versus "standardization" plague the mental hospitals. These problems arise from functional cross-purposes inherent in the conflict between instrumental and maintenance goals of the organization and in the specialized interests of different professional groups. The master goals of the mental hospital are patient care and treatment. Clearly, the entire structure of the hospital was established to implement these goals. But equally clearly, the continuation of this maintenance organization becomes a derived goal for many hospital personnel. To some degree this is necessary, for without a stabilizing organization individuation would become chaos. Life on the wards and in the hospital would become a series of encounters between conflicting prescriptions of individual therapists. But the emphasis upon organizational needs for order and stability can replace the emphasis upon individual needs of patients and therapists. The ideology of organization, developed to contain the tasks of therapy, can establish its own counterclaims for institutional survival. In this there may be detriment to the patient.

Somewhere in this dialectic between individualized attention and organizational demands an optimal stage may be reached. Presumably there is no master prescription for this optimum. It will vary from hospital to hospital, and within hospitals from time to time. Its postulated existence highlights the necessary master characteristic of mental hospital organization—*flexibility*. It needs to be a structure with a built-in "glissando" effect: capable at different times of granting many degrees of individual freedom yet maintaining organizational stability, defining intrinsic attributes of roles and tasks with sufficient clarity so that these may be performed in a broad variety of ways and yet remain functionally precise. If flexibility is the desired attribute of psychiatric hospital structure, much organizational research might profitably be focused upon the form of organization best able to produce and contain it. This problem is particularly acute in our larger mental hospitals. Their size conduces to a hierarchical, bureaucratic form of organization. Such a form, stable and able to handle complex tasks, readily becomes inflexible and unwieldly.

It is noteworthy, however, that the recent aim of structural flexibility has been in a new direction. The original goal of devising social structures that would permit staff to deal more effectively with patients is beginning to yield to the goal of finding staff structure that would best permit the good effects of patients upon each other to be maximized. The background of this changing emphasis involves changes in the approach of psychiatry and is also an effect of the size and composition of many psychiatric hospitals. The "interpersonal" emphasis of much contemporary psychiatry has underscored the sensitivity of psychiatric patients to their milieu. The therapeutic momentum of the society of patients has become an object of research and an important consideration in hospital planning. At the far pole from changing theoretical considerations, problems of practice have produced much the same emphasis. In many of our larger psychiatric hospitals, a small staff may care for many thousands of patients. Relations between staff and patients may be sporadic and limited in effects. The contacts of patients with other patients are enduring and may have a marked effect. Thus the implications of the patient social milieu of psychiatric hospitals for patient care and therapy have become a matter of practical concern and a new focus of social and psychiatric research.

Implicit in this new emphasis is a tendency to note that the assignment of mentally ill persons to medical institutions is an accident of history rather than a technical-professional necessity. In fact, in many large hospitals the burden of administration and care, and often therapy, does not rest upon physician-psychiatrists. Many of the large isolated hospitals are far closer to being true communities than they are to being hospitals. Some observers have felt that the traditional designation of mental hospitals as medical institutions is hindering their full development along new conceptual lines. They urge transfer of responsibility to nonmedical professionals. Countering this tendency is the increasing use of drugs as therapeutic aids, a trend which is clearly medical in emphasis. Perhaps the final word concerning the professional emphasis to become dominant in mental hospitals rests with developments within psychiatry itself, particularly its assimilation of ideas and techniques from the biological and the social sciences.

COMMENTARY

One of the key questions addressed by this paper concerns the ways in which the maintenance functions serve or undermine instrumental goal implementation. Maintenance functions may be overt or covert. They may serve to sustain morale and motivation or may work against them.

The paper raises an interesting question regarding the special needs for maintenance functions of staff in an institution in which the principal instrumental task of staff is providing socioemotional support to troubled people.

It is helpful to distinguish among the various kinds of authority which differ as to their source and legitimation (see Chapter 11).

Hierarchal authority is the right to influence people to behave in specified ways in an organization, and is legitimated by the position the individual holds.

Charismatic power is the ability to influence the behavior of others because of one's personal attractiveness. This power does not necessarily follow administrative authority lines (hierarchal authority) and in fact may be contrary to them. What problems might a charismatic person present to an organization?

Professional power is the ability to influence the behavior of others because of one's training, skills, and knowledge. This power does not necessarily follow administrative authority lines and may be contrary to them.

What problems and conflicts are often generated in an organization between those with hierarchal authority and those with professional power? How might these conflicts be resolved?

In many large mental hospitals, which are organized with strong departments to which all members of a discipline belong and are responsible (i.e., nursing, psychology, social work, psychiatry), communications are facilitated within a discipline and are more difficult across discipline lines. In decentralized organizations the staff is organized into multidisciplinary units with weaker departmental structures. In such organizations the communications between disciplines within a unit are facilitated.

In an interdisciplinary team the staff clearly faces the problem of definition of professional and personal roles vis-à-vis other disciplines on the team. If there are potential changes in the roles of a discipline, for example when nurses expand their skills to become individual and group psychotherapists and family counsellors, what patterns of authority (charismatic, professional, and hierarchal) may facilitate and/or impede these changes. Additionally, in times of acute stress in the work unit, shifts in use of the various kinds of authority may be observed to take place.

We must judge the extent to which the patterns of authority exercised are geared to the accomplishment of the instrumental goal of patient care in our own institution so that we can consider this issue: To what extent and in what ways does the hospital (center or program) exist for the benefit of the patient? Staff? Both?

CHAPTER 14

Social Structure and Process in Treatment

INTRODUCTION

In the previous papers in Part II you have read about the ways in which social systems impact upon individuals. It seems clear that the forces generated in group life are compelling. Some groups or organizations enable and facilitate individual learning and sense of worthwhileness. Other social groups demean the individual. These observations have led to questions about how the social environment might be deliberately structured to promote the development and nurturance of psychosocial skills. Given the opportunity to facilitate the formation of groups of patients and staff and the possibility of shaping the social structure, what kinds of people would be selected and with what inter-relationships would they be arranged?

Looking back upon the history of mental hospitals, the era of moral treatment offers an illuminating example of the use of a social setting as treatment. It was a period in which the entire social structure was deliberately manipulated for the purpose of changing human behavior. The expectation was that a strict moral environment would strengthen the personality of the ill person. The social arrangements emphasized respect for authority, self-discipline, and good habit formation. This was based on the assumption that mental illness was caused by a breakdown of moral fiber.

Understanding the causes and the basic defects or deficiencies involved in mental disorders determines what measures will be used to influence change. Current assumptions implicate psychological, biological, and social factors, and consequently therapeutic interventions include psychological, biological, and social measures.

The question addressed in this reading is: What form should so-

cial intervention take, assuming that biological and psychological ther-
apies will also be used? Every treatment setting has a social structure.
If one assumes that a common problem among the mentally ill is a
deficit of social skills, then conceivably, if he is provided a particular
kind of social system, the individual will have an opportunity to im-
prove his social interactions. The following paper presents a rationale
for utilizing the social system itself as an important element of the
therapeutic effort.

THE THERAPEUTIC COMMUNITY

Alan M. Kraft

The therapeutic community concept is based on the assumption that
the social milieu itself can be the instrument of treatment. The
realization that people change, learn, and mature as a result of their
interpersonal and social relationships and experiences is not new. It is
interwoven in the fabric of all theories of personality development.
Yet the applied use of this knowledge in the treatment of mental illness
has not been fully exploited. Its greatest application has been in the use
of individual psychotherapy, a two-person system in which one person
learns about himself through his experience with another person. The
use of the total environment with a deliberate attempt to include all
relationships for the benefit of the patient is a logical extension of this
method.

Harry Stack Sullivan [1] and the Menningers [2] were among the first
to move in this direction. The Menningers, using psychoanalytic theory,
set about to create in the hospital a favorable array of interpersonal
relationships for each patient by prescribing attitudes for the staff to
adopt. For example, the prescription of "kind firmness" by the doctor as
an attitude for all staff to assume in their interactions with a depressed patient involves manipulation of the patient's interpersonal and
social environment as part of his treatment.

In most psychiatric hospitals and children's residential treatment
centers, it has increasingly become the practice to use various aspects
of the environment, including the special talents of people and different kinds of activities, as part of the treatment program. This has
come to be known as milieu therapy, which refers to any program using
the environment or aspects of it for therapeutic purposes. The use of
the interpersonal environment may be limited or quite extensive. For
instance, a treatment program using a few hours a week of occupational

Alan M. Kraft, M.D., "The Therapeutic Community," in *American Handbook of
Psychiatry*, vol. 3, edited by Silvano Arieti, © 1966 by Basic Books, Inc., Publishers,
New York. Used by permission.

therapy could be legitimately called milieu therapy; so could an extensive and variegated activities program. Very few treatment centers are without some kind of milieu therapy program.

Definition of Therapeutic Community

The therapeutic community is a very special kind of milieu therapy in which the total social structure of the treatment unit is involved as part of the helping process. It is organized and developed in order to make available for treatment purposes all relationships and all activities in the life of the patient. It differs from other kinds of milieu therapy to the extent that it operates on the principle that all of the social and interpersonal processes in the hospital are important and relevant to the treatment of the individual. No elements are set outside the treatment, and all transactions are important as potentially therapeutic.

As no two societies of any kind are alike, so no two therapeutic communities are alike. Such groups work toward their goals in different ways, depending on the people who constitute them. A therapeutic community is a complex organization of people whose primary goal is to provide therapeutic experiences to its patients, clients, students, or inmates.

The therapeutic community is based on a conceptualization in which emotional illness is seen as an interpersonal and social phenomenon. The manifestations of mental illness are viewed in the context of the patient's relationships with other people. Intrapsychic determinants are recognized, but greater stress is laid on the interpersonal aspects of the person's functioning. The Cummings,[3] linking milieu therapy and ego psychology, state that the ego develops out of crisis resolution. They indicate that milieu therapy is effective insofar as the staff skills can be applied to helping the patient through a series of such crises in a treatment setting.

Maxwell Jones,[4] who originated the term "therapeutic community," describes it in this way:

> It would seem that in some, if not all, psychiatric conditions there is much to be learned from observing the patient in a relatively ordinary and familiar social environment so that his usual ways of relating to other people, reaction to stress, etc., can be observed. If at the same time he can be made aware of the effect of his behavior on other people and helped to understand some of the motivation underlying his actions, the situation is potentially therapeutic. This we believe to be the distinctive quality of a therapeutic community. Clearly there is the possibility of any interpersonal relationship being therapeutic or antitherapeutic. It is the introduction of trained staff personnel into the group situation together with planned collaboration of patients and staff in most, if not all, aspects of the unit life which heightens the possibility of the social experience being therapeutic.[5]

Historically, the therapeutic community bears certain resemblances to other treatment modalities of the past. For instance, it has much in common with the moral treatment [6] of the early and middle nineteenth century. The respect for human rights, the "family feeling" of hospitals, the humane consideration for patients, and the recognition of the therapeutic effects of activities are all elements shared by moral treatment and the therapeutic community. However, while its roots have many connections, it seems clear that the therapeutic community represents a departure from previous treatment methods.

Characteristics of a Therapeutic Community

Emphasis on Social and Group Interaction. The individual patient, as well as the staff member, is seen as an important member of the community or culture. It is expected that he will manifest in this treatment setting many of the very modes of interaction that characterized his relationships outside the setting. In the dyadic therapies the patient-doctor relationship is itself the arena of treatment; in the therapeutic community the arena is broadened to include all relationships. For example, the patient who isolates himself by becoming silent and withdrawn is manifesting some of his characteristic ways of relating to people. His responses to the group are available to the group for their intervention.

This differs in an important way from other kinds of settings where the primary therapeutic relationship—sometimes the only recognized therapeutic relationship—exists between the patient and his doctor. The other twenty-three hours a day typically are viewed merely as maintaining, protecting, and supporting the patient between treatments.

Focus on Communication. The network of communication receives a great deal of attention in a therapeutic community. This includes communication of all kinds, manifest and latent, verbal and nonverbal, conscious and unconscious, and at all levels—patient-patient, patient-staff, and staff-staff. The perceptual and emotional distortions of communication in all relationships are scrutinized, not just the transference and countertransference phenomena of the doctor-patient relationship.

Of great significance is the demonstration by Stanton and Schwartz [7] that there is a direct relationship between disturbed staff relationships and disturbed patient behavior. They stated explicitly what many had long suspected, that patients are acutely sensitive to staff interactions. The question is not "Should the staff share with the patients its concerns and problems regarding treatment?" but, "How much should be shared?" If the staff of a mental hospital ward is especially concerned about a suicidal patient, the patients on that unit are usually aware of this. In a therapeutic community the staff would talk to the patients about their concern and enlist their aid in helping the suicidal member of the community.

It is useless to try to exclude the patient group from knowing the problems of the staff as a staff. The patients know a great deal and sense a great deal more about staff and staff attitudes.[8] In recognition of this, the therapeutic community makes this information openly available and in doing so shares its responsibilities for treatment with patients. The patient then becomes more than a passive recipient of treatment. He has an opportunity to become a responsible participant and a contributor to his own and others' treatment processes.

Communication between the members of the therapeutic community is valuable insofar as it makes relevant information available to its members. Any information is considered relevant to the extent that it bears a relationship to the social and interpersonal processes of the unit. In order to accomplish this, the communication must be open, honest, skillful, goal-directed, and appropriately timed. The degree to which information is shared is a constant issue of discussion and scrutiny in a therapeutic community.[9]

The great attention given to an open communication network has two purposes. Almost all patients have some impairment of communication ability. They have feelings and thoughts and impulses with which they do not know how to cope. Many patients have difficulty understanding the communications of others. Making explicit much of what is implicit in a social situation helps patients to identify and express verbally what they are experiencing and to diminish perceptual distortions of communications from others.

The second purpose of open communication concerns the administrative and clinical needs of the community. It helps the staff and patients know their roles, limitations, responsibilities, and authorities. It increases their effectiveness to give them a maximum of information on which to base the decisions they must make.

Living-Learning Opportunities. All facets of the life of the patient in the social milieu are seen as presenting opportunities for a living-learning experience. The role of the staff is to use their various skills to realize these opportunities to the fullest. This culture then becomes one in which there is a favorable climate for: (1) helping the patients to gain an awareness of their feelings, thoughts, impulses, and behavior; (2) helping the patients to try their new skills in a relatively safe environment; (3) helping the patients achieve a realistic appraisal of their social and interpersonal environments, since staff and patients are able to confront members of the group with the realities of the social situation and with potentially helpful or destructive aspects of their behavior; and (4) helping each patient to increase his self-esteem.

Viewed in this way, a therapeutic community is not unlike a school for living. The "student body" is composed of those who have found themselves unable to meet the demands of everyday responsibility. The "faculty" is the staff, who have developed skills and sensitivities which enable them to teach social skills and self-understanding. The "course work" consists of the daily living situation, similar in many ways to ordinary life situations but more protective and enriched to increase learning possibilities.

Sharing Responsibilities with Patients. In such a treatment setting a value is placed on a greater sharing of responsibility with patients than is found in the usual hospital. The rationale is that by offering a greater degree of meaningful participation in the decision-making functions of the community, the staff helps prepare the patient for decision making in his life outside the hospital, and in this way helps combat the feeling of helplessness and passivity of so many patients.

The hierarchical structure so common to the mental hospital [10] does not lend itself to shared decision making involving the clinical staff, much less the patients. In the large traditional hospital the formal decision-making power lies in the administrative echelon, far removed from the clinical team which has direct contact with the patients. The growing practice of decentralization of large hospitals into smaller, more manageable clinical units, each of which has a greater degree of decision-making power, is a useful prerequisite to establishing a therapeutic community.[11] If the patients and staff are to participate together in decision making and are going to share responsibilities for their community decisions, they must be given the formal authority to do so by the central hospital authorities.

The provision by the staff of an opportunity for patients to participate with them in decision making results in an attitude or climate of mutual trust and respect between patient and staff. Psychiatric patients frequently come to treatment with the fantasy that they will be the passive recipients of "something" that will be given them or done to them. The somatic therapies and the pharmacotherapies do not require that the fantasy be destroyed. However, psychotherapy and therapeutic community treatment require that the fantasy be altered. Many patients are reluctant to give up this hope. In many cases this wish lies near the dynamic core of their difficulty. The treatment is concerned with this fantasy and its meaning to the patient. When the therapeutic culture places a value on patients assuming responsibilities, some patients find themselves in direct conflict with this demand. Many patients are distrustful of the offer of responsibility and regard it as a trick being played by the staff. It is precisely this kind of question that becomes an issue for discussion and exploration.

Patient government helps the patients fulfill their obligations and responsibilities as members of the community. To be effective, patient government must be organized and run by the patients themselves. To the extent that it is manipulated by staff for their own needs, it becomes a farce and the patients know they are being asked to pretend or to play at being involved. The responsibility and authority of patient government must be carefully spelled out. Its functions will vary from community to community. In some units patient government is a forum to receive complaints and is not expected to assume any responsibilities. Whatever its role, the formal organization of patients should be dealt with honestly and not be told it has powers it really does not have.

For patient government to be effective, the staff must trust the ultimate good judgment of the patient group and must delegate real responsibilities to it. Patients, like all other people, tend to live up to the social expectations made of them. The precise role of the patient government in the therapeutic community ideally should be worked out jointly by the staff and patients.

Patient participation in the life of the community is not limited to patient government. This particular organization deals best with the accomplishment of specific tasks and serves as a formal line of communication between the patient group and the hospital authorities. In a larger organization patient government in a representational form offers an opportunity for the representative of the patient group to deal directly with the hospital administration.

There are other functions, however, with which a formal patient government does not deal so effectively as the community meeting, which has a special usefulness. It is attended by all staff and all patients who work and live on a specific unit. It may vary in size from 15 to 100 participants, depending on the size of the unit. It is at this daily meeting that the group comes to terms with its community problems.[12] The disturbed or disturbing behavior of a patient, a suicidal patient, a staff person or patient who is leaving the community are examples of common problems dealt with by the group as community problems. This meeting is crucial to the maintenance of the open network of communications. Afterward a meeting of the staff is held at which they review the manifest and latent content and process of the meeting. They examine their own therapeutic techniques. This offers unsurpassed and unique opportunities for the staff to learn the skills it needs as therapists. This meeting presents the leader of the unit along with the other staff members the possibility of receiving a direct feedback from each other about their specific therapeutic behaviors. When viewing this as a learning situation, the members of the staff can share information with each other and learn from each other. The doctor confronts and is confronted by the other staff members and is able to receive as well as to impart information. He is able to learn as he teaches.

If there is emphasis on shared responsibility between patients and staff, there is also emphasis on shared participation in the treatment process. As a natural result of this, it frequently happens that some of the most helpful therapists are the patients themselves. There are some problems with which patients can help fellow patients more easily and at times more effectively than staff. For instance, a patient who in speaking to the group denies his responsibility for his problems and projects responsibility on others will frequently find himself confronted by fellow patients in a way that makes it difficult for him to avoid coming to grips with the problem. In such situations the staff is seldom as effective as the patients.

Inherent in this social system is a responsibility on the part of the individual to the community as well as the responsibility of the community to be therapeutic to the individual. Freedom of action is limited only by responsibility to act appropriately. Thus there are restrictions on freedom imposed by the community. Patients are not given license to act inappropriately, irresponsibly, or destructively.

If they behave in these ways there is an obligation on the part of the group to look at the meaning and the consequences of such behavior. The group applies sanctions and rewards but, more important, it helps its members learn from their behavior.

In a very real way, the community is like the outside community, since it too describes the "normal" limits of behavior. Similarly the limits of behavior in the therapeutic community are decided by the members of the community itself. Each community develops its own code of conduct, which reflects the attitudes of the group. In a great many ways the code is similar to that of the community from which the patients and staff come—the outside community. There are modifications dictated by the facts of life of an institution and by that which distinguishes the community, that its purpose is to be therapeutic. As a result the therapeutic community will have rules and regulations and its own limits of "normality." As with the outside community, it will not be true that "anything goes."

Emphasis on patient responsibility has another value. The treatment process addresses itself to the intact ego functions of each patient. It assumes that even the sickest patient is not wholly sick but rather that only parts of his ego functioning are disturbed. Each patient starts with what he has and builds from there. In the usual course of events a patient is not permitted to say, "I cannot participate in anything because I am too sick." Most therapeutic communities discourage regression by patients. Ordinarily patients are not permitted to go to bed during the day or to withdraw from all social contacts. Instead there is an expectation by the community to participate, to assume responsibility, and to interact.

Nothing that has been said should be construed as meaning that the staff is passive and that the patients run the hospital. The staff brings with it certain skills, sensitivities, and knowledge about psychodynamic, social, and interpersonal relationships. It is the staff's role to catalyze, promote, encourage, interact, and teach. They are members of the community, not bystanders.

> The fact that both staff and patients may be granted coequal rights as human beings in such a community in no way implies coequal function or role status. It cannot, for hospitals are not democracies run by elected representatives of the community, but hierarchies whose senior members are appointed to their roles of authority by extra-hospital super authorities and who carry inescapable responsibility to these super authorities for the total work of the community. Authority in the hospital is therefore both necessary and inescapable. Although powers and responsibilities may be delegated for operational purposes to other members of the community engaged for such purposes, there can never be renunciation of responsibility by the hierarchy. No amount of persuasions, group decisions, consensus seeking, joint consultation or freedom of expression can obscure this fact.[13] Authoritarianism is not the same as authority. Authority is necessary in any organization.

Role Expansion. Inevitably there must be a reassessment of their own role expectations by the staff. Staff, like patients, in such a treatment setting find themselves operating in new ways. No longer is there the usual sharp line of delineation between patients and staff.[14] Staff does not "give" treatment. Furthermore within the staff there is a diminution of the hierarchical lines which separate the disciplines. For example, it is difficult to describe a unique role for the nurse. A great deal, if not most, of what she does is similar to what the social worker, psychologist, and doctors do. Each discipline brings certain special skills and training to the setting, as well as bringing themselves as people. However, when they meet as colleagues in a therapeutic community they find they have much more in common operationally than that which differentiates them. This can be a discovery which is accompanied by great anxiety. For example, physicians on the long and tortuous road toward becoming trained psychiatrists come to enjoy a certain status with its associated privileges. It requires a high degree of ego strength on the part of the psychiatrist to face a colleague of another discipline as one therapist to another. The doctor must assume leadership more on the basis of his skills, knowledge, and abilities and less because he is called a psychiatrist.

For members of all the mental health disciplines, work in a therapeutic community requires a reexamination of the roles for which they have been trained. Training frequently has not prepared them for the jobs in which they find themselves. Fortunately, the therapeutic community (and especially the community meeting) lends itself especially well to a continuing process of inservice training.

There is one quality invariably found in a therapeutic community which may also be present in other kinds of treatment settings. This characteristic, for want of a better term, may be called *esprit de corps*. It permeates not only the staff but also the patient group. The emotional climate is one of warmth, friendliness, acceptance, and optimism. This positive group feeling is enhanced in the community that is functioning well, since the group members as individuals feel themselves to be participants in an active and productive group venture.

Elements of a Therapeutic Community

The People. The patient population may be a cross-section of the mentally ill from a specific geographic area. It may consist of a particular diagnostic grouping. It may consist of prisoners. A therapeutic community may be the treatment method in a twenty-four-hour hospital, a day hospital, a rehabilitation center, or a halfway house. There has as yet been insufficient experience to say what kinds of people are most or least likely to benefit from this kind of treatment or what kinds of settings in which this method can be effective.

The staff in a mental hospital usually consists of the traditional mental health specialists: psychiatrist, psychologists, social workers, nursing personnel, and activity therapists. Although Maxwell Jones trained a different group of people, called social therapists, this has been the exception. So long as the therapeutic community exists in a mental hospital, it is likely that the traditional disciplines will constitute the staff.

In settings outside of the hospitals, for example, schools and prisons, this is not so. Experience is as yet insufficient to determine what kinds of training will best prepare people for work in these settings.

The Organizations Within the Community.   There seems to be little structural difference between a therapeutic community and other milieu therapies in the kinds of activities available. The major difference lies in the ways they are used. Occupational therapy, work therapy, recreational therapy, patient government, are all organizations to be found in therapeutic communities.

The Physical Environment.   Ideally, the buildings that house a therapeutic community should be built in consultation with the people who will use them. In practice this almost never happens. Even when a therapeutic community moves into a brand-new building, the members of the community have little opportunity to determine the form of the new structure. The physical structure must invariably be modified to meet the needs of the group. It sets real limitations on the group, but it also challenges the ingenuity of the members of the community to make the physical plant suit their needs.

As with the social structure, the furnishings should reflect the needs and aspirations of the community. The buildings should therefore be livable and comfortable and possibly even homelike. Most therapeutic communities have open settings, but in some hospitals and in prisons they may be closed. The basic idea of shared patient responsibility is, of course, most consistent with an unlocked setting.

The Outside Community.   The goal of a therapeutic community is the successful return of its patients to the community. This purpose is best served by the establishment of close relationships between the therapeutic community and the outside community. The therapeutic community should be viewed as a part of the larger community. The staff of such a treatment center should be active members of the community in which they live. The hospital should not isolate itself by becoming self-sufficient. It should make use of community facilities, such as recreational facilities, libraries, general hospitals, and churches.

Other Treatment Methods.   The therapeutic community may be the primary, though rarely the only, treatment modality used. In other settings it may be ancillary to other treatment methods. In such centers the therapeutic community is the background and the matrix of life in the unit, but it is frequently the case that the greater emphasis is placed on individual psychotherapy as the definitive method of treatment.

The ways in which other treatment methods are used may strengthen or undermine the basic values of a therapeutic community. For example, electroshock therapy has a very legitimate use with certain kinds of patients and should be used when specifically indicated. It should not be used to control "acting-out" behavior, with which the community can and should work by use of its array of therapeutic forces.

Individual and group psychotherapy, psychodrama, pharmacotherapy, electroshock therapy, work, all can be used in a therapeutic community. In every case the use of these modalities should be planned in such a way as to enhance and articulate with the ongoing community activities.

Problems of a Therapeutic Community

1. There is no clear, conceptual model underlying the therapeutic community. The problem lies in the fact that while we have both intrapsychic and social models, a supraordinate model is required, one that transcends the existing ones.

2. While the gains in terms of personal and professional satisfaction for the staff are enormous, the lack of clear boundaries between the various professional roles and the threat of loss of professional identity are anxiety provoking.

3. "Group responsibility," unless skillfully nurtured, can become "no responsibility."

4. There is a continuing possibility that the individual patient may become lost in the concern for the group. It seems clear that in a well-functioning community there is an increased concern and respect for the individual. When patients are permitted to withdraw, to become isolated, this in itself is a problem which must be dealt with by the community.

5. The therapeutic community may teach values that are appropriate to its own culture but that might lead to difficulties if the patient were to apply these elsewhere. For instance, while a patient may be encouraged to "speak his mind" in the hospital, it may be more appropriate to "hold his tongue" when speaking to his boss outside.

6. The problems of research and program evaluation are extremely complex, because of the proliferation of the factors leading to change.

7. As few centers in this country currently offer training especially suited to functioning in a therapeutic community, it remains the function of the setting itself to train its own staff. Fortunately, the daily community meeting is an excellent living-learning experience which lends itself especially well to this training function.

NOTES

1. Harry Stack Sullivan, "Sociopsychiatric Research, Its Implications for the Schizophrenia Problem and for Mental Hygiene," *American Journal of Psychiatry* 10 (1931): 977–991.

2. W. C. Menninger, "Psychiatric Hospital Therapy Designed to Meet Unconscious Needs," *American Journal of Psychiatry* 93 (1936): 347–360, and idem, "Psychoanalytic Principles Applied to the Treatment of Hospital Patients," *Bulletin of the Menninger Clinic* 1 (1936): 35–43.

3. John Cumming and Elaine Cumming, *Ego and Milieu* (Englewood Cliffs, N.J.: Prentice-Hall, 1962).

4. Maxwell Jones, *The Therapeutic Community: A New Treatment Method in Psychiatry* (New York: Basic Books, 1953).

5. Maxwell Jones, quoted in H. A. Wilmer, *Social Psychiatry in Action* (Springfield, Ill.: Charles C Thomas, 1958).

6. J. S. Bockoven, *Moral Treatment in American Psychiatry* (New York: Springer, 1963), and Lucy D. Ozarin, "Moral Treatment and the Mental Hospital," *American Journal of Psychiatry* 111 (1954): 371–378.

7. Alfred H. Stanton and Morris S. Schwartz, *The Mental Hospital: A Study of Institutional Participation in Psychiatric Illness and Treatment* (New York: Basic Books, 1954).

8. W. Caudill et al., "Social Structure and Interaction Processes on a Psychiatric Ward," *American Journal of Orthopsychiatry* 22 (1952): 314–334.

9. W. Caudill and E. Stainbrook, "Some Covert Effects of Communication Difficulties in a Psychiatric Hospital," *Psychiatry* 17 (1954): 27–40.

10. Ivan Belknap, *Human Problems of a State Mental Hospital* (New York: McGraw-Hill, 1956), and Erving Goffman, *Asylums: Essays on the Social Situation of Mental Patients and Other Inmates* (Garden City, N.Y.: Doubleday, Anchor Books, 1961).

11. Leonardo Garcia, "The Clarinda Plan: An Ecological Approach to Hospital Organization," *Mental Hospitals* 11 (1960): 30–31.

12. Maxwell Jones, "Training in Social Psychiatry at the Ward Level," *American Journal of Psychiatry* 118 (1962): 705–708.

13. H. A. Wilmer, *Social Psychiatry in Action—A Therapeutic Community* (Springfield, Ill.: Charles C Thomas, 1958), pp. 12–13.

14. E. M. Bonn and A. M. Kraft, "The Fort Logan Mental Health Center: Genesis and Development," *Journal of the Fort Logan Mental Health Center* 1 (1963): 17–27.

COMMENTARY

The therapeutic community is a setting in which social learning and growth take place. The frame of reference is one in which emphasis is given to learning on the part of the patient—learning how to act appropriately and adaptively; learning expanded and new social roles. The acutely disturbed person is often not able to learn new social roles, and consequently may benefit less from this kind of setting. The primary task for the acutely disturbed individual is to achieve integration and stabilization.

In a comprehensive network of services, what is the place of a therapeutic community? Is it useful for all patients? Should it be limited to inpatients, day patients, or to a rehabilitation program?

It has been said that a therapeutic community often serves the personal needs and values of the staff more than the patients. One might well ask, "To what extent is it a legitimate goal for any therapeutic endeavor to serve the needs of the therapist?" Certainly therapists should enjoy and learn from their work. The therapeutic community is often in a position to address openly the question about which activities are for whose benefit. There are dilemmas of individual needs versus group needs in a therapeutic community as in all social systems. For example, if self-actualization and individuation require a person to be somewhat deviant, what are the problems for the individual and the group when there is pressure for conformity?

Every social system has the possibility of exhibiting a tyranny which allows little individuation and demands a high degree of conformity. A patient says he doesn't want to go to a group outing because he wants to read a book. One has several alternate ways to evaluate this: as an act of withdrawal, of defiance, or of regression, or as a statement of individuation.

Though the therapeutic community has been utilized for several decades, there remain some unresolved questions: What conflicts might develop when a therapeutic community is established in a setting (such as a general hospital) which is not receptive to democratization? What special requirements (skills, knowledge, personal characteristics) are made of the head of the team? What is the interplay of hierarchal, professional, and charismatic power in such a unit? What unique stresses (role, skill, and personal) are placed on the staff of such a unit? What are the unique problems of a therapeutic community in which the average length of stay is several days?

CHAPTER 15

The Primary Group At Work

INTRODUCTION

Pepper's thesis is that the interdisciplinary team *is an effective organizational unit for achieving* continuity of care. *He thus links two important concepts. Leaning heavily on primary group concepts, as discussed in Chapters 4 and 7, he advocates enhancing the sense of "we-ness" so as to help team members meet their own socioemotional needs while simultaneously enhancing efforts to carry out instrumental tasks.*

Continuity of care is presently a problem in all fields of medicine and social services. It is not a problem in those situations in which one person provides all the medical services an individual needs.

The rural general practitioner who knows each family and is the only available care giver does not have to concern himself with this issue. But most people live and work in an environment in which there is a complicated network of care givers, and in which an individual may be a client of many different services. Consider the problem of the privileged person who has his own dentist, internist, psychiatrist, surgeon, and dermatologist; each may be giving advice or prescriptions the other should know about. Or consider the multitude of underprivileged families who receive services from the social service departments, the school counselor, the family and children's service, and the pediatric or medical clinic, where frequently each service has information which would be useful to the other.

In the mental health field the solo practitioner, with deliberate effort, may try to circumvent the problem by restricting his or her work to certain techniques with certain kinds of patients. Nonetheless, practitioners should be concerned with the other relationships their patients develop with care givers, and for that reason must find ways to be kept informed about important events. Furthermore, most practitioners find they are not able themselves to provide all the kinds of mental health services which are needed, so on occasion they make referrals to colleagues of their own or allied disciplines.

In clinics, centers, and hospitals where there are congregate numbers of care givers, it is possible for each clinician to function independently, like the solo private practitioner. Yet experience has led most clinics to organize themselves into units, groups, or teams which in some way order, distribute, and share the work responsibilities. The following paper answers the question: Why?

THE TEAM: A MEANS OF ACHIEVING CONTINUITY OF CARE

Bert Pepper

The Meaning of Continuity of Care

Continuity of care is a graceless and ambiguous phrase which represents a vital and neglected principle of mental health care and treatment. Put simply, it refers to arranging mental health services so as to provide a comprehensive range of treatment services *while exposing the patient to the fewest possible changes of therapeutic personnel.* Continuity assures that the patient will not have to adjust to new staff members and lose the security of contact with those he or she has come to know and trust when a new treatment modality is initiated. Additionally, staff have an ever-growing fund of shared knowledge about each patient.

The private practice model in medicine usually provides good continuity when the family doctor remains active in treating and following patients after referral to specialists for consultation, or to a hospital for inpatient care. But public and voluntary mental health treatment programs are complex organizations, and most have evolved hierarchal structures which specialize the functions of individual staff members. As a consequence, a change in type of treatment—for example, outpatient to inpatient—usually means that the patient will have to adapt to a new therapist. More will be said later about hierarchal and horizontal organizations.

Because mental health treatment systems are so complex, several different types or models of continuity of care can be described. *Continuity by therapist* requires that the therapist not only have a full range of treatment skills, such as individual, group, family, and drug therapy, but that he or she also practice these methods wherever the patient is at any time in the treatment of the illness. Like a general medical practitioner in a rural area, such a therapist attends the patient in the clinic, the inpatient unit, or at home, as required. This kind of continuity is virtually nonexistent in most densely populated areas of the United States; it may be found in some rural areas.

Continuity by members of the treatment team implies that a multidisciplinary group of mental health professionals take responsibility for providing a full range of therapeutic modalities in the hospital, the clinic, and the home. The close working relationship among team members allows them to share information rapidly by frequent, informal, unscheduled, verbal communication. This is usually perceived by the patient and may be reassuring, encouraging him to think, "They are looking after me."

Continuity by institution can seem to occur in many mental health treatment settings—such as psychiatric hospitals with outpatient departments and community mental health centers—which have outpatient and inpatient departments operating under separate leadership, each with their own personnel. In such cases the patient may identify with and even have a positive transference to the whole institution, and assume that the elements of his or her treatment are integrated. In fact, close investigation may disclose that there is significant *discontinuity of care.* It is not infrequent to find a sense of rivalry and separateness between departments. Referral may be viewed by the staff of the receving clinical unit as possibly "dumping" a difficult, untreatable, or otherwise undesirable patient.

A review of efforts to provide continuity of care reveals that *continuity by therapist* is seldom practical in complex treatment agencies, while *continuity by institution* at best makes it difficult to provide adequately comprehensive and linked-integrated treatment. A great expenditure of effort to share information and cushion critical and traumatic transitions in the patient's treatment career is required. *Continuity by an interdisciplinary treatment team* is recommended as a practical and economical way of providing sequential and integrated services during the patient's treatment career. The advantages of team treatment will be reviewed later in this paper, and a definition of teamwork will be offered.

How Shall We Treat?

Philip May, in Chapter 28, stresses the importance of treating the transition from hospital to community care as a famliy crisis which urges the marshaling of our best resources and efforts. His studies of the outcomes of various kinds of treatment of schizophrenia lead to many pointed suggestions. One, for example, is that a home visit should be made to the family *before* the patient is discharged. Further, he urges that the patient be seen the day after release, preferably at home. May offers several good reasons for continuous care being provided by a team. For example, "The treatment strategy should center around careful integration of hospital care and aftercare. If the delivery system provides continuity of inpatient and outpatient care by the same treatment team, the transition will be easier and more effective than if care is fragmented so that a different therapist treats patients after their release."

Gruenberg [1] summarizes evidence—some of it originating even before the use of tranquilizing drugs—which indicates that severely mentally ill persons are most effectively treated when inpatient care is used for brief periods to restore basic functioning. Like May, he urges the provision of intensive treatment and support after discharge and return to the community. Gruenberg finds that the effectiveness of treatment is significantly enhanced by having:

> psychiatric services informally available from a clinical team that has had access to the full spectrum of service resources, and has consequently been able to forge a partnership with other community agencies and community professionals, to cooperate in trying to keep the patient's capacities for community life at the highest possible level. Readily available short-term in-hospital care has proven to be crucial in that regard. Such hospital care cannot be isolated from the other services, on the contrary, it is an integral part of the network of services available to the clinical team. Under these conditions, the walls between the hospital and the community are destroyed, both literally and figuratively; patients, families, clinicians and the communities service personnel flow in and out; one might say that the hospital has been "detotalized."
>
> Such a clinical team has its own patient load, which makes use of the team's hospital, outpatient clinic and emergency consultation services, and is thus able to provide help to families, medical practitioners, and social service agencies. This is the specific organizational feature of a community-care delivery system. It can be described briefly as a "unified clinical team," because the clinical team's work unites the activities of inpatient care, outpatient care, day hospitalization, night hospitalization, emergency consultation, rehabilitation, . . . community education and community relations.[2]

Gruenberg is implicitly referring to continuity of care in the above passages. Whenever we talk about unifying services, or about an interdisciplinary team which works both in the community and in the hospital, we are talking about continuous care. In view of its importance in the treatment of mentally ill persons, *providing continuity of care may well be defined as a fundamental instrumental task of mental health programs.* But there are problems in so organizing service programs, as is evident from the observation that mental health systems which offer such harmonized and sequential care are the exception, rather than the rule. There may be strong pressures from the community—often supported by staff with highly specialized training and clinical interests—to provide separate specialized services for such target groups as adolescents, alcoholics, and the elderly. Staff who have been traditionally trained may require retraining and reorientation for work on teams. A large catchment area may have to be subdivided into several smaller areas to allow for team coverage. Other obstacles to the provision of systematic, unified team care are reviewed near the end of this paper.

What Is an Interdisciplinary Team?

This paper has recommended that continuous care can usually best be achieved by an organizational structure which assigns the provision of the full range of treatment services to an interdisciplinary team. But what, indeed, is a team? Since the word has become a ubiquitous commonplace in the mental health field, it seems necessary to define the term and to review some of its current uses.

As long ago as 1965 Bowen, Marler, and Andrews noted:

. . . "There has been a tendency to term any combination of two or more people whose work in a psychiatric setting has a remote connection with that of others, and is somehow related to patients, as a psychiatric team." [3]

The ambiguity surrounding our use of the word "team" may be at least partially a result of its origins. The earliest use of the word relates to the harnessing together of two or more draft animals to pull a vehicle or farm implement—a heavy and passive object. A key word association here is *cooperation*. The most frequent general use of the word "team" today refers to organizing a group of players to compete against a similar group, as in a sport or game; here the immediate word association is *competition*. A third meaning, which seems to reflect most reasonably the use of the term in mental health, is "any group organized to work together: *a team of engineers*." [4] This definition implies the *integration of differentiated functions*.

Importantly, then, the mental health team is not simply being asked to pool brute strength to move an inanimate object, or to compete with another team. It is a *cooperating* work group which has been assigned to coordinate a set of specialized diagnostic, care, and treatment tasks. Converting the general definition to our purposes, it is suggested that the mental health team be defined as: *A collaborating interdisciplinary group of mental health personnel who coordinate their efforts and pool their skills to provide a broad spectrum of sequential care and treatment services to a defined set of patients.*

If the team is assigned responsibility for all patients residing in a defined geographic area it is usually referred to as a *geographic* or *area team*. However, other assignments are possible; for example, developing a team to serve all patients of a particular age group, such as adolescents or the elderly. Lieb and his associates [5] have described a crisis team.

Several advantages of the interdisciplinary team organization have been noted by participants and observers. As noted earlier, communications about the changing status and needs of patients being served are handled by informal verbal means, in the course of the workday; information flow tends to be easier and more rapid than may be the case when it is transmitted primarily via the written medical record. As staff members develop a sense of comfort in relying on each other, the sense of separateness between persons from different professional backgrounds may be diminished, and appropriate degrees of role interchange and blurring may take place. As team members know each other more individually they may call upon the specific human qualities of colleagues, in addition to their technical skills. When each team member discovers what he or she does best, and is accorded recognition for these skills and abilities by colleagues, a greater degree of involvement and effort of staff is seen. In addition, the easier and broader kind of communication tends to produce a more open decision-making process about patients and their treatment. As more staff members, particularly those with less professional training, see that they are meaningfully involved in important decisions, they may feel a greater sense of importance and thus work harder. All of these things combine to bring about the two major advantages of team treatment: more comprehensible and humane treatment from the patient's point of view, and elimination or reduction of the need to refer patients elsewhere.

Common Characteristics of the Mental Health Team

In many treatment settings which employ team organization the following characteristics are noted:

1. *Continuity of membership.* Members may not be readily reassigned, either permanently or temporarily, to other units of the hospital or center. Hiring or approval of new staff may be assigned to the team leadership rather than to central administration.
2. *A significant degree of programmatic (and sometimes budgetary) autonomy* assigned to the team leadership, so that authority in the facility or hospital is decentralized to the teams to some significant degree. The team ordinarily decides who needs to be admitted or discharged, and who will be treated as an outpatient, a day patient, or in some other manner.
3. *A broad interdisciplinary representation* of mental health professional skills: at least psychiatry, psychology, social work, and nursing; often occupational therapy, rehabilitation therapy, recreational therapy, volunteers, and ward staff.
4. *Leadership options.* In many cases the policy of the parent program requires that a physician or psychiatrist be the team leader. However, in some programs the team leader may be drawn from another profession because of his or her particular administrative and organizational skills, interests, and abilities. Some facilities attempt to finesse this issue by having a physician as the team leader while a nonmedical team member conducts the administrative and managerial duties under another title.

5. *Full range of diagnostic and treatment tasks assigned.* The team is usually expected to develop an individualized treatment plan for each patient, and to carry it out, monitor it, and update it as the patient's needs and conditions change, using the team's full range of capabilities.

Comparison with Departmental Hierarchal Organization

The team form of organization, with its responsibilities flowing from the community (precare, outpatient treatment, and home care) to the hospital (inpatient treatment) and back again to the community for aftercare, represents a substantial departure from the usual organization of staff and treatment responsibilities in mental health programs. Traditional organizational structure places a psychiatrist-director at the top, and utilizes chiefs—each supervising a different professional department—to whom members of their respective disciplines report directly. This structures the formal flow of authority and information among members of the same profession. As a consequence, for example, the social worker, psychiatrist, and recreational therapist who are treating a particular patient may have to create a separate and informal communication chain if they are to coordinate their treatment efforts on behalf of that patient. In effect, the profession-oriented organization of most psychiatric programs works *against* the treatment staff developing into an interdisciplinary primary work group, and may enhance rivalries, separatism, noncommunication, and poor total accountability.

In management terminology the interdisciplinary team is an example of flat, or horizontal, organization. Grouping staff by disciplines into departments whose chiefs report to the hospital director creates a hierarchal, or vertical, organization. Contemporary management experts generally encourage the development of horizontal organizations to improve communications, decision making, morale, and task sharing among staff.[6]

Continuity and Mental Health Centers

Continuity of care was elevated to great prominence in 1964 when federal regulations for the development of Comprehensive Community Mental Health Centers (CMHCs) were promulgated.[7] They stipulated that the center must "... assure continuity of care for patients." Further, they stated that "Those responsible for a patient's care within one element can, when practicable and when not clinically contraindicated, continue to care for the patient within any of the other elements." Yet when eight community mental health centers were evaluated[8] in 1969, it was found that at only two of the centers was it common for the same staff members to treat patients on inpatient, outpatient, and day treatment services. In other words, six of these federally funded centers did not offer continuity by either therapist or team. Glasscote has provided additional information on the staffing practices in these centers.[9]

A review of the above suggests that the National Institute of Mental Health staff, which developed the regulations, made continuity a recommended but not a mandatory feature of CMHCs, and that most centers ignored the suggestion, preferring their usual organizational mode.

Obstacles to the Development of Teams

As noted earlier, Gruenberg [10] uses the term "unified clinical team" to describe an interdisciplinary team which is responsible for providing continuous care in all phases of treatment. He has further indicated that such unified teams have been most successful in providing good care and treatment to seriously mentally ill persons. Nevertheless, they are the exception rather than the rule. Gruenberg suggests eight obstacles to the general establishment of unified teams:

1. *Ignorance.* Mental health administrators and professionals do not all know that continuity of care by team members is more helpful to patients.
2. *Hospital remoteness.* When the majority of inpatients were in isolated state institutions far from their home communities, continuous care was not possible. This problem is now diminishing, as suburban communities have grown up around many state hospitals, and newer hospitals are located in or near population centers.
3. *Separate administration.* Separate financing patterns are often instituted for inpatient and ambulatory care.
4. *Drug abuse.* Some may see the modern and powerful ataractic drugs as the *treatment of choice* for mental disorders, and may not recognize the important contributions of patterns of care and treatment to good outcome: "In the pre-drug period, some community care programs were able to produce results for entire communities that were similar to those now attributed to the new drugs." [11] And deteriorations appear to have continued unabated into the drug era, if no concomitant change has occurred in the service organization.[12]
5. *The specialization fetish.*
6. *Pseudoproductivity.* Production-line techniques have proven economical in the creation of large numbers of identical products assembled from identical components. However, this technique is not best for preserving a psychotic patient's functional assets, or for deciding when hospitalization must be commenced or may be terminated: "Many crucial decisions must be made on a 'try-and-see' basis. In such cases, those who do the 'trying' ought to be able to 'see.' If the person who decides to send a patient home is different from the person who sees the result, neither is able to learn from the decision that has been made for the patient." [13]
7. *Teaching isolated from service.*
8. *Research isolated from service.*

Administraive territoriality is another obstacle. Persons in positions of authority, including hospital and clinic directors, are often unwilling voluntarily to decentralize their authority to team leaders. All sorts of rationalizations—and valid reasons—are available: Who will bear ultimate medicolegal responsibility? Is there anyone competent to be the team leader? Similarly, the chief of each professional department may enumerate all kinds of reasons, valid and invalid, which argue against members of the staff reporting to the team leader instead of to him or her directly. In some cases this problem has been dealt with by making the discipline chief a team leader; this, in effect, continues his or her authority, but shifts its locus and functions. In other cases, particularly where only physicians have been chosen to lead teams, the various discipline heads have been left in place, sometimes with little to do. In other situations staff is required to report dually, to the team leader for day-to-day supervision and to the chief of service for "professional and technical supervision." This has sometimes worked, but at other times it has produced a disruptive power struggle between team leaders and discipline heads. Team members may be uncertain as to which work group they should join.

The Experience of Being a Team Leader

Persons who have become team leaders have described their work as satisfying, demanding, exciting, challenging, exhausting, and *managerial* in nature. Despite the fact that they usually come to the role with a background of training and experience in clinical areas, they soon find they are required to function primarily as administrators. Since few mental health professionals have been well trained in managerial skills, some unified teams have failed to function well because the members were unable to coordinate their efforts to meet the needs of their patients while also meeting their own socioemotional needs.

Summary

Experience with the use of unified interdisciplinary teams replacing discipline-oriented staffing arrangements has generally been found to improve patient care and treatment. The changeover usually results in temporary discomfort and confusion as staff learn to define and work in their new role configurations. However, an esprit de corps and sense of "we-ness" develops, and many find that they enjoy a higher degree of work satisfaction, in no small measure because they can see the improved care and treatment being provided the patients.

The changeover frequently leads to a decreased average length of inpatient stay, more rapid initiation of active treatment after hospital admission, the use of a wider variety of treatment modalities in a harmonized manner, and a greater degree of individualized programming. In brief, it tends to shift programs from custody and care to active treatment. Of course, no form or organization can make up for a severe deficiency or total lack of staff resources. A severely understaffed facility will fail to meet its patients' care and treatment needs, no matter how the available staff are assigned. But it is this writer's thesis that, measure for measure, a well-organized interdisciplinary team will continuously deliver the greatest return on resources invested.

NOTES

1. E. M. Gruenberg, "Obstacles to Optimal Psychiatric Service Delivery Systems," *Psychiatric Quarterly* 46, no. 4 (1972): 483–496.
2. Ibid., pp. 484–485.
3. W. T. Bowen, D. D. Marler, and L. Androes, "The Psychiatric Team: Myth and Mystique," *American Journal of Psychiatry* 122 (December 1965): 687–690.
4. *American Heritage Dictionary of the English Language, s.v.* "team."
5. J. Lieb, I. Lipsitch, and A. Slaby, *The Crisis Team: A Handbook for the Mental Health Professional* (New York: Harper & Row, 1973).
6. W. G. Bennis and P. E. Slater, *The Temporary Society* (New York: Harper & Row, 1968).
7. *Federal Register* (Washington, D.C.: Government Printing Office, May 1964).
8. R. N. Glasscote et al., *The Community Mental Health Center: An Interim Appraisal* (Washington, D.C.: American Psychiatric Association, 1969).
9. R. N. Glasscote and J. E. Gudeman, *The Staff of the Mental Health Center: A Field Study* (Washington, D.C.: American Psychological Association, 1969).
10. Gruenberg, "Obstacles."
11. T. C. Smith, W. H. Bower, and C. M. Wignall, "Influence of Policy and Drugs on Colorado State Hospital Population," *Archives of General Psychiatry* 12 (1965): 352–362.
12. Paul H. Hoch et al., "Observations on the British Open Hospitals," *Mental Hospitals* 8 (1957): 5–15.
13. Gruenberg, "Obstacles," p. 491.

COMMENTARY

Although clinicians find working in teams effective, certain real problems are commonly encountered.
   1. The definition of specialist-generalist roles. Members of different disciplines bring special skills, orientations, values, and legal authorities. Across the entire spectrum of knowledge and skills available in the team, the various disciplines share a great deal, and find that many of their clinical activities are not to be uniquely performed by one discipline. Yet there are differences, and it is inevitably an issue the members of the team must resolve in order for them to work together. Which tasks are generalists' and which are specialized? How are these to be defined? How delegated?
   2. Integrated or coordinated functioning. The question here is really the degree of teamwork members of the team will utilize. Will the unit operate as does a basketball team in which each member's

effectiveness requires that he or she have a wide range of the relevant skills, and each functions in a highly integrated way with others on the team? Or is it more like an airliner crew in which the pilot, engineer, and navigator each have an essential, highly specialized, but partial function which is contributing to the task? Perhaps the reader can recall examples of each from his/her own clinical work experience.

3. Shared responsibility.   *Where several members of a team work with the same patient, questions often arise: Whose patient is it? Is it the team's? The psychotherapist's? The physician's? The rehabilitation therapist's? Often each clinician feels it is his/her patient, and this can give rise to covert conflict among team members unless dealt with.*

From the patient's perspective this phenomenon may be perceived as a confusing array of persons who had influence on his treatment. The flexibility of a team, the shared roles, the group decision making will often appear to a person who is not confused to be a chaotic situation. The confused and disorganized person may be unable to deal at all with such complexities and may indeed require a simpler therapeutic network. How is a team to be helpful to patients as they sort out the authority and other role relationships of the team?

4. Leadership.   *It is not unusual for patterns of leadership to arise which enable individual members of a team to assume leadership responsibilities for different kinds of functions. This leads to shifts in leadershp from time to time as the task shifts. For example, one person may be able to lead the group in its thinking about rehabilitation; another may be especially knowledgeable about work with families; another does well when there is a crisis with a disturbed patient and is able to lead the staff group at such a time. The critical question may be whether the chief of the unit and the members of the team are able to live comfortably with shifting leadership without considering this a threat to authority.*

5. Decision making.   *The manner in which decisions are made and the degree of participation by team members is almost always an important issue (see Chapters 11 and 14).*

Two questions might be asked about Pepper's thesis. Do you agree with his point that continuity of care is an essential element of any treatment plan? If it is, do you agree that the team is an effective means of achieving the goal? Given the problems which a team approach entails, the reader may well ask, "Is it worth the trouble?" Teams are so complex and create so many problems of their own, wouldn't it be more beneficial to patients if each clinician had his/her own patients and worked autonomously? It might be a useful exercise to debate this issue.

PART III

ISSUES OF DEVIANCE, LABELING, AND SOCIAL CONTROL

CHAPTER 16

Issues of Deviance, Labeling, and Social Control

Alfred Dean

> Sometimes I aint sho who's got ere a right
> to say when a man is crazy and when he
> ain't. Sometimes I think it ain't none of us
> pure crazy and ain't none of us pure sane
> until the balance of us talks him that-a-
> way. It's like it ain't so much what a fel-
> low does, but it's the way the majority of
> folks is looking at him when he does it.
> —William Faulkner, As I Lay Dying

With penetrating and earthy simplicity Faulkner captures the focus of Part III—the processes by which mental illness and deviance are labeled and dealt with. It is no accident that we are concerned at once with the labeling of both *mental illness* and *deviance*. In the eyes of psychiatrists and layman alike, the two are often interrelated, overlapping, or even indistinguishable.

Within the historical spectrum of convergent interests and mutual influence between psychiatry and the social sciences, the focus upon the phenomena of deviance, labeling, and social control is a distinctly central and contemporary topic. The vigor of attention brought to these subjects—attested in the selected articles—parallels that which had previously been brought to the sociological examination of psychiatric institutions. It is as if a glimpse in these directions opened new windows, offering fresh observations and perspectives rich in implication. Indeed, these sociological topics bear upon some of the most consequential issues in modern psychiatry. In this introduction we will delineate these concepts and issues in an effort to provide for a clearer appreciation of the papers which follow.

Elements of Labeling

One significant dimension of the process of labeling is that it is part of a process of creating *conceptions* of reality. Like all words, labels are shorthand expressions for concepts, which in turn are symbolic tools for comprehending or constructing "reality." *Depressed, lovesick, weird, gay, homosexual, sick, evil, bum*—all of these are variant constructs of reality.

The history of man's attempt to grasp his universe of experience and thereby to explain, predict, and control events has inevitably involved the use of concepts. This is as true of prehistoric man as of a space-age scientist. In an age of empiricism, even those whose work depends upon science may forget that facts do not speak for themselves. It is concepts, conceptual frameworks, and theories that serve to *select, organize,* and *explain* our observations. Most of all, it is our perspective of the facts that determine our courses of action.

The process of codifying *reality* (illness, deviance, or otherwise)— whether undertaken by scientists or ordinary men—is a cultural and social process. The "construction of reality" involves the creation of a shared language and symbol system, shared experiences, and social persuasion through authority, power, or other means. To be sure, the rules of reality construction in science are distinct in certain respects.

What psychiatrists call "mental illness" has always posed difficult scientific problems, and the scientific status of these "realities" is rather low. We know that ordinary men in various cultures—including modern America—have not ordinarily recognized even the most severe psychiatric disturbance as such. Many, if not all, cultures have their distinct concepts of the abnormal. Every society has defined illness partly with reference to scientific or empirical knowledge and partly with reference to other belief systems. Where clear, reliable, and effective knowledge falls short, there is a proliferation of professional and public concepts— as is the case with psychiatric disturbances.

The study of the American public's conceptions of mental illness, or those of various subgroups of Americans, probably has a history briefer than that of our youngest reader.[1] We may note that mental illness confronts the public in a range of behaviors unrecognized as pathognomonic—fluctuating, ambiguous, but predominately defined within normative and normal frames of reference. To put the matter differently, the *specialized* conceptions of mental illness held by professionals are not widely disseminated, whatever their role as *special defining agents* for the community. A recent article in *Better Homes and Gardens* bears timely testimony to the public's interested confusion about the nature of mental illness.[2]

In the public view, it may be said, "mental illness is deviance." Deviance is behavior which violates group rules. To be sure, the situation becomes more complex. Not all behavior is socially regulated. In Chapter 19 Becker considers some of the factors which influence social reactions to deviance. In Chapter 21 Dean examines the varieties of deviance associated with mental illness.

Discerning Normality as a Scientific Issue

The problem of discerning normality is a scientific as well as a public problem. Professional judgments regarding the existence of psycho-pathology usually are made with reference to *conceptions* of normal behavior, thoughts, and feelings, rather than on the basis of identifiable biological disorder. This elemental fact raises challenging questions: Where do we obtain our standards of normal behavior? Are our conceptions culture bound? Can we judge the normality of individuals from different cultures—even those similar to our own?

In effect, the utilization of arbitrary and inconsistent norms of abnormality, the absence of universally applicable criteria of abnormality, raise questions about the very concept of psychopathology, not to mention classifications of psychiatric disorders. It would seem that an adequate theory of psychiatric disorders must address these issues, no matter how convinced we are that in the real world of work such things as delusions, mania, and hallucinations are observable events.

Functions and Dysfunctions of the Medical Model

Somewhat related to the above problems are those associated with the "medical model." Psychiatry developed as a medical specialty. Freud brought a medical lexicon to the description, analysis, and treatment of a newly identified class of psychological or psychobiological phenomena. Still, it is doubtful that he regarded them as within the existing purview of "disease." His use of the term "psychopathology" had reference to essentially psychological processes, regardless of how they were mediated by the biological system. Today the term is sometimes used indiscriminately to refer to symbolic disturbances which *may* have an organic basis as well as to functional disturbances.

There can be little doubt that terminological laissez faire and hence analytical confusion is an important contributor to current lively debates about "What is mental illness?" To be sure, the sheer difficulty of conceiving "mind-body" relationships and severe limitations in empirical knowledge about such relationshps have also been a source of terminological and analytical confusion. However, there also appear to be historical and ideological roots to the perpetuation of these shadowy and medically cloaked concepts.

The term "mental illness" seems to have been a humanistically motivated attempt to relabel individuals whose "strange" or deviant behavior might better be regarded as somehow naturalistically disordered. Whatever scientific, practical, or social value this metaphor may have had, it has also generated problems in each of these areas, as Szasz points out in Chapter 17.

The term "myth" refers to a fiction or distortion which is purveyed by a group to serve social purposes. Szasz suggests that the illness concept serves to obscure the recognition by patients and families that problems stem from interpersonal conflicts, ethical dilemmas, and so on. In later publications Szasz, Scheff, and others have suggested, similarly, that psychiatrists have wittingly or unwittingly utilized the medical model for social, economic, or political purposes.

Apart from these possible myth functions, the medical model has dominated and obscured the conceptualization of psychiatric disturbances. The self-conscious clarification and discrimination of biological, psychological, and sociological factors, and their interactions in what is termed "mental illness," remains a central task in theory and practice.

That the preceding scientific issues have down-to-earth as well as theoretical implications is dramatically evidenced in several papers. Jewell reports the case of a Navaho man diagnosed as catatonic schizophrenic who spent over eighteen months in a psychiatric hospital.[3] The events which pressed him into the hospital are a telling illustration of the sociology of labeling. But his delayed discharge reflects an even more disturbing problem in psychiatric theory and the structure of the hospital. Jewell's research casts serious doubt on the existence of psychosis in this patient. In a recent study using pseudopatients, Rosenhan documents and analyzes the inability of highly trained professionals to discriminate the sane from the insane (Chapter 20).

Impact of Mental Illness upon the Family

In his analysis of illness and the role of the physician, Parsons writes:

> The phenomena of physical and mental illness and their counteraction are more intimately connected with the general equilibrium of the social system than is generally supposed. . . . The physician is not merely the person responsible for the care of a special class of "problem cases." He stands at a strategic point in the general balance of forces in the society of which he is a part.[4]

In the strict medical sense, illness is a biological event which hopefully, with treatment, can be reversed. Parsons argues that illness also implies disturbances in the structure and functions of the *social system* in which it occurs, since the sick person is unable to perform his normal social roles. He thus regards illness as a special form of *deviant behavior* resulting in social disequilibrium. In this sense the physician is fundamentally a social therapist as surely as he is a biological engineer.

Cross-cultural studies offer dramatic evidence of the social problems associated with illness. Sick, weak, or deformed infants were often subjected to infanticide. Similarly, the elderly were sometimes abandoned to die or expected to commit suicide. In American society our isolation, institutionalization, and abandonment of the elderly stems significantly from the fact that they have been deprived of useful roles in family, community, and society. Alternatively, their integration into these groupings is problematic due to other sociocultural patterns. Thus role failure is a serious problem for the individual as well as the group.

Mental illness can lead to role failure common to other illnesses, such as inability to work, irritability, and argumentativeness. However, mental illness may also lead to more exotic or strange forms of deviance. The significance and variability of societal reactions to psychotics are dramatized by two polar responses: their burning as witches and their elevation to saints or shamans. Just as the human body will react to an illness (treated or untreated), so will the social system respond to deviance. The social behavior of sick persons, the social consequences and social reactions to illness should thus be matters of central concern to social scientists as areas where existing knowledge might be applied and new knowledge acquired. Indeed, over the past twenty years the development of research and theory so focused, as well as changes in the treatment of severe mental illness, have confirmed the importance of this area of inquiry and application.

With the development of community psychiatry, new questions arose or became more prominent concerns for mental health professionals. The questions were variations on one theme: How well would patients fare in the community? How well would they function in their social roles with the assistance of psychoactive drugs and available professional help? What degree of tolerance, acceptance, and support would patients receive from family, community, and society? Would patients be pressured to return to the hospital or flee back for asylum?

For social scientists these questions became somewhat rephrased: What kind of deviant behavior would these patients exhibit? In what kinds of sociocultural groups would their behavior be more or less acceptable? What factors will affect tolerance for deviance? Will the social expectations of family and community be appropriate and constructive? Under what conditions will disturbed persons and families seek professional help? While pursuing these practical questions, social scientists were gaining new information and generating new theories about deviance, conflict, social control, and change in human groups.

The families of psychiatric patients have been an important unit of observation in these studies, since the family experiences the impact of mental illness most directly and effects most consequential social reactions. Sociological studies of the family's confrontation with mental illness have important implications for clinical as well as community psychiatry. In part, some of these studies continue to document the importance of understanding the familial context of the patient's disturbances—a long-recognized truism, but one which has been insufficiently developed in psychiatric theory and practice. Among the newer insights provided by these studies are the importance of repairing social relationships and restoring social organization as a therapeutic task; the role of social crises as a precipitant of treatment efforts; and conflicting definitions of the situation which may undermine treatment relationships.

Institutions of Social Control

Since psychiatric disturbances are often associated with asocial or antisocial behavior, the mental health professions have become entangled in communal and societal structures which strive to preserve the social order and to deal with offenses against it. Every society develops institutionalized arrangements for dealing with deviance. Complex urban industrial societies have evolved remarkable monuments to the problems of maintaining social order—in a morass of legal, judicial, and correctional institutions as massive and awesome as the columns supporting the Supreme Court. In recent years serious criticisms have been leveled at laws dealing with the mentally ill and at psychiatry's relationship to the law.

However, the law is only one instrument of social control, and psychiatry is implicated in the regulation of deviance quite apart from the law. In a very real sense, psychiatry has played two institutional roles in the structure of society: treatment and social control. Recently the compatibility and propriety of these two roles have been questioned on multiple grounds—legal, ethical, humanitarian, and therapeutic. Our purpose in this chapter is not to consider the details of these controversies, since they are partly provided in Chapter 29. Rather, hopefully, the concepts and observations presented here may offer a sharper understanding of these professional and social issues.

The ability to affix the labels of "sick" or "deviant" to behavior is a demonstration of social power, since it effectively defines the nature, sources, and consequences of nonnormative behavior. Thus viewed, labeling is part of the "political" or "power" processes which occur in all human groups. Similarly, psychiatrists in their roles as labelers of illness and deviance are so empowered by family, community, and society and, in turn, unmistakably enter the political structures and processes within these groups. More broadly, the ability to influence social behavior or the social system of values, beliefs, norms, and role relationships is to exercise social power.

Power is built into every social system in the form of authority. For example, a father has the right to discipline his child, but the child has the right to be cared for. Yet power may be gathered and exercised by means which are not legitimated and structured, that is, not *institutionalized* in the system. For example, a child may exercise power over his parents by refusing to eat, feigning illness, or withdrawing affection.

Within the arena of labeling, deviance, and social control, both institutionalized and noninstitutionalized power are brought into play. The nature of social power should be understood by therapists to comprehend not only their patients, but their own roles vis-à-vis family, community, and society.

When used to support the status quo, labeling is one mechanism of *social control*—a device for restoring or maintaining the social order. Labeling may also be used to effect social change, and is only one means of social persuasion. It is necessary to examine other ways in which behavior is effectively sanctioned, influenced, and controlled. As Kitsuse states:

> A sociological theory of deviance must focus specifically upon the interactions which not only define behaviors as deviant but also organize and activate the application of sanctions by individuals, groups, or agencies. For in modern society, the socially significant differentiation of deviants from the non-deviant population is increasingly contingent upon circumstances of situation, place, social and personal biography, and the bureaucratically organized activities of agencies of control.[5]

In 1964 Scheff described the role of court-appointed psychiatrists in involuntary commitment proceedings.[6] He found that in the face of uncertainty there was a strong presumption of illness by the court and court psychiatrists. In recent years involuntary commitment, the legal rights of mental patients, and the right to treatment have become major issues at the juncture of psychiatry and the law. Current action in these areas is partially in response to belatedly recognized problems. However, many of these changes reflect broader societal movements, as in civil rights and social welfare. In Chapter 29 Pepper provides a detailed examination of these matters in the context of "The Treatment System as Social Policy."

Even when not directly linked to the legal system, psychiatric concepts and practices may serve social control functions. If, for example, an individual's expression of deviant behavior or ideas may be facilely regarded as an expression of madness, attributable to unknown biochemical processes or personality problems, arguments and action may be advanced for treating or controlling him or her. Similarly, if psychiatric disturbances are implicitly or expressly regarded as having their sources *within the individual* rather than in the environment, treatment or action will be so directed. In both of these examples psychiatric concepts lend themselves to the labeling and regulation of deviance and to maintenance of the status quo. Some of the papers which follow (Chapters 17, 18, 21, 29) argue that these examples are not hypothetical, and that in other less obvious ways as well, psychiatry has served as a conservative defense for the public order.

Now what had been declared at the outset of this chapter may be more fully sensed—that the papers which follow are provocative indeed. Mental health professionals recognize that, for individuals, consequential issues are emotional issues. Growth requires self-examination and evaluation, and so it may be said of professions.

Secondary Deviance

Having pointed to the scientific and social foundations of labeling, and to its consequences, it remains to consider its psychological impact. How does social identification influence psychological identity? From the early roots of social psychology in the works of Cooley and Mead to the present time, there has been conviction that an individual's self-concepts are molded by social response. Does labeling an individual as mentally ill contribute to the manifestations of mental illness? There is some evidence, however unsophisticated, that this might well be so.

Certainly there is related evidence that labeling may have a prophetic effect in the production of stuttering, delinquency and criminality, mental retardation, drug addiction, and conformity to racial stereotypes.[7] These otherwise disparate observations seem linked by the powerful social psychological principle of labeling.

In essence, the concept of secondary deviance suggests that labeling and other social responses to deviance may serve to perpetuate or reinforce it. Perhaps the best-known example is criminal behavior. Prisons are settings in which offenders are informally, though systematically, socialized into criminal subcultures. Similarly, upon re-entry into society the criminal record may continue to be "carried" and thus lead to difficulty in getting jobs and to social distrust. This social and psychological situation has been known to foster a vicious circle.

Certainly the concept of secondary deviance is inadequate. The labeling of deviance often inhibits further deviance just as surely as it sometimes reinforces it. Further research is required to determine more precisely the conditions under which it leads in one direction or the other. Nonetheless, the implications of this concept must be considered with reference to labeling individuals as mentally ill. There is evidence that, once affixed, the label may become "stuck." An individual's past, present, and future behavior may become subjected to interpretation in this framework. Clinicians should be invited to explore these phenomena in the articles which follow and in their own work.

NOTES

1. In 1955 Clausen and various associates published a set of pioneering papers exploring how families identify and cope with severe mental illness. The authors indicate that there had been virtually no prior research on this subject. See John Clausen and Marian Radke Yarrow, issue eds., "The Impact of Mental Illness on the Family," *Journal of Social Issues* 11, no. 4 (Spring 1955): 6–11.

2. Gerald M. Knox (with Lillian Rothman), "Mental Illness: Facts You Should Have Clear In Your Own Mind," *Better Homes and Gardens,* August 1973, pp. 20–26.

3. Donald P. Jewell, "A Case of a 'Psychotic' Navaho Indian Male," *Human Organization* 11, no. 1 (1952): 32–36.

4. Talcott Parsons, "Illness and the Role of the Physician: A Sociological Perspective," in *Personality In Nature, Society, and Culture,* ed. Clyde Kluckhohn and Henry A. Murray (New York: Knopf, 1954), p. 609.

5. John J. Kitsuse, "Societal Reactions to Deviant Behavior: Problems of Theory and Method," *Social Problems* 9 (Winter 1962): 247–257.

6. Thomas J. Scheff, "Screening Mental Patients," in *Deviance: The Interactionist Perspective,* ed. Earl Rubington and Martin S. Weinberg (London: Collier-Macmillan, 1968), pp. 172–185.

7. For an examination of the concept of secondary deviance and relevant studies, see Edwin M. Lement, *Human Deviance, Social Problems, and Social Control* (Englewood Cliffs, N.J.: Prentice-Hall, 1967).

CHAPTER 17

Challenging the Medical Model

INTRODUCTION

Thomas Szasz issued his historic challenge to the medical model of psychiatry in 1960. His works have been a major force since then in debates on the legitimacy of the "mental illness" concept. Although there had been several earlier critics of the uses of psychiatry by society, none had so effectively attacked the validity and meaningfulness of the very term "mental illness."

The paper which follows represents the first published use of Szasz' now-famous title, "The Myth of Mental Illness." [1] *His challenging analysis of the concept of mental illness, coupled with a stinging critique of the ways in which the concept has become operational, is heard frequently in contemporary discussions.*

Recent debate about the validity and value of the mental illness concept has stimulated the development of alternative conceptual models. These variously challenge, augment, or try to supplant the medical model. The majority of psychiatrists today probably basically still support the medical-mental illness model, while some also concede the validity and usefulness of the social, educational, and behavior modification models in addition. Many psychiatrists are attempting to combine elements of these approaches in a pragmatic manner in order best to benefit their patients. Nonmedical mental health workers such as social workers and psychologists may differ and prefer to eschew the medical model in favor of a social or behavioral approach which places their own professional skills in a central position. While there are exceptions, the general composition of the opposing camps supports the observation that "where you stand depends on where you sit."

Szasz must be credited with having been a major force in expand-

ing professional views and attitudes toward the composition of mental disorders, allowing more room for the social, environmental, and other nonmedical factors to be given due weight and consideration. In order to gain an audience in the first place it was probably essential for him to oversimplify the issues and overstate his position. Many who generally support his thesis believe that there is room for a medical component in a full range of treatment efforts.

It may be helpful to view the following paper in its historical context. Szasz and several other thinkers and researchers on the subject of mental disorder were at work independently in the period 1959–1962. The mental hospital of the day was under attack by Goffman [2] *as being a "total institution"; by Barton* [3] *for producing "institutional neurosis"; by Gruenberg* [4] *for producing cases of "social breakdown syndrome"; by the Joint Commission on Mental Illness and Health,* [5] *which was calling for a major reorganization of services; and by Birnbaum,* [6] *who was calling for the patient's "right to treatment." It took the efforts of these and many other critics to begin to melt the glacier of the large mental hospital, at first producing only little rivulets.*

Szasz' later writings include strident criticisms of the motivation as well as the conduct of those who practice within the medical-mental illness model. This has led to many ad hominem counterattacks which have diverted the field from a sufficiently thoughtful and substantive analysis of this important issue. "The Myth of Mental Illness" was selected for this book in the hope that its relatively non-pejorative presentation will encourage the reader to consider the issue on its merits.

NOTES

1. "The Myth of Mental Illness" was originally published in the *American Psychologist* in 1960. Szasz used the same title again a year later for a book on the same subject.

2. Erving Goffman, *Asylums* (Garden City, N.Y.: Doubleday, Anchor Books, 1961).

3. Russell Barton, "Consideration, Clinical Features and Differential Diagnosis of Institutional Neurosis," Third World Congress of Psychiatry, Montreal, *Proceedings* 2 (June 1961): 890–895.

4. Ernest M. Gruenberg, Richard Kasius, and Matthew Huxley, "Objective Appraisal of Deterioration in a Group of Long-Stay Hospital Patients," *Milbank Memorial Fund Quarterly* 40 (1962): 90–100.

5. Joint Commission on Mental Illness and Health, *Action for Mental Health* (New York: Basic Books, 1961).

6. Morton Birnbaum, "The Right to Treatment," *American Bar Association Journal* 46 (1960).

THE MYTH OF MENTAL ILLNESS

Thomas S. Szasz

My aim in this essay is to raise the question "Is there such a thing as mental illness?" and to argue that there is not. Since the notion of mental illness is extremely widely used nowadays, inquiry into the ways in which this term in employed would seem to be especially indicated. Mental illness, of course, is not literally a "thing"—or physical object— and hence it can "exist" only in the same sort of way in which other theoretical concepts exist. Yet, familiar theories are in the habit of posing, sooner or later—at least to those who come to believe in them—as "objective truths" (or "facts"). During certain historical periods, explanatory conceptions such as deities, witches, and microorganisms appeared not only as theories but as self-evident *causes* of a vast number of events. I submit that today mental illness is widely regarded in a somewhat similar fashion, that is, as the cause of innumerable diverse happenings. As an antidote to the complacent use of the notion of mental illness—whether as a self-evident phenomenon, theory, or cause—let us ask this question: "What is meant when it is asserted that someone is mentally ill?"

In what follows I shall describe briefly the main uses to which the concept of mental illness has been put. I shall argue that this notion has outlived whatever usefulness it might have had and that it now functions merely as a convenient myth.

Mental Illness as a Sign of Brain Disease

The notion of mental illness derives its main support from such phenomena as syphilis of the brain or delirious conditions—intoxications, for instance—in which persons are known to manifest various peculiarities or disorders of thinking and behavior. Correctly speaking, however, these are diseases of the brain, not of the mind. According to one school of thought, *all* so-called mental illness is of this type. The assumption is made that some neurological defect, perhaps a very subtle one, will ultimately be found for all the disorders of thinking and behavior. Many contemporary psychiatrists, physicians, and other scientists hold this view. This position implies that people *cannot* have troubles—expressed

Thomas S. Szasz, "The Myth of Mental Illness," *American Psychologist*, XV, 1960, pp. 113–118. Copyright © 1960 by the American Psychological Association. Reproduced by permission.

in what are *now called* "mental illnesses"—because of differences in personal needs, opinions, social aspirations, values, and so on. *All problems in living* are attributed to physicochemical processes which in due time will be discovered by medical research.

"Mental illnesses" are thus regarded as basically no different than all other diseases (that is, of the body). The only difference, in this view, between mental and bodily diseases is that the former, affecting the brain, manifest themselves by means of mental symptoms, whereas the latter, affecting other organ systems (for example, the skin, liver, etc.), manifest themselves by means of symptoms referable to those parts of the body. This view rests on and expresses what are, in my opinion, two fundamental errors.

In the first place, what central nervous system symptoms would correspond to a skin eruption or a fracture? It would *not* be some emotion or complex bit of behavior. Rather, it would be blindness or a paralysis of some part of the body. The crux of the matter is that a disease of the brain, analogous to a disease of the skin or bone, is a neurological defect, and not a problem in living. For example, a *defect* in a person's visual field may be satisfactorily explained by correlating it with certain definite lesions in the nervous system. On the other hand, a person's *belief*—whether this be a belief in Christianity, in Communism, or in the idea that his internal organs are "rotting" and that his body is, in fact, already "dead"—cannot be explained by a defect or disease of the nervous system. Explanations of this sort of occurrence—assuming that one is interested in the belief itself and does not regard it simply as a "symptom" or expression of something else that is *more interesting*—must be sought along different lines.

The second error in regarding complex psychosocial behavior, consisting of communications about ourselves and the world about us, as mere symptoms of neurological functioning is *epistemological*. In other words, it is an error pertaining not to any mistakes in observation or reasoning, as such, but rather to the way in which we organize and express our knowledge. In the present case, the error lies in making a symmetrical dualism between mental and physical (or bodily) symptoms, a dualism which is merely a habit of speech and to which no known observations can be found to correspond. Let us see if this is so. In medical practice, when we speak of physical disturbances, we mean either signs (for example, a fever) or symptoms (for example, pain). We speak of mental symptoms, on the other hand, when we refer to a patient's *communications about himself, others, and the world about him*. He might state that he is Napoleon or that he is being persecuted by the Communists. These would be considered mental symptoms *only* if the observer believed that the patient was *not* Napoleon or that he was *not* being persecuted by the Communists. This makes it apparent that the statement that "X is a mental symptom" involves rendering a judgment. The judgment entails, moreover, a covert comparison or matching of the patient's ideas, concepts, or beliefs with those of the observer and the society in which they live. The notion of mental symptom is therefore inextricably tied to the *social* (including *ethical*) *context* in which it is made in much the same way as the notion of bodily symptom is tied to an *anatomical* and *genetic context*.[1]

To sum up what has been said thus far: I have tried to show that for those who regard mental symptoms as signs of brain disease, the concept of mental illness is unnecessary and misleading. For what they mean is that people so labeled suffer from diseases of the brain, and, if that is what they mean, it would seem better for the sake of clarity to say that and not something else.

Mental Illness as a Name for Problems in Living

The term "mental illness" is widely used to describe something which is very different than a disease of the brain. Many people today take it for granted that living is an arduous process. Its hardship for modern man, moreover, derives not so much from a struggle for biological survival as from the stresses and strains inherent in the social intercourse of complex human personalities. In this context, the notion of mental illness is used to identity or describe some feature of an individual's so-called personality. Mental illness—as a deformity of the personality, so to speak—is then regarded as the *cause* of the human disharmony. It is implicit in this view that social intercourse between people is regarded as something *inherently harmonious,* its disturbance being due solely to the presence of "mental illness" in many people. This is obviously fallacious reasoning, for it makes the abstraction "mental illness" into a *cause*, even though this abstraction was created in the first place to serve only as a shorthand expression for certain types of human behavior. It now becomes necessary to ask: "What kinds of behavior are regarded as indicative of mental illness, and by whom?"

The concept of illness, whether bodily or mental, implies *deviation from some clearly defined norm.* In the case of physical illness, the norm is the structural and functional integrity of the human body. Thus, although the desirability of physical health, as such, is an ethical value, what health *is* can be stated in anatomical and physiological terms. What is the norm deviation from which is regarded as mental illness? This question cannot be easily answered. But whatever this norm might be, we can be certain of only one thing: namely, that it is a norm that must be stated in terms of *psychosocial, ethical,* and *legal* concepts. For example, notions such as "excessive repression" or "acting out an unconscious impulse" illustrate the use of psychological concepts for judging (so-called) mental health and illness. The idea that chronic hostility, vengefulness, or divorce are indicative of mental illness would be illustrations of the use of ethical norms (that is, the desirability of love, kindness, and a stable marriage relationship). Finally, the widespread psychiatric opinion that only a mentally ill person would commit homicide illustrates the use of a legal concept as a norm of mental health. The norm from which deviation is measured whenever one speaks of a mental illness is a *psychosocial and ethical one*. Yet, the remedy is sought in terms of *medical* measures which—it is hoped and assumed—are free from wide differences of ethical value. The definition of the disorder and the terms in which its remedy are sought are therefore at serious odds with one another. The practical significance of this covert conflict between the alleged nature of the defect and the remedy can hardly be exaggerated.

Having identified the norms used to measure deviations in cases of mental illness, we will now turn to the question: "Who defines the norms and hence the deviation?" Two basic answers may be offered: (1) It may be the person himself (that is, the patient) who decides that he deviates from a norm. For example, an artist may believe that he suffers from a work inhibition, and he may implement this conclusion by seeking help *for* himself from a psychotherapist. (2) It may be someone other than the patient who decides that the latter is deviant (for example, relatives, physicians, legal authorities, society generally, etc.). In such a case a psychiatrist may be hired by others to do something *to* the patient in order to correct the deviation.

These considerations underscore the importance of asking the question "Whose agent is the psychiatrist?" and of giving a candid answer to it.[2] The psychiatrist (psychologist or nonmedical psychotherapist), it now develops, may be the agent of the patient, of the relatives, of the school, of the military services, of a business organization, of a court of law, and so forth. In speaking of the psychiatrist as the agent of these persons or organizations, it is not implied that his values concerning norms, or his ideas and aims concerning the proper nature of remedial action, need to coincide exactly with those of his employer. For example, a patient in individual psychotherapy may believe that his salvation lies in a new marriage; his psychotherapist need not share this hypothesis. As the patient's agent, however, he must abstain from bringing social or legal force to bear on the patient which would prevent him from putting his beliefs into action. If his *contract* is with the patient, the psychiatrist (psychotherapist) may disagree with him or stop his treatment, but he cannot engage others to obstruct the patient's aspirations. Similarly, if a psychiatrist is engaged by a court to determine the sanity of a criminal, he need not fully share the legal authorities' values and intentions in regard to the criminal and the means available for dealing with him. But the psychiatrist is expressly barred from stating, for example, that it is not the criminal who is "insane" but the men who wrote the law on the basis of which the very actions that are being judged are regarded as "criminal." Such an opinion could be voiced, of course, but not in a courtroom, and not by a psychiatrist who makes it his practice to assist the court in performing its daily work.

To recapitulate: In actual contemporary social usage, the finding of a mental illness is made by establishing a deviance in behavior from certain psychosocial, ethical, or legal norms. The judgment may be made, as in medicine, by the patient, the physician (psychiatrist), or others. Remedial action, finally, tends to be sought in a therapeutic—or covertly medical—framework, thus creating a situation in which *psychosocial, ethical,* and/or *legal deviations* are claimed to be correctable by (so-called) *medical action.* Since medical action is designed to correct only medical deviations, it seems logically absurd to expect that it will help solve problems whose very existence had been defined and established on nonmedical grounds. I think that these considerations may be fruitfully applied to the present use of tranquilizers and, more generally, to what might be expected of drugs of whatever type in regard to the amelioration or solution of problems in human living.

The Role of Ethics in Psychiatry

Anything that people *do*—in contrast to things that *happen* to them [3]—takes place in a context of value. In this broad sense, no human activity is devoid of ethical implications. When the values underlying certain activities are widely shared, those who participate in their pursuit may lose sight of them altogether. The discipline of medicine, both as a pure science (for example, research) and as a technology (for example, therapy), contains many ethical considerations and judgments. Unfortunately, these are often denied, minimized, or merely kept out of focus, for the ideal of the medical profession as well as of the people whom it serves seems to be having a system of medicine (allegedly) free of ethical value. This sentimental notion is expressed by such things as the doctor's willingness to treat and help patients irrespective of their religious or political beliefs, whether they are rich or poor, etc. While there may be some grounds for this belief—albeit it is a view that is not impressively true even in these regards—the fact remains that ethical considerations encompass a vast range of human affairs. Making the practice of medicine neutral in regard to some specific issues of value need not, and cannot, mean that it can be kept free from all such values. The practice of medicine is intimately tied to ethics, and the first thing that we must do, it seems to me, is to try to make this clear and explicit. I shall let this matter rest here, for it does not concern us specifically in this essay. Lest there be any vagueness, however, about how or where ethics and medicine meet, let me remind the reader of such issues as birth control, abortion, suicide, and euthanasia as only a few of the major areas of current ethicomedical controversy.

Psychiatry, I submit, is very much more intimately tied to problems of ethics than is medicine. I use the word "psychiatry" here to refer to that contemporary discipline which is concerned with *problems in living* (and not with disease of the brain, which are problems for neurology). Problems in human relations can be analyzed, interpreted, and given meaning only within given social and ethical contexts. Accordingly, it *does* make a difference—arguments to the contrary notwithstanding—what the psychiatrist's socioethical orientations happen to be, for these will influence his ideas on what is wrong with the patient, what deserves comment or interpretation, in what possible directions change might be desirable, and so forth. Even in medicine proper, these factors play a role, as, for instance, in the divergent orientations which physicians, depending on their religious affiliations, have toward such things as birth control and therapeutic abortion. Can anyone really believe that a psychotherapist's ideas concerning religious belief, slavery, or other similar issues play no role in his practical work? If they do make a difference, what are we to infer from it? Does it not seem reasonable that we ought to have different psychiatric therapies—each expressly recognized for the ethical positions which they embody—for, say, Catholics and Jews, religious persons and agnostics, democrats and communists, white supremacists and Negroes, and so on? Indeed, if we look at how psychiatry is actually practiced today (especially in the United States), we find that people do seek psychiatric help in accordance with their social status and ethical beliefs.[4] This should really not surprise us more than being told that practicing Catholics rarely frequent birth control clinics.

The foregoing position which holds that contemporary psychotherapists deal with problems in living, rather than with mental illnesses and their cures, stands in opposition to a currently prevalent claim, according to which mental illness is just as "real" and "objective" as bodily illness. This is a confusing claim since it is never known exactly what is meant by such words as "real" and "objective." I suspect, however, that what is intended by the proponents of this view is to create the idea in the popular mind that mental illness is some sort of disease entity, like an infection or a malignancy. If this were true, one could *catch* or *get* a "mental illness," one might *have* or *harbor* it, one might *transmit* it to others, and finally one could get *rid* of it. In my opinion, there is not a shred of evidence to support this idea. To the contrary, all the evidence is the other way and supports the view that what people now call mental illnesses are for the most part *communications* expressing unacceptable ideas, often framed, moreover, in an unusual idiom. The scope of this essay allows me to do no more than mention this alternative theoretical approach to this problem.[5]

This is not the place to consider in detail the similarities and differences between bodily and mental illnesses. It shall suffice for us here to emphasize only one important difference between them: namely, that whereas bodily disease refers to public, physicochemical occurrences, the notion of mental illness is used to codify relatively more private, sociopsychological happenings of which the observer (diagnostician) forms a part. In other words, the psychiatrist does not stand *apart* from what he observes, but is, in Harry Stack Sullivan's apt words, a "participant observer." This means that he is *committed* to some picture of what he considers reality—and to what he thinks society considers reality—and he observes and judges the patient's behavior in the light of these considerations. This touches on our earlier observation that the notion of mental symptom itself implies a comparison between observer and observed, psychiatrist and patient. This is so obvious that I may be charged with belaboring trivialities. Let me therefore say once more that my aim in presenting this argument was expressly to criticize and counter a prevailing contemporary tendency to deny the moral aspects of psychiatry (and psychotherapy) and to substitute for them allegedly value-free medical considerations. Psychotherapy, for example, is being widely practiced as though it entailed nothing other than restoring the patient from a state of mental sickness to one of mental health. While it is generally accepted that mental illness has something to do with man's social (or interpersonal) relations, it is paradoxically maintained that problems of values (that is, of ethics) do not arise in this process.[6] Yet, in one sense, much of psychotherapy may revolve around nothing other than the elucidation and weighing of goals and values—many of which may be mutually contradictory—and the means whereby they might best be harmonized, realized, or relinquished.

The diversity of human values and the methods by means of which they may be realized is so vast, and many of them remain so unacknowledged, that they cannot fail but lead to conflicts in human relations. Indeed, to say that human relations at all levels—from mother to child, through husband and wife, to nation and nation—are fraught with stress, strain, and disharmony is, once again, making the obvious explicit. Yet, what may be obvious may be also poorly understood. This I think is the case here. For it seems to me that—at least in our scientific theories of behavior—we have failed to *accept* the simple fact that human relations are inherently fraught with difficulties and that to make them even relatively harmonious requires much patience and hard work. I submit that the idea of mental illness is now being put to work to obscure certain difficulties which at present may be inherent—not that they need be unmodifiable—in the social intercourse of persons. If this is true, the concept functions as a disguise, for instead of calling attention to conflicting human needs, aspirations, and values, the notion of mental illness provides an amoral and impersonal "thing" (an "illness") as an explanation for *problems in living*.[7] We may recall in this connection that not so long ago it was devils and ,witches who were held responsible for men's problems in social living. The belief in mental illness, as something other than man's trouble in getting along with his fellow man, is the proper heir to the belief in demonology and witchcraft. Mental illness exists or is "real" in exactly the same sense in which witches existed or were "real."

Choice, Responsibility, and Psychiatry

While I have argued that mental illnesses do not exist, I obviously did not imply that the social and psychological occurrences to which this label is currently being attached also do not exist. Like the personal and social troubles which people had in the Middle Ages, they are real enough. It is the labels we give them that concern us and, having labeled them, what we do about them. While I cannot go into the ramified implications of this problem here, it is worth noting that a demonologic conception of problems in living gave rise to therapy along theological lines. Today, a belief in mental illness implies—nay, requires—therapy along medical or psychotherapeutic lines.

What is implied in the line of thought set for here is something quite different. I do not intend to offer a new conception of "psychiatric illness" nor a new form of "therapy." My aim is more modest and yet also more ambitious. It is to suggest that the phenomena now called mental illnesses be looked at afresh and more simply, that they be removed from the category of illnesses, and that they be regarded as the expressions of man's struggle with the problem of *how* he should live. The last-mentioned problem is obviously a vast one, its enormity reflecting not only man's inability to cope with his environment, but even more his increasing self-reflectiveness.

By problems in living, then, I refer to that truly explosive chain reaction which began with man's fall from divine grace by partaking of the fruit of the tree of knowledge. Man's awareness of himself and of the world about him seems to be a steadily expanding one, bringing in its wake an ever larger *burden of understanding* (an expression borrowed from Susanne Langer).[8] *This burden, then, is to be expected and must not be misinterpreted.* Our only *rational* means for lightening it is *more understanding*, and appropriate *action* based on such understanding. This main alternative lies in acting as though the burden were not what in fact we perceive it to be and taking refuge in an outmoded theological view of man. In the latter view, man does not fashion his life and much of his world about him, but merely lives out his fate in a world created by superior beings. This may logically lead to pleading nonresponsibility in the face of seemingly unfathomable problems and difficulties. Yet, if man fails to take increasing responsibility for his actions, individually as well as collectively, it seems unlikely that some higher power or being would assume this task and carry this burden for him. Moreover, this seems hardly the proper time in human history for obscuring the issue of man's responsibility for his actions by hiding it behind the skirt of an all-explaining conception of mental illness.

Conclusions

I have tried to show that the notion of mental illness has outlived whatever usefulness it might have had and that it now functions merely as a convenient myth. As such, it is a true heir to religious myths in general and to the belief in witchcraft in particular; the role of all these belief-systems was to act as *social tranquilizers*, thus encouraging the hope that mastery of certain specific problems may be achieved by means of substitutive (symbolic-magical) operations. The notion of mental illness thus serves mainly to obscure the everyday fact that life for most people is a continuous struggle, not for biological survival, but for a "place in the sun," "peace of mind," or some other human value. For man aware of himself and of the world about him, once the needs for preserving the body (and perhaps the race) are more or less satisfied, the problem arises as to what he should do with himself. Sustained adherence to the myth of mental illness allows people to avoid facing this problem, believing that mental health, conceived as the absence of mental illness, automatically insures the making of right and safe choices in one's conduct of life. But the facts are all the other way. It is the making of good choices in life that others regard, retrospectively, as good mental health!

The myth of mental illness encourages us, moveover, to believe in its logical corollary: that social intercourse would be harmonious, satisfying, and the secure basis of a "good life" were it not for the disrupting influences of mental illness or "psychopathology." The potentiality for universal human happiness, in this form at least, seems to me but another example of the I-wish-it-were-true type of fantasy. I do believe that human happiness or well-being on a hitherto unimaginably large scale, and not just for a select few, is possible. This goal could be achieved, however, only at the cost of many men, and not just a few being willing and able to tackle their personal, social, and ethical conflicts. This means having the courage and integrity to forego waging battles on false fronts, finding solutions for substitute problems—for instance, fighting the battle of stomach acid and chronic fatigue instead of facing up to a marital conflict.

Our adversaries are not demons, witches, fate, or mental illness. We have no enemy whom we can fight, exorcise, or dispel by "cure." What we do have are *problems in living*—whether these be biologic, economic, political, or sociopsychological. In this essay I was concerned only with problems belonging in the last-mentioned category, and within this group mainly with those pertaining to moral values. The field to which modern psychiatry addresses itself is vast, and I made no effort to encompass it all. My argument was limited to the proposition that mental illness is a myth, whose function it is to disguise and thus render more palatable the bitter pill of moral conflicts in human relations.

NOTES

1. T. S. Szasz, *Pain and Pleasure: A Study of Bodily Feelings* (New York: Basic Books, 1957), and idem, "The Problem of Psychiatric Nosology: A Contribution to a Situational Analysis of Psychiatric Operations," *American Journal of Psychiatry* 114 (1957): 405–413.
2. T. S. Szasz, "Malingering: 'Diagnosis' or Social Condemnation?" *AMA Archives of Neurological Psychiatry* 76 (1956): 432–443, and idem, "Psychiatry, Ethics, and the Criminal Law," *Columbia Law Review* 58 (1958): 183–198.
3. R. S. Peters, *The Concept of Motivation* (London: Routledge & Kegan Paul, 1958).
4. A. B. Hollingshead and F. C. Redlich, *Social Class and Mental Illness* (New York: Wiley, 1958).

5. T. S. Szasz, "On the Theory of Psychoanalytic Treatment," *International Journal of Psychoanalysis* 38 (1957): 166–182.

6. Freud went so far as to say: "I consider ethics to be taken for granted. Actually I have never done a mean thing" (E. Jones, *The Life and Work of Sigmund Freud*, vol. 3 [New York: Basic Books, 1957], p. 247). This surely is a strange thing to say for someone who has studied man as a social being as closely as did Freud. I mention it here to show how the notion of "illness" (in the case of psychoanalysis, "psychopathology," or "mental illness") was used by Freud—and by most of his followers—as a means for classifying certain forms of human behavior as falling within the scope of medicine, and hence (by fiat) outside that of ethics!

7. T. S. Szasz, "Moral Conflict and Psychiatry," *Yale Review* 49 (1959): 555–566.

8. S. K. Langer, *Philosophy in a New Key* (New York: Mentor, 1953).

COMMENTARY

The first paragraph of Szasz' paper contains the key to understanding and utilizing his ideas: Mental illness is a theoretical concept. A concept has no actual or physical existence. Key questions about its usefulness are: Does it help us to organize data so that they become coherent? Does it have predictive value? Is it contradicted by available data which cannot be fitted into the conceptual scheme? *These questions must be answered before we can respond fully to the question Szasz labels as "key":* Is the concept of mental illness frequently pressed into service to maintain certain social-ethical values of the community, by exerting social control (labeled psychiatric treatment) over individuals who behave differently or unpredictably? *All of the chapters in the present part address this issue, as does Chapter 29.*

Critics of Szasz note that he deals with mental illness as a single, unitary concept and set of phenomena, synonymous with problems in living. *They ask whether his arguments and description apply to the full panoply of symptoms, signs, and behaviors which are collectively defined and treated as mental illness. For example, since the typical thought pattern of many persons who are labeled schizophrenic responds to phenothiazine drugs, can this be seen as parallel to a dermatologist treating a variety of inflammatory skin outbreaks with cortisone?*

In practice, mental illness is also a label which is widely applied to persons exhibiting and experiencing a wide range of emotions, physiological and psychological processes, and behaviors. Some label themselves to gain attention, sympathy, or protection from their own self-destructive impulses. Others are labeled by members of their community who seek to control or exclude them. Still others gain the "mentally ill" label because they exhibit acute and drastic alterations in lifelong personality and behavior patterns; sometimes they are additionally labeled acute schizophrenic psychosis, postpartum depression, involutional depressive psychosis, or acute manic psychosis. Is mental illness a myth for some of them? For all?

CHAPTER 18

Schizophrenia: Disease or Label?

INTRODUCTION

In the following paper sociologist Thomas Scheff offers a critique of the use of the label "schizophrenia" as a psychiatric-medical diagnosis. He begins by suggesting a disarmingly simple experiment which cannot fail to captivate while it simultaneously makes the reader conscious of the "public order"—something which is usually invisible, but always pervasive in person-to-person situations. Once we become conscious of it, we quickly become aware that, like the air we breathe, social pressure is invisible, essential, and constantly acting upon each of us. It shapes our perceptions of others and of ourselves, and cues our social conduct.

In the preceding chapter we considered Thomas Szasz' sharp attack on the concept of mental illness and use of the medical model. Like Szasz, Scheff finds that "mental illness" is neither valid nor specific. A chief proponent of labeling theory, Scheff suggests that this affords, at the least, a fresh perspective on the medical model.

Labeling theory suggests that certain behaviors are labeled by society as deviant because they defy societal rules of conduct. In contrast, when society does not call an action deviant it implies that such behavior is normal and unexceptional. A key extension of this concept is the notion that transitory behaviors may be made permanent by the labeling process. For example, a child who is labeled "bad" by his teacher in the classroom may thereafter be stereotyped in that role by tacit agreement among the teacher, the other students, and the subject individual; he may thus be encouraged to continue to behave badly in order to fulfill his role.

SCHIZOPHRENIA AS IDEOLOGY

Thomas J. Scheff

In lieu of beginning this paper with a (necessarily) abstract discussion of a concept, *the public order,* I shall invite the reader to consider a *gedanken* experiment that will illustrate its meaning. Suppose in your next conversation with a stranger, instead of looking at his eyes or mouth, you scrutinize his ear. Although the deviation from ordinary behavior is slight (involving only a shifting of the direction of gaze a few degrees, from the eyes to an ear), its effects are explosive. The conversation is disrupted almost instantaneously. In some cases, the subject of this experiment will seek to save the situation by rotating to bring his eyes into your line of gaze; if you continue to gaze at his ear, he may rotate through a full 360 degrees. Most often, however, the conversation is irretrievably damaged. Shock, anger, and vertigo are experienced not only by the "victim" but, oddly enough, by the experimenter himself. It is virtually impossible for either party to sustain the conversation, or even to think coherently, as long as the experiment continues.

The point of this experiment is to suggest the presence of a public order that is all-pervasive, yet taken almost completely for granted. During the simplest kinds of public encounter, there are myriad understandings about comportment that govern the participants' behavior—understandings governing posture, facial expression, and gestures, as well as the content and form of the language used. In speech itself, the types of conformity are extremely diverse and include pronunciation; grammar and syntax; loudness, pitch, and phrasing; and aspiration. Almost all of these elements are so taken for granted that they "go without saying" and are more or less invisible, not only to the speakers but to society at large. These understandings constitute part of our society's assumptive world, the world that is thought of as normal, decent, and possible.

The probability that these understandings are, for the most part, arbitrary to a particular historical culture (is shaking hands or rubbing noses a better form of greeting?) is immaterial to the individual member of society whose attitude of everyday life is, *whatever is, is right.* There is a social, cultural, and interpersonal status quo whose existence is felt only when abrogated. Since violations occur infrequently, and since the culture provides no very adequate vocabulary for talking about either the presence or abuse of its invisible understandings, such deviations are considered disruptive and disturbing. The society member's loyalty to his culture's unstated conventions is unthinking but extremely intense.

Thomas J. Scheff, "Schizophrenia as Ideology," *Schizophrenia Bulletin,* issue 2, Fall 1970, pp. 15–19. Used by permission.

The sociologist Mannheim referred to such intense and unconscious loyalty to the status quo as *ideological*. Ideology, in this sense, refers not only to the defense of explicit political or economic interests but, much more broadly, to a whole world view or perspective on what reality is. As a contrast to the ideological view, Mannheim cited the *utopian* outlook, which tends "to shatter, either partially or wholly, the order of things prevailing at the time." [1] The attitude of everyday life, which is ideological, is transfixed by the past and the present; the possibility of a radically different scheme of things, or revolutionary changes in custom and outlook, is thereby rejected. The utopian perspective, by contrast, is fixed on the future; it rejects the status quo with abrupt finality. *Social change* arises out of the clash of the ideological and utopian perspectives.

Residual Rule Violations

It is the thesis of this paper that the concepts of mental illness in general—and schizophrenia in particular—are not neutral, value-free, scientifically precise terms but, for the most part, the leading edge of an ideology embedded in the historical and cultural present of the white middle class of Western societies. The concept of illness and its associated vocabulary—symptoms, therapies, patients, and physicians—reify and legitimate the prevailing public order at the expense of other possible worlds. The medical model of disease refers to culture-free processes that are independent of the public order; a case of pneumonia or syphilis is pretty much the same in New York or New Caledonia. [2]

Most of the "symptoms" of mental illness, however, are of an entirely different nature. Far from being culture free, such "symptoms" are themselves offenses against implicit understandings of particular cultures. Every society provides its members with a set of explicit norms—understandings governing conduct with regard to such central institutions as the state, the family, and private property. Offenses against these norms have conventional names; for example, an offense against property is called "theft," and an offense against sexual propriety is called "perversion." As we have seen above, however, the public order also is made up of countless unnamed understandings. "Everyone knows," for example, that during a conversation one looks at the other's eyes or mouth, but not at his ear. For the convenience of the society, offenses against these unnamed residual understandings are usually lumped together in a miscellaneous, catchall category. If people reacting to an offense exhaust the conventional categories that might define it (e.g., theft, prostitution, and drunkenness), yet are certain that an offense has been committed, they may resort to this residual category. In earlier societies, the residual category was witchcraft, spirit possession, or possession by the devil; today, it is mental illness. The symptoms of mental illness are, therefore, violations of residual rules.

To be sure, some residual-rule violations are expressions of under-lying physiological processes: the hallucinations of the toxic psychoses and the delusions associated with general paresis, for example. Perhaps future research will identify further physiological processes that lead to violations of residual rules. For the present, however, the key attri-butes of the medical model have yet to be established and verified for the major mental illnesses. There has been no scientific verification of the cause, course, site of pathology, uniform and invariant signs and symp-toms, and treatment of choice for almost all of the conventional, "func-tional" diagnostic categories. Psychiatric knowledge in these matters rests almost entirely on unsystematic clinical impressions and profes-sional lore. It is quite possible, therefore, that many psychiatrists' and other mental health workers' "absolute certainty" about the cause, site, course, symptoms, and treatment of mental illness represents an ideo-logical reflex, a spirited defense of the present social order.

Residue of Residues

Viewed as offenses against the public order, the symptoms of schizo-phrenia are particularly interesting. Of all the major diagnostic cate-gories, the concept of schizophrenia (although widely used by psychia-trists in the United States and in those countries influenced by American psychiatric nomenclature) is the vaguest and least clearly defined. Such categories as obsession, depression, and mania at least have a vernacu-lar meaning. Schizophrenia, however, is a broad gloss; it involves, in no very clear relationship, ideas such as "inappropriateness of affect," "impoverishment of thought," "inability to be involved in meaningful human relationships," "bizarre behavior" (e.g., delusions and hallucina-tions), "disorder of speech and communication," and "withdrawal."

These very broadly defined symptoms can be redefined as offenses against implicit social understandings. The appropriateness of emo-tional expression is, after all, a cultural judgment. Grief is deemed appropriate in our society at a funeral, but not at a party. In other cul-tures, however, such judgments of propriety may be reversed. With re-gard to thought disorder, cultural anthropologists have long been at pains to point out that ways of thought are fundamentally different in different societies. What constitutes a meaningful human relationship, anthropologists also report, is basically different in other times and places. Likewise, behavior that is bizarre in one culture is deemed tolerable or even necessary in another. Disorders of speech and commu-nication, again, can be seen as offenses against culturally prescribed rules of language and expression. Finally, the notion of "withdrawal" as-sumes a cultural standard concerning the degree of involvement and the amount of distance between the individual and those around him.

The broadness and vagueness of the concept of schizophrenia sug-gest that it may serve as the residue of residues. As diagnostic categories such as hysteria and depression have become conventionalized names for residual rule breaking, a need seems to have developed for a still more generalized, miscellaneous diagnostic category. If this is true, the schizophrenic explores not only "inner space" (Ronald Laing's phrase) but also the normative boundaries of his society.

These remarks should not be taken to suggest that there is no internal experience associated with "symptomatic" behavior; the individual with symptoms *does* experience distress and suffering, or under some conditions, exhilaration and freedom. The point is, however, that public, consensual "knowledge" of mental illness is based, by and large, on knowledge not of these internal states but of their overt manifestations. When a person goes running down the street naked and screaming, lay and professional diagnosticians alike assume the existence of mental illness within that person—even though they have not investigated his internal state. Mental health procedure and the conceptual apparatus of the medical model posit internal states, but the events actually observed are external.

Labeling Theory

A point of view which is an alternative to the medical model, and which acknowledges the culture-bound nature of mental illness, is afforded by labeling theory in sociology.[3] Like the evidence supporting the medical model, which is uneven and in large measure unreliable, the body of knowledge in support of the labeling theory of mental illness is by no means weighty or complete enough to prove its correctness.[4] But even though labeling theory is hypothetical, its use may afford perspective— if only because it offers a viewpoint that, along a number of different dimensions, is diametrically opposed to the medical model.

The labeling theory of deviance, when applied to mental illness, may be presented as a series of nine hypotheses:

1. Residual rule breaking arises from fundamentally diverse sources (i.e., organic, psychological, situations of stress, volitional acts of innovation or defiance).
2. Relative to the rate of treated mental illness the rate of unrecorded residual rule breaking is extremely high.
3. Most residual rule breaking is "denied" and is of transitory significance.
4. Stereotyped imagery of mental disorder is learned in early childhood.
5. The stereotypes of insanity are continually reaffirmed, inadvertently, in ordinary social interaction.
6. Labeled deviants may be rewarded for playing the stereotyped deviant role.
7. Labeled deviants are punished when they attempt the return to conventional roles.
8. In the crisis occurring when a residual rule breaker is publicly labeled, the deviant is highly suggestible and may accept the label.
9. Among residual rule breakers, labeling is the single most important cause of careers of residual deviance.

The evidence relevant to these hypotheses is reviewed in the author's *Being Mentally Ill.*[5]

According to labeling theory, the societal reaction is the key process that determines outcome in most cases of residual rule breaking. That reaction may be either denial (the most frequent reaction) or labeling. Denial is to "normalize" the rule breaking by ignoring or rationalizing it ("boys will be boys"). The key hypothesis in labeling theory is that, when residual rule breaking is denied, the rule breaking will generally be transitory (as when the stress causing rule breaking is removed; e.g., the cessation of sleep deprivation). compensated for, or channeled into some socially acceptable form. If, however, labeling occurs (i.e., the rule breaker is segregated as a stigmatized deviant), the rule breaking which would otherwise have been terminated, compensated for, or channeled may be stabilized; thus, the offender, through the agency of labeling, is launched on a career of "chronic mental illness." Crucial to the production of chronicity, therefore, are the contingencies (often external to the deviants) that give rise to labeling rather than denial; e.g., the visibility of the rule breaking, the power of the rule breaker relative to persons reacting to his behavior, the tolerance level of the community, and the availability in the culture of alternative channels of response other than labeling (among Indian tribes, for example, involuntary trance states may be seen as a qualification for a desirable position in the society, such as that of shaman).

"Schizophrenia"—A Label

On the basis of the foregoing discussion, it would seem likely that labeling theory would prove particularly strategic for facilitating the investigation of schizophrenia. Schizophrenia is the single most widely used diagnosis for mental illness in the United States, yet the cause, site, course, and treatment of choice are unknown, or the subject of heated and voluminous controversy. Moreover, there is some evidence that the reliability of diagnosis of schizophrenia is quite low. Finally, there is little agreement on whether a disease entity of schizophrenia even exists, what constitutes schizophrenia's basic signs and symptoms if it *does* exist, and how these symptoms are to be reliably and positively identified in the diagnostic process. Because of the all but overwhelming uncertainties and ambiguities inherent in its definition, "schizophrenia" is an appellation, or "label," which may be easily applied to those residual rule breakers whose deviant behavior is difficult to classify.

In this connection, it is interesting to note the perfectly enormous anomaly of classification procedures in most schizophrenia research. The hypothetical cause of schizophrenia, the independent variable in the research design—whether it is a physiological, biochemical, or psychological attribute—is measured with considerable attention to reliability, validity, and precision. I have seen reports of biochemical research in which the independent variable is measured to two decimal places. Yet the measurement of the dependent variable, the diagnosis of schizophrenia, is virtually ignored. The precision of the measurement, obviously, is virtually nil, since it represents at best an ordinal scale, or, much more likely, a nominal scale. In most studies, the reliability and validity of the diagnosis receives no attention at all: An experimental group is assembled by virtue of hospital diagnoses—leaving the measurement of the dependent variable to the mercy of the obscure vagaries of the process of psychiatric screening and diagnosis. Labeling theory should serve at least to make this anomaly visible to researchers in the field of schizophrenia.

More broadly, the clash between labeling theory and the medical and psychological models of mental illness may serve to alert researchers to some of the fundamental assumptions that they may be making in setting up their research. Particular reference should be made to the question of whether they are unknowingly aligning themselves with the social status quo; for example, by accepting unexamined the diagnosis of schizophrenia, they may be inadvertently providing the legitimacy of science to what is basically a social value judgment. For the remainder of this paper, I wish to pursue this point—the part that medical science may be playing in legitimating the status quo.

As was earlier indicated, there is a public order which is continually reaffirmed in social interaction. Each time a member of the society conforms to the stated or unstated cultural expectations of that society, as when he gazes at the eyes of the person with whom he is in conversation, he is helping to maintain the social status quo. Any deviation from these expectations, however small and regardless of its motivation, may be a threat to the status quo, since most social change occurs through the gradual erosion of custom.

Since all social orders are, as far as we know, basically arbitrary, a threat to society's fundamental customs impels its conforming members to look to extrasocial sources of legitimacy for the status quo. In societies completely under the sway of a single, monolithic religion, the source of legitimacy is always supernatural. Thus, during the Middle Ages, the legitimacy of the social order was maintained by reference to God's commands, as found in the Bible and interpreted by the Catholic Church. The Pope was God's deputy, the kings ruled by divine right, the particular cultural form that the family happened to take at the time—the patrilocal, monogamous, nuclear family—was sanctified by the church, and so on.

In modern societies, however, it is increasingly difficult to base legitimacy upon appeals to supernatural sources. As complete, unquestioning religious faith has weakened, one very important new source of legitimacy has emerged: In the eyes of laymen, modern science offers the kind of absolute certainty once provided by the church. The institution of medicine is in a particularly strategic position in this regard, since the physician is the only representative of science with whom the average man associates. To the extent that medical science lends its name to the labeling of nonconformity as mental illness, it is giving legitimacy to the social status quo. The mental health researcher may protest that he is interested not in the preservation of the status quo but in a scientific question: "What are the causes of mental illness?" According to the argument given here, however, his question is loaded—like, "When did you stop beating your wife?" or, more to the point, "What are the causes of witchcraft?" [6] Thus, a question about causality may also be ideological, in Mannheim's sense, in that it reaffirms current social beliefs, if only inadvertently.

NOTES

1. K. Mannheim, *Ideology and Utopia* (London: Routledge & Kegan Paul, 1936).

2. For criticism of the medical model from psychiatric, psychological, and sociological perspectives, see E. Goffman, *Asylums* (Garden City, N.Y.: Doubleday, Anchor Books, 1961); R. Laing, *The Politics of Experience* (New York: Pantheon, 1967); E. M. Lemert, *Social Pathology* (New York: McGraw-Hill, 1951); T. J. Scheff, *Being Mentally Ill: A Sociological Theory* (Chicago: Aldine, 1966); T. S. Szasz, *The Myth of Mental Illness* (New York: Hoeber-Harper, 1961); and L. P. Ullman and L. Krasner, *A Psychological Approach to Abnormal Behavior* (Englewood Cliffs, N.J.: Prentice-Hall, 1969).

3. For a general statement of this theory, see H. Becker, *Outsiders* (New York: Free Press, 1963).

4. Useful supporting material can be found in M. Balint, *The Doctor, the Patient, and the Illness* (New York: International Universities Press, 1957); R. Laing and A. Esterson, *Sanity, Madness and the Family* (London: Tavistock, 1964); Lemert, *Social Pathology;* T. J. Scheff, *Mental Illness and Social Processes* (New York: Harper & Row, 1967); and S. P. Spitzer and N. K. Denzin, *The Mental Patient: Studies in the Sociology of Deviance* (New York: McGraw-Hill, 1968).

5. Scheff, *Being Mentally Ill.*

6. For a comparison of the treatment of witches and the mentally ill, see T. S. Szasz, *The Manufacture of Madness* (New York: Harper & Row, 1970).

COMMENTARY

Scheff makes the point that much past research on schizophrenia failed to develop and utilize a replicable and explicitly defined set of classification criteria. It may be argued that more recent research reports seem to be heeding this admonition to some degree: It is no longer standard to have the experimental group defined simply by all members having received a diagnosis of schizophrenia at some time in the past, usually on admission to a mental hospital.

The paper offers an interesting theoretical basis for therapeutic efforts in noting that when rule breaking is denied or ignored it will generally be transitory: "If, however, labeling occurs . . . the rule breaking . . . may be stabilized; thus, the offender, through the agency of labeling, is launched on a career of 'chronic mental illness.'" This thesis fits well with the recommendation offered by behavioral psychology that the therapist (or family) seek to extinguish negative behaviors by not attending to them.

The crux of Scheff's thesis gains added interest when placed in counterpoint to current research results. Over the last several years researchers from various disciplines—from the psychologic to the biochemical to the genetic—have strongly suggested that there are biochemical-heredo-genetic factors of significance in the etiology of schizophrenia. Can all of this be reconciled? It may be hypothesized that schizophrenia is an organic disorder, but that its specific expressions might well be culturally determined to a significant degree. Like such medical illnesses as liver cancer and hypertension, it might differ in its patterns of incidence and expression in various cultures.

Scheff's observation that schizophrenia is a vague, unreliable concept and one which is defined with reference to culturally variable social behavior raises social and ethical issues as well as scientific and diagnostic ones. It implies that people who are simply different from the norm or from cultural conceptions of the norm may be easily labeled as schizophrenic. Does this happen? Is there a sufficient risk of this happening to imply a need for social and legal safeguards? What kinds of safeguards might be devised?

Cannot Scheff's paper be regarded as a threat to the status quo? If so, what kinds of responses might it elicit? Do societies differ in the extent to which they encourage or tolerate deviance?

Scheff presents labeling theory as a set of intriguing hypotheses. What evidence can be mounted to affirm or negate them—or more likely, to suggest the conditions under which they hold? Can they be tested?

CHAPTER 19

Deviance:

An Interactionist Perspective

INTRODUCTION

All social groups, whatever their size or complexity, from nations to families, develop measures which influence the behaviors of members in order to confine the limits of these behaviors. Extremes of behavior are discouraged; conformity is rewarded. The desired behaviors are shaped to conform to the shared beliefs, values, and norms. Social groups use a variety of means to achieve this conformity, such as coercion (imprisonment), economic rewards or punishments, and social ostracism or praise.

Deviance is the term used to describe behavior which goes beyond the social group's accepted range. Every social group experiences deviance and develops measures to control it. There is a rich literature concerned with how deviance develops, why particular persons become deviant, and how deviance is managed.

This paper by Becker deals with another interesting and important facet of deviance, particularly for mental health clinicians, namely what is involved in the labeling process. Why are some behaviors called deviant and others not? Some rule-breaking behaviors are more susceptible to the label of deviance than others. Degrees of reward and punishment vary. Certain conditions must exist if rule-breaking behavior is to be called deviant. The author also describes some of the consequences to the individual of having been labeled deviant. One of the issues upon which this paper will shed light is the grey zone of human behavior between accepted idiosyncrasy and bizarre dyssocial behavior. One may be considered a sign of distinction and an asset; the other is often considered an indiscretion or breakdown and leads to further social isolation. Yet descriptively the distinction may

*be imperceptible. The label of deviance, as the paper will point out, is
not absolute, but is situational and interactive. It depends partly on
the behavior, but it also depends upon who does it and what the consequences are to the* labeler.

ON LABELING OUTSIDERS

Howard S. Becker

One day an outbreak of wailing and a great commotion told me that a
death had occurred somewhere in the neighborhood. I was informed that
Kima'i, a young lad of my acquaintance, of sixteen or so, had fallen from
a coco-nut palm and killed himself. . . . I found that another youth had
been severely wounded by some mysterious coincidence. And at the funeral there was obviously a general feeling of hostility between the village
where the boy died and that into which his body was carried for burial.

Only much later was I able to discover the real meaning of these
events. The boy had committed suicide. The truth was that he had broken
the rules of exogamy, the partner in his crime being his maternal cousin,
the daughter of his mother's sister. This had been known and generally
disapproved of but nothing was done until the girl's discarded lover, who
had wanted to marry her and who felt personally injured, took the initiative. This rival threatened first to use black magic against the guilty
youth, but this had not much effect. Then one evening he insulted the
culprit in public—accusing him in the hearing of the whole community
of incest and hurling at him certain expressions intolerable to a native.

For this there was only one remedy; only one means of escape remained to the unfortunate youth. Next morning he put on festive attire
and ornamentation, climbed a coco-nut palm and addressed the community, speaking from among the palm leaves and bidding them fare-
well. He explained the reasons for his desperate deed and also launched
forth a veiled accusation against the man who had driven him to his
death, upon which it became the duty of his clansmen to avenge him.
Then he wailed aloud, as is the custom, jumped from a palm some sixty
feet high and was killed on the spot. There followed a fight within the
village in which the rival was wounded; and the quarrel was repeated
during the funeral. . . .

If you were to inquire into the matter among the Trobrianders, you
would find . . . that the natives show horror at the idea of violating the
rules of exogamy and that they believe that sores, disease, and even
death might follow clan incest. This is the ideal of native law, and in
moral matters it is easy and pleasant strictly to adhere to the ideal—
when judging the conduct of others or expressing an opinion about conduct in general.

When it comes to the application of morality and ideals to real life, however, things take on a different complexion. In the case described it was obvious that the facts would not tally with the ideal of conduct. Public opinion was neither outraged by the knowledge of the crime to any extent, nor did it react directly—it had to be mobilized by a public statement of the crime and by insults being hurled at the culprit by an interested party. Even then he had to carry out the punishment himself. . . . Probing further into the matter and collecting concrete information, I found that the breach of exogamy—as regards intercourse and not marriage—is by no means a rare occurrence, and public opinion is lenient, though decidedly hypocritical. If the affair is carried on *sub rosa* with a certain amount of decorum, and if no one in particular stirs up trouble— "public opinion" will gossip, but not demand any harsh punishment. If, on the contrary, scandal breaks out—everyone turns against the guilty pair and by ostracism and insults one or the other may be driven to suicide.[1]

You can commit clan incest and suffer from no more than gossip as long as no one makes a public accusation; but you will be driven to your death if the accusation is made. The point is that the response of other people has to be regarded as problematic. Just because one has committed an infraction of a rule does not mean that others will respond as though this has happened. (Conversely, just because one has not violated a rule does not mean that he may not be treated, in some circumstances, as though he had.)

The degree to which other people will respond to a given act as deviant varies greatly. Several kinds of variation seem worth noting. First of all, there is variation over time. A person believed to have committed a given "deviant" act may at one time be responded to much more leniently than he would be at some other time. The occurrence of "drives" against various kinds of deviance illustrates this clearly. At various times, enforcement officials may decide to make an all-out attack on some particular kind of deviance, such as gambling, drug addiction, or homosexuality. It is obviously much more dangerous to engage in one of these activities when a drive is on than at any other time. (In a very interesting study of crime news in Colorado newspapers, Davis found that the amount of crime reported in Colorado newspapers showed very little association with actual changes in the amount of crime taking place in Colorado. And, further, that people's estimate of how much increase there had been in crime in Colorado was associated with the increase in the amount of crime news but not with any increase in the amount of crime.) [2]

The degree to which an act will be treated as deviant depends also on who commits the act and who feels he has been harmed by it. Rules tend to be applied more to some persons than others. Studies of juvenile delinquency make the point clearly. Boys from middle-class areas do not get as far in the legal process when they are apprehended as do boys from slum areas. The middle-class boy is less likely, when picked up by the police, to be taken to the station; less likely when taken to the station to be booked; and it is extremely unlikely that he will be convicted and sentenced.[3] This variation occurs even though the original infraction of the rule is the same in the two cases. Similarly, the law is differentially applied to Negroes and whites. It is well known that a Negro believed to have attacked a white woman is much more likely to be punished than a white man who commits the same offense; it is only slightly less well known that a Negro who murders another Negro is much less likely to be punished than a white man who commits murder.[4] This, of course, is one of the main points of Sutherland's analysis of white-collar crime: crimes committed by corporations are almost always prosecuted as civil cases, but the same crime committed by an individual is ordinarily treated as a criminal offense.[5]

Some rules are enforced only when they result in certain consequences. The unmarried mother furnishes a clear example. Vincent [6] points out that illicit sexual relations seldom result in severe punishment or social censure for the offenders. If, however, a girl becomes pregnant as a result of such activities the reaction of others is likely to be severe. (The illicit pregnancy is also an interesting example of the differential enforcement of rules on different categories of people. Vincent notes that unmarried fathers escape the severe censure visited on the mother.)

Why repeat these commonplace observations? Because, taken together, they support the proposition that deviance is not a simple quality, present in some kinds of behavior and absent in others. Rather, it is the product of a process which involves responses of other people to the behavior. The same behavior may be an infraction of the rules at one time and not at another; may be an infraction when committed by one person, but not when committed by another; some rules are broken with impunity, others are not. In short, whether a given act is deviant or not depends in part on the nature of the act (that is, whether or not it violates some rule) and in part on what other people do about it.

Some people may object that this is merely a terminological quibble, that one can, after all, define terms any way he wants to and that if some people want to speak of rule-breaking behavior as deviant without reference to the reactions of others they are free to do so. This, of course, is true. Yet it might be worthwhile to refer to such behavior as *rule-breaking behavior* and reserve the term *deviant* for those labeled as deviant by some segment of society. I do not insist that this usage be followed. But it should be clear that insofar as a scientist uses "deviant" to refer to any rule-breaking behavior and takes as his subject of study only those who have been *labeled* deviant, he will be hampered by the disparities between the two categories.

If we take as the object of our attention behavior which comes to be labeled as deviant, we must recognize that we cannot know whether a given act will be categorized as deviant until the response of others has occurred. Deviance is not a quality that lies in behavior itself, but in the interaction between the person who commits an act and those who respond to it. . . .

In any case, being . . . branded as deviant has important consequences for one's further social participation. . . . The most important consequence is a drastic change in the individual's public identity. Committing the improper act and being publicly caught at it place him in a new status. He has been revealed as a different kind of person from the kind he was supposed to be. He is labeled a "fairy," "dope fiend," "nut" or "lunatic," and treated accordingly.

In analyzing the consequences of assuming a deviant identity let us make use of Hughes' distinction between master and auxiliary status traits.[7] Hughes notes that most statuses have one key trait which serves to distinguish those who belong from those who do not. Thus the doctor, whatever else he may be, is a person who has a certificate stating that he has fulfilled certain requirements and is licensed to practice medicine; this is the master trait. As Hughes points out, in our society a doctor is also informally expected to have a number of auxiliary traits: most people expect him to be upper middle class, white, male, and Protestant. When he is not there is a sense that he has in some way failed to fill the bill. Similarly, though skin color is the master status trait determining who is Negro and who is white, Negroes are informally expected to have certain status traits and not to have others; people are surprised and find it anomalous if a Negro turns out to be a doctor or a college professor. People often have the master status trait but lack some of the auxiliary, informally expected characteristics; for example, one may be a doctor but be female or Negro.

Hughes deals with this phenomenon in regard to statuses that are well thought of, desired, and desirable (noting that one may have the formal qualifications for entry into a status but be denied full entry because of lack of the proper auxiliary traits), but the same process occurs in the case of deviant statuses. Possession of one deviant trait may have a generalized symbolic value, so that people automatically assume that its bearer possesses other undesirable traits allegedly associated with it.

To be labeled a criminal one need only commit a single criminal offense, and this is all the term formally refers to. Yet the word carries a number of connotations specifying auxiliary traits characteristic of anyone bearing the label. A man who has been convicted of housebreaking and thereby labeled criminal is presumed to be a person likely to break into other houses; the police, in rounding up known offenders for investigation after a crime has been committed, operate on this premise. Further, he is considered likely to commit other kinds of crimes as well, because he has shown himself to be a person without "respect for the law." Thus, apprehension for one deviant act exposes a person to the likelihood that he will be regarded as deviant or undesirable in other respects.

There is one other element in Hughes' analysis we can borrow with profit: the distinction between master and subordinate statuses.[8] Some statuses, in our society as in others, override all other statuses and have a certain priority. Race is one of these. Membership in the Negro race, as socially defined, will override most other status considerations in most other situations; the fact that one is a physician or middle class or female will not protect one from being treated as a Negro first and any of these other things second. The status of deviant (depending on the kind of deviance) is this kind of master status. One receives the status as a result of breaking a rule, and the identification proves to be more important than most others. One will be identified as a deviant first, before other identifications are made.

NOTES

1. Bronislaw Malinowski, *Crime and Custom in Savage Society* (New York: Humanities Press, 1926), pp. 77–80. Reprinted by permission of Humanities Press and Routledge & Kegan Paul, Ltd.
2. F. James Davis, "Crime News in Colorado Newspapers," *American Journal of Sociology* 57 (January 1952): 325–330.
3. See Albert K. Cohen and James F. Short, Jr., "Juvenile Delinquency," in *Contemporary Social Problems*, ed. Robert K. Merton and Robert A. Nisbet (New York: Harcourt, Brace, 1961), p. 87.
4. See Harold Garfinkel, "Research Note on Inter- and Intra-Racial Homicides," *Social Forces* 27 (May 1949): 369–381.
5. Edwin H. Sutherland, "White Collar Criminality," *American Sociological Review* 5 (February 1940): 1–12.
6. Clark Vincent, *Unmarried Mothers* (New York: Free Press, 1961), pp. 3–5.
7. Everett C. Hughes, "Dilemmas and Contradictions of Status," *American Journal of Sociology* 50 (March 1945): 353–359.
8. Ibid.

COMMENTARY

Becker indicates that deviance is more complex than merely the performance of some kind of unacceptable behavior. Every society, every social group constructs rules for behavior, some written, some unwritten. Deviance is the transgression of these rules. But the rules are not always sharply defined, nor are they evenly interpreted. Some transgressions are forgiven or overlooked, some treated harshly. It is not only the act itself, but also the context in which it occurs and the reaction of others to it that determine the extent to which it is labeled as deviant. Deviance is not an absolute quality, nor a quality which resides in the person or in the behavior. It is relative and interactional.

There are consequences to being labeled deviant, for once an individual carries that identification it tends to override other roles he may have in the eyes of others. Thus the title "mental patient," once attached to an individual, may well influence judgments made about all of his or her behavior.

There are some important implications of these observations to the mental health disciplines. For example, consider the labels "eccentric" and "mentally ill." Does the application of these labels depend upon such factors as the degree of deviance, the status of the person, and the context in which the person acts?

To some extent mental health workers tend to interpret behavior as "sick" which in other circumstances might be observed without special note. It is worthwhile to examine interactions in which "clinical" expectations influence judgment of a patient's adaptive behavior which might otherwise have been considered within expected bounds (see Chapter 20). The paper questions the extent to which the diagnostic process leads clinicians to focus on maladaptive behavior and to overlook competent constructive behavior. This same phenomenon of interpreting behavior as deviant takes place in families as well.

Clinicians may ask themselves about the extent to which they interpret patients' behavior as symptomatic when under other circumstances they would not. Is this good clinical acumen? Or is it situational bias? In what ways are diagnostic signs which depend on behavioral descriptions able to be freed from situational and interactive influences? In what ways are the meaning, value, reliability, and validity of psychiatric diagnoses affected?

CHAPTER 20

Impeaching the Diagnostic Process

INTRODUCTION

In Chapter 12 you read about the experience of a sociologist who, unbeknown to the staff, had himself admitted as a patient to a psychiatric ward. He described the social interactions on the ward from the perspective of a patient who voluntarily participated in treatment.

Rosenhan, in this selection, examines hospitalization from still another perspective, raising some disturbing questions about psychiatric diagnosis and the labeling process. It is an article which makes us pause to think about ways in which mental health professionals arrive at diagnoses and how diagnoses are used by professionals.

The paper reports a study in which a number of normal individuals had themselves admitted to a mental hospital by falsely reporting they were experiencing hallucinations. Rosenhan describes some of the experiences of these pseudopatients. He is critical of the diagnostic process, attacking its validity.

The paper is a dramatic presentation. It has been used in an attack not only on psychiatric diagnoses, but also on hospitalization— and even more broadly upon psychiatry itself.

This controversial paper has been widely criticized in the psychiatric literature. Yet it is important because it raises important questions. Whether or not you agree with its conclusions, it is worth reading. Be prepared to be stimulated to thoughtful reflection.

The paper deals with two related issues. The major part, and the more provocative one, is concerned with the diagnostic process. The second issue is that of the stigma attached to a person called "mentally ill."

ON BEING SANE IN INSANE PLACES

David L. Rosenhan

If sanity and insanity exist, how shall we know them?

The question is neither capricious nor itself insane. However much we may be personally convinced that we can tell the normal from the abnormal, the evidence is simply not compelling. It is commonplace, for example, to read about murder trials wherein eminent psychiatrists for the defense are contradicted by equally eminent psychiatrists for the prosecution on the matter of the defendant's sanity. More generally, there are a great deal of conflicting data on the reliability, utility, and meaning of such terms as "sanity," "insanity," "mental illness," and "schizophrenia." [1] Finally, as early as 1934, Benedict suggested that normality and abnormality are not universal.[2] What is viewed as normal in one culture may be seen as quite aberrant in another. Thus, notions of normality and abnormality may not be quite as accurate as people believe they are.

To raise questions regarding normality and abnormality is in no way to question the fact that some behaviors are deviant or odd. Murder is deviant. So, too, are hallucinations. Nor does raising such questions deny the existence of the personal anguish that is often associated with "mental illness." Anxiety and depression exist. Psychological suffering exists. But normality and abnormality, sanity and insanity, and the diagnoses that flow from them may be less substantive than many believe them to be.

At its heart, the question of whether the sane can be distinguished from the insane (and whether degrees of insanity can be distinguished from each other) is a simple matter: Do the salient characteristics that lead to diagnoses reside in the patients themselves or in the environments and contexts in which observers find them? From Bleuler, through Kretchmer, through the formulators of the recently revised *Diagnostic and Statistical Manual* of the American Psychiatric Association, the belief has been strong that patients present symptoms, that those symptoms can be categorized, and, implicitly, that the sane are distinguishable from the insane. More recently, however, this belief has been questioned. Based in part on theoretical and anthropological, legal, and therapeutic ones, the view has grown that psychological categorization of mental illness is useless at best and downright harmful, misleading, and pejorative at worst. Psychiatric diagnoses, in this view, are in the minds of the observers and are not valid summaries of characteristics displayed by the observed.[3]

David L. Rosenhan, "On Being Sane in Insane Places, *Science*, CLXXIX, January 19, 1973, pp. 150–158. Copyright © the American Association for the Advancement of Science. Used by permission.

Gains can be made in deciding which of these is more nearly accurate by getting normal people (that is, people who do not have, and have never suffered, symptoms of serious psychiatric disorders) admitted to psychiatric hospitals and then determining whether they were discovered to be sane and, if so, how. If the sanity of such pseudopatients were always detected, there would be prima facie evidence that a sane individual can be distinguished from the insane context in which he is found. Normality (and presumably abnormality) is distinct enough that it can be recognized wherever it occurs, for it is carried within the person. If, on the other hand, the sanity of the pseudopatients were never discovered, serious difficulties would arise for those who support traditional modes of psychiatric diagnoses. Given that the hospital staff was not incompetent, that the pseudopatient had been behaving as sanely as he had been outside of the hospital, and that it had never been previously suggested that he belonged in a psychiatric hospital, such an unlikely outcome would support the view that psychiatric diagnosis betrays little about the patient but much about the environment in which an observer finds him.

This article describes such an experiment. Eight sane people gained secret admission to twelve different hospitals.[4] Their diagnostic experiences constitute the data of the first part of this article; the remainder is devoted to a description of their experiences in psychiatric institutions. Too few psychiatrists and psychologists, even those who have worked in such hospitals, know what the experience is like. They rarely talk about it with former patients, perhaps because they distrust information coming from the previously insane. Those who have worked in psychiatric hospitals are likely to have adapted so thoroughly to the settings that they are insensitive to the impact of that experience. And while there have been occasional reports of researchers who submitted themselves to psychiatric hospitalization,[5] these researchers have commonly remained in the hospitals for short periods of time, often with the knowledge of the hospital staff. It is difficult to know the extent to which they were treated like patients or like research colleagues. Nevertheless, their reports about the inside of the psychiatric hospital have been valuable. This article extends those efforts.

Pseudopatients and Their Settings

The eight pseudopatients were a varied group. One was a psychology graduate student in his twenties. The remaining seven were older and "established." Among them were three psychologists, a pediatrician, a psychiatrist, a painter, and a housewife. Three pseudopatients were women, five were men. All of them employed pseudonyms, lest their alleged diagnoses embarrass them later. Those who were in mental health professions alleged another occupation in order to avoid the special attentions that might be accorded by staff, as a matter of courtesy or caution, to ailing colleagues.[6] With the exception of myself (I was the first pseudopatient and my presence was known to the hospital administrator and chief psychologist and, so far as I can tell, to them alone), the presence of pseudopatients and the nature of the research program was not known to the hospital staffs.[7]

The settings were similarly varied. In order to generalize the findings, admission into a variety of hospitals was sought. The twelve hospitals in the sample were located in five different states on the East and West coasts. Some were old and shabby, some were quite new. Some were research-oriented, others not. Some had good staff-patient ratios, others were quite understaffed. Only one was a strictly private hospital. All of the others were supported by state or federal funds or, in one instance, by university funds.

After calling the hospital for an appointment, the pseudopatient arrived at the admissions office complaining that he had been hearing voices. Asked what the voices said, he replied that they were often unclear, but as far as he could tell they said "empty," "hollow," and "thud." The voices were unfamiliar and were of the same sex as the pseudopatient. The choice of these symptoms was occasioned by their apparent similarity to existential symptoms. Such symptoms are alleged to arise from painful concerns about the perceived meaninglessness of one's life. It is as if the hallucinating person were saying, "My life is empty and hollow." The choice of these symptoms was also determined by the *absence* of a single report of existential psychoses in the literature.

Beyond alleging the symptoms and falsifying name, vocation, and employment, no further alterations of person, history, or circumstances were made. The significant events of the pseudopatient's life history were presented as they had actually occurred. Relationships with parents and siblings, with spouse and children, with people at work and in school, consistent with the aforementioned exceptions, were described as they were or had been. Frustrations and upsets were described along with joys and satisfactions. These facts are important to remember. If anything, they strongly biased the subsequent results in favor of detecting sanity, since none of their histories or current behaviors were seriously pathological in any way.

Immediately upon admission to the psychiatric ward, the pseudopatient ceased simulating *any* symptoms of abnormality. In some cases, there was a brief period of mild nervousness and anxiety, since none of the pseudopatients really believed that they would be admitted so easily. Indeed, their shared fear was that they would be immediately exposed as frauds and greatly embarrassed. Moreover, many of them had never visited a psychiatric ward; even those who had, nevertheless had some genuine fears about what might happen to them. Their nervousness, then, was quite appropriate to the novelty of the hospital setting, and it abated rapidly.

Apart from that short-lived nervousness, the pseudopatient behaved on the ward as he "normally" behaved. The pseudopatient spoke to patients and staff as he might ordinarily. Because there is uncommonly little to do on a psychiatric ward, he attempted to engage others in conversation. When asked by staff how he was feeling, he indicated that he was fine, that he no longer experienced symptoms. He responded to instructions from attendants, to calls for medication (which was not swallowed), and to dining-hall instructions. Beyond such activities as were available to him on the admissions ward, he spent his time writing down his observations about the ward, its patients, and the staff. Initially these notes were written "secretly," but as it soon became clear that no one much cared, they were subsequently written on standard tablets of paper in such public places as the dayroom. No secret was made of these activities.

The pseudopatient, very much as a true psychiatric patient, entered a hospital with no foreknowledge of when he would be discharged. Each was told that he would have to get out by his own devices, essentially by convincing the staff that he was sane. The psychological stresses associated with hospitalization were considerable, and all but one of the pseudopatients desired to be discharged almost immediately after being admitted. They were, therefore, motivated not only to behave sanely, but to be paragons of cooperation. That their behavior was in no way disruptive is confirmed by nursing reports, which have been obtained on most of the patients. These reports uniformly indicate that the patients were "friendly," "cooperative," and "exhibited no abnormal indications."

The Normal Are Not Detectably Sane

Despite their public "show" of sanity, the pseudopatients were never detected. Admitted, except in one case, with a diagnosis of schizophrenia,[8] each was discharged with a diagnosis of schizophrenia "in remission." The label "in remission" should in no way be dismissed as a formality, for at no time during any hospitalization had any question been raised about any pseudopatient's simulation. Nor are there any indications in the hospital records that the pseudopatient's status was suspect. Rather, the evidence is strong that, once labeled schizophrenic, the pseudopatient was stuck with that label. If the pseudopatient was to be discharged, he must naturally be "in remission"; but he was not sane, nor, in the institution's view, had he ever been sane.

The uniform failure to recognize sanity cannot be attributed to the quality of the hospitals, for, although there were considerable variations among them, several are considered excellent. Nor can it be alleged that there was simply not enough time to observe the pseudopatients. Length of hospitalization ranged from seven to fifty-two days, with an average of nineteen days. The pseudopatients were not, in fact, carefully observed, but this failure clearly speaks more to traditions within psychiatric hospitals than to lack of opportunity.

Finally, it cannot be said that the failure to recognize the pseudo-patients' sanity was due to the fact that they were not behaving sanely. While there was clearly some tension present in all of them, their daily visitors could detect no serious behavioral consequences— nor, indeed, could other patients. It was quite common for the patients to "detect" the pseudopatients' sanity. During the first three hospitalizations, when accurate counts were kept, 35 of a total of 118 patients on the admissions ward voiced their suspicions, some vigorously. "You're not crazy. You're a journalist, or a professor [referring to the continual note taking]. You're checking up on the hospital." While most of the patients were reassured by the pseudopatient's insistence that he had been sick before he came in but was fine now, some continued to believe that the pseudopatient was sane throughout his hospitalization.[9] The fact that the patients often recognized normality when staff did not raises important questions.

Failure to detect sanity during the course of hospitalization may be due to the fact that physicians operate with a strong bias toward what statisticians call the type 2 error.[10] This is to say that physicians are more inclined to call a healthy person sick (a false positive, type 2) than a sick person healthy (a false negative, type 1). The reasons for this are not hard to find: It is clearly more dangerous to misdiagnose illness than health. Better to err on the side of caution, to suspect illness even among the healthy.

But what holds for medicine does not hold equally well for psychiatry. Medical illnesses, while unfortunate, are not commonly pejorative. Psychiatric diagnoses, on the contrary, carry with them personal, legal, and social stigmas.[11] It was therefore important to see whether the tendency toward diagnosing the sane insane could be reversed. The following experiment was arranged at a research and teaching hospital whose staff had heard these findings but doubted that such an error could occur in their hospital. The staff was informed that at some time during the following three months, one or more pseudopatients would attempt to be admitted into the psychiatric hospital. Each staff member was asked to rate each patient who presented himself at admissions or on the ward according to the likelihood that the patient was a pseudopatient. A 10-point scale was used, with a 1 and 2 reflecting high confidence that the patient was a pseudopatient.

Judgments were obtained on 193 patients who were admitted for psychiatric treatment. All staff who had had sustained contact with or primary responsibility for the patient—attendants, nurses, psychiatrists, physicians, and psychologists—were asked to make judgments. Forty-one patients were alleged, with high confidence, to be pseudopatients by at least one member of the staff. Twenty-three were considered suspect by at least one psychiatrist. Nineteen were suspected by one psychiatrist *and* one other staff member. Actually, no genuine pseudopatient (at least from my group) presented himself during this period.

The experiment is instructive. It indicates that the tendency to designate sane people as insane can be reversed when the stakes (in this case, prestige and diagnostic acumen) are high. But what can be said of the nineteen people who were suspected of being "sane" by one psychiatrist and another staff member? Were these people truly "sane," or was it rather the case that in the course of avoiding the type 2 error the staff tended to make more errors of the first sort—calling the crazy "sane"? There is no way of knowing. But one thing is certain: Any diagnostic process that lends itself so readily to massive errors of this sort cannot be a very reliable one.

The Stickiness of Psychodiagnostic Labels

Beyond the tendency to call the healthy sick—a tendency that accounts better for diagnostic behavior on admission than it does for such behavior after a lengthy period of exposure—the data speak to the massive role of labeling in psychiatric assessment. Having once been labeled schizophrenic, there is nothing the pseudopatient can do to overcome the tag. The tag profoundly colors others' perceptions of him and his behavior.

From one viewpoint, these data are hardly surprising, for it has long been known that elements are given meaning by the context in which they occur. Gestalt psychology made this point vigorously, and Asch [12] demonstrated that there are "central" personality traits (such as "warm" versus "cold") which are so powerful that they markedly color the meaning of other information in forming an impression of a given personality.[13] "Insane," "schizophrenic," "manic-depressive," and "crazy" are probably among the most powerful of such central traits. Once a person is designated abnormal, all of his other behaviors and characteristics are colored by that label. Indeed, that label is so powerful that many of the pseudopatients' normal behaviors were overlooked entirely or profoundly misinterpreted. Some examples may clarify this issue.

Earlier I indicated that there were no changes in the pseudopatient's personal history and current status beyond those of name, employment, and, where necessary, vocation. Otherwise, a veridical description of personal history and circumstances was offered. Those circumstances were not psychotic. How were they made consonant with the diagnosis of psychosis? Or were those diagnoses modified in such a way as to bring them into accord with the circumstances of the pseudopatient's life, as described by him?

As far as I can determine, diagnoses were in no way affected by the relative health of the circumstances of a pseudopatient's life. Rather, the reverse occurred: The perception of his circumstances was shaped entirely by the diagnosis. A clear example of such translation is found in the case of a pseudopatient who had had a close relationship with his mother but was rather remote from his father during his early childhood. During adolescence and beyond, however, his father became a close friend, while his relationship with his mother cooled. His present relationship with his wife was characteristically close and warm. Apart from occasional angry exchanges, friction was minimal. The children had rarely been spanked. Surely there is nothing especially pathological about such a history. Indeed, many readers may see a similar pattern in their own experiences, with no markedly deleterious consequences. Observe, however, how such a history was translated in the psychopathological context, this from the case summary prepared after the patient was discharged:

> This white 39-year-old male . . . manifests a long history of considerable ambivalence in close relationships, which begins in early childhood. A warm relationship with his mother cools during his adolescence. A distant relationship to his father is described as becoming very intense. Affective stability is absent. His attempts to control emotionality with his wife and children are punctuated by angry outbursts and, in the case of the children, spankings. And while he says that he has several good friends, one senses considerable ambivalence embedded in those relationships also. . . .

The facts of the case were unintentionally distorted by the staff to achieve consistency with a popular theory of the dynamics of a schizophrenic reaction.[14] Nothing of an ambivalent nature had been described in relations with parents, spouse or friends. To the extent that ambivalence could be inferred, it was probably not greater than is found in all human relationships. It is true the pseudopatient's relationships with his parents changed over time, but in the ordinary context that would hardly be remarkable—indeed, it might very well be expected. Clearly, the meaning ascribed to his verbalizations (that is, ambivalence, affective instability) was determined by the diagnosis: schizophrenia. An entirely different meaning would have been ascribed if it were known that the man was "normal."

All pseudopatients took extensive notes publicly. Under ordinary circumstances, such behavior would have raised questions in the minds of observers, as, in fact, it did among patients. Indeed, it seemed so certain that the notes would elicit suspicion that elaborate precautions proved needless. The closest any staff member came to questioning these notes occurred when one pseudopatient asked his physician what kind of medication he was receiving and began to write down the response. "You needn't write it," he was told gently. "If you have trouble remembering, just ask me again."

If no questions were asked of the pseudopatients, how was their writing interpreted? Nursing records for three patients indicate that the writing was seen as an aspect of their pathological behavior. "Patient engages in writing behavior" was the daily nursing comment on one of the pseudopatients who was never questioned about his writing. Given that the patient is in the hospital, he must be psychologically disturbed. And given that he is disturbed, continuous writing must be a behavioral manifestation of that disturbance, perhaps a subset of the compulsive behaviors that are sometimes correlated with schizophrenia.

One tacit characteristic of psychiatric diagnosis is that it locates the sources of aberration within the individual and only rarely within the complex of stimuli that surrounds him. Consequently, behaviors that are stimulated by the environment are commonly misattributed to the patient's disorder. For example, one kindly nurse found a pseudopatient pacing the long hospital corridors. "Nervous, Mr. X?" she asked. "No, bored," he said.

The notes kept by pseudopatients are full of patient behaviors that were misinterpreted by well-intentioned staff. Often enough, a patient would go "berserk" because he had, wittingly or unwittingly, been mistreated by, say, an attendant. A nurse coming upon the scene would rarely inquire even cursorily into the environmental stimuli of the patient's behavior. Rather, she assumed that his upset derived from his pathology, not from his present interactions with other staff members. Occasionally, the staff might assume that the patient's family (especially when they had recently visited) or other patients had stimulated the outburst. But never were the staff found to assume that one of themselves or the structure of the hospital had anything to do with a patient's behavior. One psychiatrist pointed to a group of patients who were sitting outside the cafeteria entrance half an hour before lunchtime. To a group of young residents he indicated that such behavior was characteristic of the oral-acquisitive nature of the syndrome. It seemed not to occur to him that there were very few things to anticipate in a psychiatric hospital besides eating.

A psychiatric label has a life and an influence of its own. Once the impression has been formed that the patient is schizophrenic, the expectation is that he will continue to be schizophrenic. When a sufficient amount of time has passed, during which the patient has done nothing bizarre, he is considered to be in remission and available for discharge. But the label endures beyond discharge, with the unconfirmed expectation that he will behave as a schizophrenic again. Such labels, conferred by mental health professionals, are as influential on the patient as they are on his relatives and friends, and it should not surprise anyone that the diagnosis acts on all of them as a self-fulfilling prophecy. Eventually, the patient himself accepts the diagnosis, with all of its surplus meanings and expectations, and behaves accordingly.[15]

The inferences to be made from these matters are quite simple. Much as Zigler and Phillips have demonstrated that there is enormous overlap in the symptoms presented by patients who have been variously diagnosed,[16] so there is enormous overlap in the behaviors of the sane and the insane. The sane are not "sane" all of the time. We lose our tempers "for no good reason." We are occasionally depressed or anxious, again for no good reason. And we may find it difficult to get along with one or another person—again for no reason that we can specify. Similarly, the insane are not always insane. Indeed, it was the impression of the pseudopatients while living with them that they were sane for long periods of time—that the bizarre behaviors upon which their diagnoses were allegedly predicted constituted only a small fraction of their total behavior. If it makes no sense to label ourselves permanently depressed on the basis of an occasional depression, then it takes better evidence than is presently available to label all patients insane or schizophrenic on the basis of bizarre behaviors or cognitions. It seems more useful, as Mischel [17] has pointed out, to limit our discussions to *behaviors*, the stimuli that provoke them, and their correlates.

It is not known why powerful impressions of personality traits, such as "crazy" or "insane," arise. Conceivably, when the origins of and stimuli that give rise to a behavior are remote or unknown, or when the behavior strikes us as immutable, trait labels regarding the *behaver* arise. When, on the other hand, the origins and stimuli are known and available, discourse is limited to the behavior itself. Thus, I may hallucinate because I am sleeping, or I may hallucinate because I have ingested a peculiar drug. These are termed sleep-induced hallucinations, or dreams, and drug-induced hallucinations, respectively. But when the stimuli to my hallucinations are unknown, that is called craziness, or schizophrenia—as if that inference were somehow as illuminating as the others.

The Experience of Psychiatric Hospitalization

The term "mental illness" is of recent origin. It was coined by people who were humane in their inclinations and who wanted very much to raise the station of (and the public's sympathies toward) the psychologically disturbed from that of witches and "crazies" to one that was akin to the physically ill. And they were at least partially successful, for the treatment of the mentally ill *has* improved considerably over the years. But while treatment has improved, it is doubtful that people really regard the mentally ill in the same way that they view the physically ill. A broken leg is something one recovers from, but mental illness allegedly endures forever.[18] A broken leg does not threaten the observer, but a crazy schizophrenic? There is by now a host of evidence that attitudes toward the mentally ill are characterized by fear, hostility, aloofness, suspicion, and dread.[19] The mentally ill are society's lepers.

That such attitudes infect the general population is perhaps not surprising, only upsetting. But that they affect the professionals—attendants, nurses, physicians, psychologists, and social workers—who treat and deal with the mentally ill is more disconcerting, both because such attitudes are self-evidently pernicious and because they are unwitting. Most mental health professionals would insist that they are sympathetic toward the mentally ill, that they are neither avoidant nor hostile. But it is more likely that an exquisite ambivalence characterizes their relations with psychiatric patients, such that their avowed impulses are only part of their entire attitude. Negative attitudes are there too and can easily be detected. Such attitudes should not surprise us. They are the natural offspring of the labels patients wear and the places in which they are found.

Consider the structure of the typical psychiatric hospital. Staff and patients are strictly segregated. Staff have their own living space, including their dining facilities, bathrooms, and assembly places. The glassed quarters that contain the professional staff, which the pseudo-patients came to call "the cage," sit out on every dayroom. The staff emerge primarily for caretaking purposes—to give medication, to conduct a therapy or group meeting, to instruct or reprimand a patient. Otherwise, staff keep to themselves, almost as if the disorder that afflicts their charges is somehow catching.

So much is patient-staff segregation the rule that, for four public hospitals in which an attempt was made to measure the degree to which staff and patients mingle, it was necessary to use "time out of the staff cage" as the operational measure. While it was not the case that all time spent out of the cage was spent mingling with patients (attendants, for example, would occasionally emerge to watch television in the dayroom), it was the only way in which one could gather reliable data on time for measuring.

The average amount of time spent by attendants outside of the cage was 11.3 percent (range, 3 to 52 percent). This figure does not represent only time spent mingling with patients, but also includes time spent on such chores as folding laundry, supervising patients while they shave, directing ward cleanup, and sending patients to off-ward activities. It was the relatively rare attendant who spent time talking with patients or playing games with them. It proved impossible to obtain a "percent mingling time" for nurses, since the amount of time they spent out of the cage was too brief. Rather, we counted instances of emergence from the cage. On the average, daytime nurses emerged from the cage 11.5 times per shift, including instances when they left the ward entirely (range, 4 to 39 times). Late afternoon and night nurses were even less available, emerging on the average 9.4 times per shift (range, 4 to 41 times). Data on early morning nurses, who arrived usually after midnight and departed at 8 A.M., are not available because patients were asleep during most of this period.

Physicians, especially psychiatrists, were even less available. They were rarely seen on the wards. Quite commonly, they would be seen only when they arrived and departed, with the remaining time being spent in their offices or in the cage. On the average, physicians emerged on the ward 6.7 times per day (range, 1 to 17 times). It proved difficult to make an accurate estimate in this regard, since physicians often maintained hours that allowed them to come and go at different times.

The hierarchical organization of the psychiatric hospital has been commented on before,[20] but the latent meaning of that kind of organization is worth noting again. Those with the most power have least to do with patients, and those with the least power are most involved with them. Recall, however, that the acquisition of role-appropriate behaviors occurs mainly through the observation of others, with the most powerful having the most influence. Consequently, it is understandable that attendants not only spend more time with patients than do any other members of the staff—that is required by their station in the hierarchy—but also, insofar as they learn from their superiors' behavior, spend as little time with patients as they can. Attendants are seen mainly in the cage, which is where the models, the action, and the power are.

I turn now to a different set of studies, these dealing with staff response to patient-initiated contact. It has long been known that the amount of time a person spends with you can be an index of your significance to him. If he initiates and maintains eye contact, there is reason to believe that he is considering your requests and needs. If he pauses to chat or actually stops and talks, there is added reason to infer that he is individuating you. In four hospitals, the pseudopatient approached the staff member with a request which took the following form: "Pardon me, Mr. [or Dr. or Mrs.] X, could you tell me when I will be eligible for grounds privileges?" (or ". . . when I will be presented at the staff meeting?" or ". . . when I am likely to be discharged?"). While the content of the question varied according to the appropriateness of the target and the pseudopatient's (apparent) current needs, the form was always a courteous and relevant request for information. Care was taken never to approach a particular member of the staff more than once a day, lest the staff member become suspicious or irritated. In examining these data, remember that the behavior of the pseudopatients was neither bizarre nor disruptive. One could indeed engage in good conversation with them.

The data for these experiments are shown in Table 1, separately for physicians (column 1) and for nurses and attendants (column 2). Minor differences among these four institutions were overwhelmed by the degree to which staff avoided continuing contacts that patients had initiated. By far, their most common response consisted of either a brief response to the question, offered while they were "on the move" and with head averted, or no response at all.

The encounter frequently took the following bizarre form: (pseudopatient) "Pardon me, Dr. X. Could you tell me when I am eligible for grounds privileges?" (physician) "Good morning, Dave. How are you today?" (Moves off without waiting for a response.)

It is instructive to compare these data with data recently obtained at Stanford University. It has been alleged that large and eminent universities are characterized by faculty who are so busy that they have no time for students. For this comparison, a young lady approached individual faculty members who seemed to be walking purposefully to some meeting or teaching engagement and asked them the following six questions.

1. "Pardon me, could you direct me to Encina Hall?" (At the medical school: ". . . to the Clinical Research Center?").
2. "Do you know where Fish Annex is?" (There is no Fish Annex at Stanford).
3. "Do you teach here?"

TABLE 1

Self-initiated Contact by Pseudopatients with Psychiatrists and Nurses and Attendants, Compared to Contact with Other Groups

Contact	Psychiatric Hospitals		University Campus (Non-medical)	University Medical Center Physicians		
	(1) Psychi-atrists	(2) Nurses and Attend-ants	(3) Faculty	(4) "Looking for a Psychi-atrist"	(5) "Looking for an Internist"	(6) No Additional Comment
Responses						
Moves on, head averted (%)	71	88	0	0	0	0
Makes eye contact (%)	23	10	0	11	0	0
Pauses and chats (%)	2	2	0	11	0	10
Stops and talks (%)	4	0.5	100	78	100	90
Mean number of questions answered (out of 6)	*	*	6	3.8	4.8	4.5
Respondents (No.)	13	47	14	18	15	10
Attempts (No.)	185	1283	14	18	15	10

* Not applicable.

4. "How does one apply for admission to the college?" (At the medical school: ". . . to the medical school?").
5. "Is it difficult to get in?"
6. "Is there financial aid?"

Without exception, as can be seen in Table 1 (column 3), all of the questions were answered. No matter how rushed they were, all respondents not only maintained eye contact, but stopped to talk. Indeed, many of the respondents went out of their way to direct or take the questioner to the office she was seeking, to try to locate "Fish Annex," or to discuss with her the possibilities of being admitted to the university.

Similar data, also shown in Table 1 (columns 4, 5, and 6), were obtained in the hospital. Here, too, the young lady came prepared with six questions. After the first question, however, she remarked to eighteen of her respondents (column 4), "I'm looking for a psychiatrist," and to fifteen others (column 5), "I'm looking for an internist." Ten other respondents received no inserted comment (column 6). The general degree of cooperative responses is considerably higher for these university groups than it was for pseudopatients in psychiatric hospitals. Even so, differences are apparent within the medical school setting.

Once having indicated that she was looking for a psychiatrist, the degree of cooperation elicited was less than when she sought an internist.

Powerlessness and Depersonalization

Eye contact and verbal contact reflect concern and individuation; their absence, avoidance and depersonalization. The data I have presented do not do justice to the rich daily encounters that grew up around matters of depersonalization and avoidance. I have records of patients who were beaten by staff for the sin of having initiated verbal contact. During my own experience, for example, one patient was beaten in the presence of other patients for having approached an attendant and told him, "I like you." Occasionally, punishment meted out to patients for misdemeanors seemed so excessive that it could not be justified by the most radical interpretations of psychiatric canon. Nevertheless, they appeared to go unquestioned. Tempers were often short. A patient who had not heard a call for medication would be roundly excoriated, and the morning attendants would often wake patients with, "Come on, you m——f——s, out of bed!"

Neither anecdotal nor "hard" data can convey the overwhelming sense of powerlessness which invades the individual as he is continually exposed to the depersonalization of the psychiatric hospital. It hardly matters *which* psychiatric hospital—the excellent public ones and the very plush private hospital were better than the rural and shabby ones in this regard, but, again, the features that psychiatric hospitals had in common overwhelmed by far their apparent differences.

Powerlessness was evident everywhere. The patient is deprived of many of his legal rights by dint of his psychiatric commitment.[21] He is shorn of credibility by virtue of his psychiatric label. His freedom of movement is restricted. He cannot initiate contact with the staff, but may only respond to such overtures as they make. Personal privacy is minimal. Patient quarters and possessions can be entered and examined by any staff member, for whatever reason. His personal history and anguish is available to any staff member (often including the "grey lady" and "candy striper" volunteer) who chooses to read his folder, regardless of their therapeutic relationship to him. His personal hygiene and waste evacuation are often monitored. The water closets may have no doors.

At times, depersonalization reached such proportions that pseudopatients had the sense that they were invisible, or at least unworthy of account. Upon being admitted, I and other pseudopatients took the initial physical examinations in a semipublic room, where staff members went about their own business as if we were not there.

On the ward, attendants delivered verbal and occasionally serious physical abuse to patients in the presence of other observing patients, some of whom (the pseudopatients) were writing it all down. Abusive behavior, on the other hand, terminated quite abruptly when other staff members were known to be coming. Staff are credible witnesses. Patients are not.

A nurse unbuttoned her uniform to adjust her brassiere in the presence of an entire ward of viewing men. One did not have the sense that she was being seductive. Rather, she didn't notice us. A group of staff persons might point to a patient in the dayroom and discuss him animatedly, as if he were not there.

One illuminating instance of depersonalization and invisibility occurred with regard to medications. All told, the pseudopatients were administered nearly 2,100 pills, including Elavil, Stelazine, Compazine, and Thorazine, to name but a few. (That such a variety of medications should have been administered to patients presenting identical symptoms is itself worthy of note.) Only two were swallowed. The rest were either pocketed or deposited in the toilet. The pseudopatients were not alone in this. Although I have no precise records on how many patients rejected their medications, the pseudopatients frequently found the medications of other patients in the toilet before they deposited their own. As long as they were cooperative, their behavior and the pseudopatients' own in this matter, as in other important matters, went unnoticed throughout.

Reactions to such depersonalization among pseudopatients were intense. Although they had come to the hospital as participant observers and were fully aware that they did not "belong," they nevertheless found themselves caught up in and fighting the process of depersonalization. Some examples: A graduate student in psychology asked his wife to bring his textbooks to the hospital so he could "catch up on his homework"—this despite the elaborate precautions taken to conceal his professional association. The same student, who had trained for quite some time to get into the hospital, and who had looked forward to the experience, "remembered" some drag races that he had wanted to see on the weekend and insisted that he be discharged by that time. Another pseudopatient attempted a romance with a nurse. Subsequently, he informed the staff that he was applying for admission to graduate school in psychology and was very likely to be admitted, since a graduate professor was one of his regular hospital visitors. The same person began to engage in psychotherapy with other patients—all of this as a way of becoming a person in an impersonal environment.

The Sources of Depersonalization

What are the origins of depersonalization? I have already mentioned two. First are attitudes held by all of us toward the mentally ill—including those who treat them—attitudes characterized by fear, distrust, and horrible expectations on the one hand, and benevolent intentions on the other. Our ambivalence leads, in this instance as in others, to avoidance.

Second, and not entirely separate, the hierarchical structure of the psychiatric hospital facilitates depersonalization. Those who are at the top have least to do with patients, and their behavior inspires the rest of the staff. Average daily contact with psychiatrists, psychologists, residents, and physicians combined ranged from 3.9 to 25.1 minutes, with an overall mean of 6.8 (six pseudopatients over a total of 129 days of hospitalization). Included in this average are time spent in the admissions interview, ward meetings in the presence of a senior staff member, group and individual psychotherapy contacts, case presentation conferences, and discharge meetings. Clearly, patients do not spend much time in interpersonal contact with doctoral staff. And doctoral staff serve as models for nurses and attendants.

There are probably other sources. Psychiatric installations are presently in serious financial straits. Staff shortages are pervasive, staff time at a premium. Something has to give, and that something is patient contact. Yet, while financial stresses are realities, too much can be made of them. I have the impression that the psychological forces that result in depersonalization are much stronger than the fiscal ones and that the addition of more staff would not correspondingly improve patient care in this regard. The incidence of staff meetings and the enormous amount of record keeping on patients, for example, have not been as substantially reduced as has patient contact. Priorities exist, even during hard times. Patient contact is not a significant priority in the traditional psychiatric hospital, and fiscal pressures do not account for this. Avoidance and depersonalization may.

Heavy reliance upon psychotropic medication tacitly contributes to depersonalization by convincing staff that treatment is indeed being conducted and that further patient contact may not be necessary. Even here, however, caution needs to be exercised in understanding the role of psychotropic drugs. If patients were powerful rather than powerless, if they were viewed as interesting individuals rather than diagnostic entities, if they were socially significant rather than social lepers, if their anguish truly and wholly compelled our sympathies and concerns, would we not *seek* contact with them, despite the availability of medications? Perhaps for the pleasure of it all?

The Consequences of Labeling and Depersonalization

Whenever the ratio of what is known to what needs to be known approaches zero, we tend to invent "knowledge" and assume that we understand more than we actually do. We seem unable to acknowledge that we simply don't know. The needs for diagnosis and remediation of behavioral and emotional problems are enormous. But rather than acknowledge that we are just embarking on understanding, we continue to label patients "schizophrenic," "manic-depressive," and "insane," as if in those words we had captured the essence of understanding. The facts of the matter are that we have known for a long time that diagnoses are often not useful or reliable, but we have nevertheless continued to use them. We now know that we cannot distinguish insanity from sanity. It is depressing to consider how that information will be used.

Not merely depressing, but frightening. How many people, one wonders, are sane but not recognized as such in our psychiatric institutions? How many have been needlessly stripped of their privileges of citizenship, from the right to vote and drive to that of handling their own accounts? How many have feigned insanity in order to avoid the criminal consequences of their behavior, and, conversely, how many would rather stand trial than live interminably in a psychiatric hospital—but are wrongly thought to be mentally ill? How many have been stigmatized by well-intentioned, but nevertheless erroneous, diagnoses? On the last point, recall again that a "type 2 error" in psychiatric diagnosis does not have the same consequences it does in medical diagnosis. A diagnosis of cancer that has been found to be in error is cause for celebration. But psychiatric diagnoses are rarely found to be in error. The label sticks, a mark of inadequacy forever.

Finally, how many patients might be "sane" outside the psychiatric hospital but seem insane in it—not because craziness resides in them, as it were, but because they are responding to a bizarre setting, one that may be unique to institutions which harbor nether people? Goffman [22] calls the process of socialization to such institutions "mortification"—an apt metaphor that includes the processes of depersonalization that have been described here. And while it is impossible to know whether the pseudopatients' responses to these processes are characteristic of all inmates—they were, after all, not real patients— it is difficult to believe that these processes of socialization to a psychiatric hospital provide useful attitudes or habits of response for living in the "real world."

Summary and Conclusions

It is clear that we cannot distinguish the sane from the insane in psychiatric hospitals. The hospital itself imposes a special environment in which the meanings of behavior can easily be misunderstood. The consequences to patients hospitalized in such an environment— the powerlessness, depersonalization, segregation, mortification, and self-labeling—seem undoubtedly countertherapeutic.

I do not, even now, understand this problem well enough to perceive solutions. But two matters seem to have some promise. The first concerns the proliferation of community mental health facilities, of crisis intervention centers, of the human potential movement, and of behavior therapies that, for all of their own problems, tend to avoid psychiatric labels, to focus on specific problems and behaviors, and to retain the individual in a relatively nonpejorative environment. Clearly, to the extent that we refrain from sending the distressed to insane places, our impressions of them are less likely to be distorted. (The risk of distorted perceptions, it seems to me, is always present, since we are much more sensitive to an individual's behaviors and verbalizations than we are to the subtle contextual stimuli that often promote them. At issue here is a matter of magnitude. And, as I have shown, the magnitude of distortion is exceedingly high in the extreme context that is a psychiatric hospital.)

The second matter that might prove promising speaks to the need to increase the sensitivity of mental health workers and researchers to the *Catch* 22 position of psychiatric patients. Simply reading materials in this area will be of help to some such workers and researchers. For others, directly experiencing the impact of psychiatric hospitalization will be of enormous use. Clearly, further research into the social psychology of such total institutions will both facilitate treatment and deepen understanding.

I and the other pseudopatients in the psychiatric setting had distinctly negative reactions. We do not pretend to describe the subjective experiences of true patients. Theirs may be different from ours, particularly with the passage of time and the necessary process of adaptation to one's environment. But we can and do speak to the relatively more objective indices of treatment within the hospital. It could be a mistake, and a very unfortunate one, to consider that what happened to us derived from malice or stupidity on the part of the staff. Quite the contrary, our overwhelming impression of them was of people who really cared, who were committed, and who were uncommonly intelligent. Where they failed, as they sometimes did painfully, it would be more accurate to attribute those failures to the environment in which they, too, found themselves than to personal callousness. Their perceptions and behavior were controlled by the situation, rather than being motivated by a malicious disposition. In a more benign environment, one that was less attached to global diagnosis, their behaviors and judgments might have been more benign and effective.

NOTES

1. P. Ash, "The Reliability of Psychiatric Diagnoses," *Journal of Abnormal Social Psychology* 44 (1949): 272–276; A. T. Beck, "Reliability of Psychiatric Diagnoses: 1. A Critique of Systematic Studies," *American Journal of Psychiatry* 119 (1962): 210–216; A. T. Boisen, "Types of Dementia Praecox—A Study in Psychiatric Classification," *Psychiatry* 2 (1938): 233–236; N. Kreitman, "The Reliability of Psychiatric Diagnosis," *Journal of Mental Science* 107 (1961): 876–886; idem et al., "The Reliability of Psychiatric Assessment: An Analysis," ibid., p. 887–908; H. O. Schmitt and C. P. Fonda, "The Reliability of Psychiatric Diagnoses: A New Look." *Journal of Abnormal Social Psychology* 52 (1956): 262–267; and W. Seeman, "Psy-

chiatric Diagnosis," *Journal of Nervous and Mental Disease* 118 (1935): 541–544. For an analysis of these artifacts and summaries of the disputes, see J. Zubin, "Classification of the Behavior Disorders," *Annual Review of Psychology* 18 (1967): 373–406, and L. Phillips and J. G. Draguns, "Classification of the Behavior Disorders," ibid. 22 (1971): 447–482.

2. R. Benedict, "Anthropology and the Abnormal," *Journal of General Psychology* 10 (1934): 59–82.

3. See in this regard H. Becker, *Outsiders: Studies in the Sociology of Deviance* (New York: Free Press, 1963); B. M. Braginsky, D. D. Braginsky, and K. Ring, *Methods of Madness: The Mental Hospital as a Last Resort* (New York: Holt, Rinehart, 1969); G. M. Crocetti and P. V. Lemkau, "On Rejection of the Mentally Ill," *American Sociological Review* 30 (1965): 577–578; E. Goffman, *Behavior in Public Places* (New York: Free Press, 1964); R. D. Laing, *The Divided Self: A Study of Sanity and Madness* (Chicago: Quadrangle, 1960); D. L. Phillips, "Rejection: A Possible Consequence of Seeking Help for Mental Disorders," *American Sociological Review* 28 (1963): 963–972; T. R. Sarbin, " 'Schizophrenia' Is a Myth, Born of Metaphor, Meaningless," *Psychology Today* 6 (1972): 18–27; E. Schur, "Reactions to Deviance: A Critical Assessment," *American Journal of Sociology* 75 (1969): 309; T. Szasz, *Law, Liberty, and Psychiatry* (New York: Macmillan, 1963); and idem, *The Myth of Mental Illness: Foundations of a Theory of Mental Illness* (New York: Hoeber-Harper, 1963). For a critique of some of these views, see W. R. Gove, "Societal Reaction as an Explanation of Mental Illness: An Evaluation," *American Sociological Review* 35 (1970): 873–884. See also E. Goffman, *Asylums* (Garden City, N.Y.: Doubleday-Anchor, 1961), and T. J. Scheff, *Being Mentally Ill: A Sociological Theory* (Chicago: Aldine, 1966).

4. Data from a ninth pseudopatient are not incorporated in this report because, although his sanity went undetected, he falsified aspects of his personal history, including his marital status and parental relationships. His experimental behaviors therefore were not identical to those of the other pseudopatients.

5. A. Barry, *Bellevue is a State of Mind* (New York: Harcourt Brace, 1971); I. Belknap, *Human Problems of a State Mental Hospital* (New York: McGraw-Hill, 1956); W. Caudill et al., "Social Structure and Interaction Processes on a Psychiatric Ward," *American Journal of Orthopsychiatry* 22 (1952): 314–334, and in abridged form chap. 12 of this book; A. R. Goldman, R. H. Bohr, and T. A. Steinberg, "On Posing as Mental Patients: Reminiscences," *Professional Psychology* 1 (1970): 427–434; and "Learning by 'Living-In' An Acute Hospital Ward," by Don A. Rockwell, M.D., *Roche Report* 1, no. 13 (1971): 8.

6. Beyond the personal difficulties that the pseudopatient is likely to experience in the hospital, there are legal and social ones that, combined, require considerable attention before entry. For example, once admitted to a psychiatric institution, it is difficult, if not impossible, to be discharged in short notice, state law to the contrary notwithstanding. I was not sensitive to these difficulties at the outset of the project, nor to the personal and situational emergencies that can arise, but later a writ of habeas corpus was prepared for each of the entering pseudopatients and an attorney was kept "on call" during every hospitalization. I am grateful to John Kaplan and Robert Bartels for legal advice and assistance in these matters.

7. However distasteful such concealment is, it was a necessary first step to examining these questions. Without concealment, there would have been no way to know how valid these experiences were; nor was there any other way of knowing whatever detections occurred were a tribute to the diagnostic acumen of the staff or to the hospital's rumor network. Obviously, since my concerns are general ones that cut across individual hospitals and staffs, I have respected their anonymity and have eliminated clues that might lead to their identification.

8. Interestingly, of the twelve admissions, eleven were diagnosed as schizophrenic and one, with the identical symptomatology, as manic-depressive psychosis. This diagnosis has a more favorable prognosis, and it was given by the only private hospital in our sample. On the relations between social class and psychiatric diagnosis, see A. B. Hollingshead and F. C. Redlich, *Social Class and Mental Illness: A Community Study* (New York: Wiley, 1958).

9. It is possible, of course, that patients have quite broad latitudes in diagnosis and therefore are inclined to call many people sane, even those whose behavior is patently aberrant. However, although we have no hard data on this matter, it was our distinct impression that this was not the case. In many instances, patients not only singled us out for attention, but came to imitate our behaviors and styles.

10. Scheff, *Being Mentally Ill*.

11. J. Cumming and E. Cumming, "On the Stigma of Mental Illness," *Com-*

munity Mental Health 1 (1965): 135–143; A. Farina and K. Ring, "The Influence of Perceived Mental Illness on Interpersonal Relations," *Journal of Abnormal Psychology* 70 (1965): 47–51; H. E. Freeman and O. G. Simmons, *The Mental Patient Comes Home* (New York: Wiley, 1963); W. J. Johannsen, "Attitudes Toward Mental Patients," *Mental Hygiene* 53 (1969): 218–228; and A. S. Linsky, "Who Shall Be Excluded: The Influence of Personal Attributes in Community Reaction to the Mentally Ill," *Social Psychiatry* 5 (1970): 166–171.

12. S. E. Asch, "Forming Impressions of Personality," *Journal of Abnormal Social Psychology* 41 (1946): 258–290, and idem, *Social Psychology* (Englewood Cliffs, N.J.: Prentice-Hall, 1952).

13. See also I. N. Mensh and J. Wishner, "Forming Impressions of Personality: Further Evidence," *Journal of Personality* 16 (1947): 188–191; J. Wishner, "Reanalysis of 'Impressions of Personality,'" *Psychological Review* 67 (1960): 96–112; J. S. Bruner and R. Tagiuri, "The Perception of People," in *Handbook of Social Psychology*, ed. G. Lindzey, vol. 2 (Cambridge, Mass.: Addison-Wesley, 1954), pp. 634–654; and J. S. Bruner, D. Shapiro, and R. Tagiuri, "The Meaning of Traits in Isolation and in Combination," in *Person Perception and Interpersonal Behavior*, ed. R. Tagiuri and L. Patrullo (Stanford, Calif.: Stanford University Press, 1958), pp. 277–288.

14. For an example of a similar self-fulfilling prophecy, in this instance dealing with the "central" trait of intelligence, see R. Rosenthal and L. Jacobson, *Pygmalion in the Classroom* (New York: Holt, Rinehart, 1968).

15. Scheff, *Being Mentally Ill.*

16. E. Zigler and L. Phillips, "Psychiatric Diagnosis and Symptomatology," *Journal of Abnormal and Social Psychology* 63 (1961): 69–75. See also R. K. Freudenberg and J. P. Robertson, "Symptoms in Relation to Psychiatric Diagnosis and Treatment," *American Medical Association Archives of Neurology and Psychiatry* 76 (1956): 14–22.

17. W. Mischel, *Personality and Assessment* (New York: Wiley, 1968).

18. The most recent and unfortunate instance of this tenet is that of Senator Thomas Eagleton.

19. T. R. Sarbin and J. C. Mancuso, "Failure of a Moral Enterprise: Attitude of the Public Toward Mental Illness," *Journal of Clinical Consulting Psychology* 35 (1970): 159–173; T. R. Sarbin, "On the Futility of the Proposition That Some People Be Labeled 'Mentally Ill,'" *Journal of Consulting Psychology* 31 (1967): 447–453; and J. C. Nunnally, Jr., *Popular Conceptions of Mental Health* (New York: Holt, Rinehart, 1961).

20. A. H. Stanton and M. S. Schwartz, *The Mental Hospital: A Study of Institutional Participation in Psychiatric Illness and Treatment* (New York: Basic Books, 1954).

21. D. B. Wexler and S. E. Scoville, "The Administration of Psychiatric Justice: Theory and Practice in Arizona," *Arizona Law Review* 13 (1971): 1–259.

22. Goffman, *Asylums.*

COMMENTARY

The author concludes from his data, "It is clear that we cannot distinguish the sane from the insane in psychiatric hospitals." This broad statement is a dramatic challenge to both the validity and reliability of psychiatric diagnoses. This assertion, however overdrawn and criticized,[1] should not be dismissed. It is clear that the very nature of personal experience is de facto subjective and may be misrepresented to a clinician. It is also clear that the unsuspecting clinician will tend to take as valid the reports of his patients about their thoughts and feelings. Clinicians are easily deceived when there is no apparent motive to misrepresent.

But the clinical evaluation of a patient involves more than a report of his personal experience. We know very little about the part of the evaluation process at the hospitals referred to in this paper that dealt with the psychiatric history and mental status examination. We have no information about what thinking went into the evaluation. The process of clinical evaluation, which should result in more than a diagnostic label, should be based on more than a person's statements that he heard a voice.

While we may question the skills of the examiners or even be embarrassed by their gullibility, it is also essential to recognize a very serious problem with the process of diagnosis which results from the pressures of the context in which the process takes place. There is the pressure not to underdiagnose, not to miss a serious disorder and thereby harm a patient. The clinician's competence is less likely to be challenged for overdiagnosis than for underdiagnosis. A variety of additional pressures in society and in the profession call forward this tendency on the part of the examiner to overdiagnose, to evaluate the illness as more rather than less serious.

This same contextual pressure leads clinicians to misinterpret appropriate behavior. In all the hospitals in the experiment there was a common thread. The staffs and the "patients" were trapped by the preconception that mental patients behave in strange ways and are not to be responded to in the same way "normal" people are. This led in at least one instance to the construction of a post hoc explanation of a "schizophrenic" history. It led skilled staff to misinterpret taking of notes as a symptom. It led to confusion and inability to distinguish between anxiety and boredom. We are challenged to understand the genesis of this behavior on the part of a clinical staff without discounting it as being due entirely to naïveté.

The article also makes the point that the role of patient is experienced in a forceful way as being powerless, demeaning, and dehumanizing, and that these are antitherapeutic effects. It seems that in spite of the best intentions and skills of staff, mental hospitals have the strong and pressing potential to discourage personal growth, development of self-esteem, and the learning of useful social roles. Hospital social systems have the potential to be harmful as well as helpful, and too often they may be injurious in these ways.

This article has been widely criticized. The reader is referred to a representative critique published in two volumes of the Bulletin of the Menninger Clinic.[2]

While the Rosenhan study should be evaluated like any other— on the strength and limitations of its observations and inferences— mental health professionals may also profitably examine it simply in terms of its applicability to their own setting. Such "self-examination," like that which we hopefully conduct with our clients, need not be accusative or destructive.

This exploration might be guided by the following questions: Do we selectively perceive the aberrant or pathological behavior of patients? Are we inclined to label appropriate behavior as inappropriate? Do we help patients to discriminate between normal and abnormal behavior? Do we wittingly or unwittingly depreciate, depersonalize, or stigmatize patients? What efforts may be made to obviate the kinds of untoward staff attitudes and behavior depicted by Rosenhan?

NOTES

1. Sewart Hiltner, "Comment on 'On Being Sane in Insane Places,' " *Bulletin of the Menninger Clinic* 37, no. 6 (November 1973): 633–636; Charles Hofling, " 'On Being Sane in Insane Places,' Rhetoric or Logic," *Bulletin of the Menninger Clinic* 37, no. 6 (November 1973): 631–633; Philip Holzman, "Comments on D. Rosenhan's 'On Being Sane in Insane Places,' " *Bulletin of the Menninger Clinic,* 37, no. 6 (November 1973): 629–630; Alan Kraft, "Diagnosis: Evaluation or Label," *Bulletin of the Menninger Clinic,* 37, no. 6 (November 1973): 636–638; Frederick Shectman, "On Being Misinformed by Misleading Arguments," *Bulletin of the Menninger Clinic* 37, no. 5 (September 1973): 523–525; Robert S. Wallerstein, "Discussion of Rosenhan's 'On Being Sane in Insane Places,' " *Bulletin of the Menninger Clinic* 37, no. 5 (September 1973): 526–530; George Weiderman, "Psychiatric Disease: Fiction or Reality," *Bulletin of the Menninger Clinic* 37, no. 5 (September 1973): 519–522.

2. Ibid.

CHAPTER 21

Treatment and the Family System

INTRODUCTION

In one way or another, the helping professions and laymen alike recognize the family as a unique human grouping which is of central significance to its members. Despite testimonials to its importance, there is considerable evidence that the family is neglected as a unit of observation, analysis, and intervention. Moreover, even when the family is examined there has been some tendency to regard it simply as an aggregate of interacting personalities rather than as a socio-cultural system. In this paper Dean provides additional basic data and concepts which may enhance the clinician's sociological perspective of the structure and functions of the American family.

Pointing to some central elements of family sociology, Dean refers to families with whom clinicians are familiar—families faced with psychiatric disturbances. Utilizing revealing case material, he demonstrates that such families represent natural experiments in the processes of social organization, deviance, and disorganization, and thus serve to dramatize the distinct sociological properties of families.

As has been noted in our examination of the primary group, the family is central in fulfilling profound and multiple needs of individuals. Properly understood, mediated, and mobilized, the patient's family may become a powerful ally in treatment efforts. Yet as Parsons theoretically suggests, and Dean's paper documents, illness and deviance disrupt the structure and functions of the family. Dean indicates that the specific role networks of the patient serve to determine the kinds of behavior which will be experienced as problematic and the ability of the family to cope with deviance. He examines the "treatment" efforts of patients and family members—often initiated despite the denial of mental illness—as one type of effort employed to restore group functioning.

Among numerous pointedly relevant observations, Dean describes the increased primacy of the nuclear family in middle-class society. The upwardly mobile conjugal family which has given up the restrictions and supports of the extended family has taken an enormous burden on itself. The smaller, nuclear family has undertaken the task of fulfilling substantial portions of the socioemotional needs of its members. In other times and in other cultures there have been strong cross-generational relationships and supports, as well as intraconjugal family supports. Often in the contemporary nuclear family there is a sense of privacy, autonomy, and self-sufficiency. This phenomenon has concentrated important functions having to do with tension release, nurturance, and conflict resolution within the relatively small family unit.

The author also illustrates the application of sociology to such clinical concerns as the case history, social diagnosis, and social therapy. This paper thus abundantly exemplifies our concern with integrating social science into the real work of mental health professionals.

MENTAL ILLNESS AND
FAMILY HOMEOSTASIS [1]

Alfred Dean

Research into the public's reactions to psychiatric disturbances has developed largely over the past twenty years, and many of these studies are focused on the families of disturbed individuals. They rest on the reasonable assumptions that it is the family which most directly receives the impact of symptomatic and deviant behavior; which must struggle with identifying psychiatric disturbance and appropriate sources of help; which is the context of many of the patient's principal strivings; and which is the setting to which the patient will return after the "treatment hour" or hospitalization. In each instance the family's response may be more or less constructive.

This is an area of inquiry addressed to substantially practical questions: What factors facilitate or defer early recognition of psychiatric disturbance and recourse to professional help? What factors shape treatment relationships and render them more or less effective? What is the impact upon family members and the family system—with what implications for therapeutic intervention? What factors influence the ability of the chronically ill to remain in the commuity? [2] An understanding of such questions and the data which may inform them requires a deep appreciation of the nature and consequences of *deviance, labeling,* and *social control.* It is partly for this reason that we have chosen to consider such families in these terms.

I am also concerned here with the need to extend our discussion in this book of the family as a social system.[3] This implies a double task: further understanding of the *family* as a unique type of human group, and further understanding of its *systemic properties.* The study of families faced with psychiatric problems is a useful vehicle to such knowledge, because they represent "natural experiments" in the processes of social organization and disorganization. Just as the study of physical disorders exposes "normal" structures and functions by identifying "malfunctions," so does the study of disrupted social systems. What child has not discovered this avenue of understanding, as in tinkering with a discarded clock or broken toy?

Our examination of key sociological concepts has necessarily emphasized those elements which give order and stability to group life. Deviance, conflict, disorganization, and change are also ubiquitous social phenomena which have particular relevance to the mental health field. Moreover, in our review of some research findings we will attempt to demonstrate that the ostensibly antithetical elements of social organization and disorganization are best understood as two sides of the same coin: the currency of social life. Like the individual and the group, they illuminate each other.

As in the dissection of an organic form, such an examination implies a varied review of structures and functions. In order to undertake a bounded task and give it coherence and direction, the unifying emphasis of this paper is on the *disequilibrating* consequences of deviance and on the processes of *reequilibration.* This is analagous to a preoccupation with the processes by which a living organism responds to threats to its vital functions and its integrity.

The most central, defining feature of any social system is that it is an *organized entity* with differentiated, interdependent parts, including cultural roles, values, and beliefs. All systems exhibit *structure* and *function.* For present purposes we may consider these terms as analogous to the anatomy and physiology of the human animal. As noted earlier, social systems take on their particular forms in an apparent effort to satisfy individual and collective "needs."

Deviant behavior is traditionally defined as any rule-breaking behavior. The rules of a particular group are most effectively conceived as attached to specific statuses, roles, and social situations. Among the most familiar experiences of social life is learning that such rules exist, and that their transgression leads to powerful, punitive responses. Like the child, we often learn about the norms by unwittingly committing deviant acts. In time we learn to search for cues to appropriate behavior, a process which rarely may be self-conscious, as in new social situations.

These facts seem clear and verifiable enough, but it is necessary to go beyond them. Why do the rules exist? When and why do transgressions become a problem? Why do people express disapproval, frustration, or anger at individuals who don't conform to expectations? The approach we will take here to each of these questions is to propose that deviance implies the failure to fulfill some function of the social system —that it disrupts structural elements and threatens the *integrity of the system as a whole*. I shall refer broadly to these structural-functional disturbances as a process of *disequilibration*. The following case study of one family's confrontation with psychiatric disturbances will be used to illustrate and amplify the nature and implications of these propositions.

The patient, Mrs. Susan Nelson, is a forty-nine-year-old housewife. Over a period of five years she exhibited a progressive history of severe depression, nervousness, and use of alcohol. She has been married to her husband, Dewey, for a period of thirty years. He is employed as a contract engineer for a manufacturing company. His job requires him to travel, and he is typically home on weekends.

The Nelsons live in a rather exclusive residential area in one of Minnesota's larger cites. They belong to an Episcopalian church in their community. Mrs. Nelson has been quite active in a number of social and community welfare activities.

Mr. Nelson is a graduate of a prestigeful State University. Mrs. Nelson has a high school education. Among their social commitments is membership in a country club associated with the residential area in which they live. On the basis of income, occupation, and residential location as well as social activities, this family would probably be described as upper-middle to lower-middle class within our social system.

The Nelson's have two children: a twenty-one-year-old son, Bill, who attends State University, and a seventeen-year-old daughter, Stephanie, a junior in high school. Mrs. Nelson is the youngest of four children, two of whom have died within the past five years. Her father died about twelve years ago, and her mother died within the past two years. One remaining sibling lives in Wisconsin.

Family Form and Function-Equilibrium

One characteristic of American family structure exhibited by this family is its emphasis on the conjugal or nuclear family, which consists of husband, wife, and their children. The "primacy" of the conjugal family has a number of aspects. In part it means that loyalties and responsibilities are attached to the conjugal family in contrast to the extended family. It also means the family values its independence from the extended families of orientation. Sociologists believe that the independence of the conjugal family (a rather unusual pattern viewed cross-culturally) is importantly a function of the economic structure of American society. We are now a society of urbanized, hired employees, in contrast to a time when the family was a unit of economic production —such as yesteryear's farm family or "business families." The primacy of the American conjugal family is born in part of necessity.

It is also believed that the emphasis on the nuclear family is closely related to the emphasis on social mobility in American society. The "American Dream" has always been for succeeding generations of family members to move up the socioeconomic ladder. The conjugal family has its bags packed, and it moves vertically. It is not to be hampered by ties to family, community, or tradition.

In each of these respects the Nelson family fit the general pattern. They moved from the towns of their families of orientation and maintained ties of "safe distance." They did not have or make occasions to see members of the extended family frequently, but did respond to various types of emergencies, particularly those of illness or death; such events figured prominently in the symptomatic history of the patient.

The activities of the Nelson family reflected their middle-class background. They valued social mobility, hard work, security, and education. Mr. Nelson placed a heavy emphasis on his job, career, and "success." Participation in social activities and community affairs was part of the same value-belief complex.

The middle-class conjugal family places a premium on family life. It is also *filialcentric*, that is, its activities, values, and motives attach special importance to children. In part, this emphasis on the children involves the transmission of class-related values which are reflected in its attempts to see that they get a "proper" education.

The primacy of the conjugal family is also related to its emphasis on fulfilling deep-seated emotional needs, as for security, affection, and other emotional responses. The cult of romantic love in American society is a symbol of the exclusiveness, uniqueness, and depth with which the *companionship marriage* is viewed. This is virtually regarded as its raison d'être. Some sociologists have identified the family as the major institutional form of tension reduction in American society.[4] These varied functions have been termed *expressive functions*. Perhaps no other society has ever expected so much personal fulfillment from the nuclear family, a fact which is probably reflected in our high rates of marriage, divorce, and remarriage.

The evidence indicates that both Mr. and Mrs. Nelson found their relationship reasonably satisfactory until Mrs. Nelson began to show signs of depression, anxiety, and increased drinking. Both indicate that they were compatible and had a satisfactory sexual relationship. In the context of her illness, Mrs. Nelson reported that she did not doubt that her husband loved her, but that he had probably never been adequately demonstrative. She also allowed that, in retrospect, she had always resented his job to some degree. However, she had never before regarded either as a particular problem.

There also was apparently a good parent-children relationship. Mrs. Nelson regarded her relationship to them, and especially to her daughter, as very gratifying.

The *division of labor* in the family is another major plane in its organization of roles. It is an *instrumental system*, a system of roles that are designed to fulfill certain tasks associated with the group's adaptation to its environment. The instrumental system is "economic" in its broadest sense.

In the Nelson family the division of labor was organized around traditional, familiar lines. As the husband-father, Mr. Nelson was regarded as the principal "breadwinner." As noted earlier, the instrumental roles which he assumed were also in pursuit of the social class values of mobility and life style. Mr. Nelson entered his job during the depression and became successful.

Mrs. Nelson assumed the role of housewife-mother. The evidence suggests she played her roles rather successfully, and placed a great premium on them. The structure of the family in American society has historically been decisively shaped by the husband's occupation. In this particular family Mr. Nelson's job meant that Mrs. Nelson assumed an even heavier burden in her responsibilities for managing the home, social life, and child rearing. In support of her husband's career, it was also her responsibility to act as hostess for her husband's business associates and clients. Mrs. Nelson had apparently performed well in each of these roles—until she began to exhibit her symptoms.

We have described two major axes in the organization of this family, and how it reflected the American family pattern.[5] It seems that this system functioned rather well. It was a system of roles, values, and beliefs that had a certain integrity, coherence, and stability. It was a system in equilibrium, fulfilling numerous biologic, psychologic, and social functions. Next we shall see how this system became disrupted and disorganized.

The following summary of problematic events will serve as a reference for discussion.

Symptomatology

Mrs. Nelson exhibited severe depression, anxiety, and alcohol abuse. These symptoms were apparently fairly sudden in onset and showed a progressive history over a five-year period. While their manifestation became more frequent over time, they were subject to significant periods of exacerbation and remission. Mrs. Nelson also obliquely communicated the possibility that she might commit suicide, and on one occasion took an overdose of tranquilizers. These symptoms were prominent expressions of her disturbance; they were also the features of her behavior which most clearly captured the attention and intervention efforts of various clinicians. For these reasons, and due to the necessary limitations and emphases of this paper, they may be regarded as a capsule statement of her symptomatology.

We do not wish to imply that we regard her depression, anxiety, and excessive drinking as her only symptoms—or even that they were her most crucial or revealing problems. Other forms of problematic and diagnostically relevant behavior are documented in the following pages. We do wish to make a distinction between "illness" or *illness behavior* and *social behavior*. In the following section Mrs. Nelson's behavior is examined with reference to the sociocultural system in which it occurred. Her behavior is analyzed into various types of socially problematic or deviant behavior which represent a breakdown in the antecedent structures and functions of the family system.[6]

Deviance and Disequilibrium

Instrumental role failure. Mrs. Nelson's anxiety, depression, and excessive drinking were associated with a number of forms of instrumental role failure. She neglected her "household responsibilities" such as cooking and cleaning. Mrs. Nelson also reported neglecting the needs of her teenage daughter, describing her actions as "sins of omission." She began to decline to participate in quasi-social activities associated with her husband's work. She also withdrew from social and community activities and was denied participation by her husband because of her excessive drinking.

Mrs. Nelson also exhibited a pattern of making long distance telephone calls when she was drinking, which her husband described as "a tremendous expense."

In addition to the *loss of functions,* or their *imposition on others,* Mrs. Nelson's behavior imposed a new set of instrumental tasks upon the family. Mr. Nelson had to monitor her behavior by calling home and checking with his wife or daughter to see how she was doing. When drinking she was withdrawn and would not eat. She was also moody, demanding, and argumentative. The fact that Mr. Nelson was away much of the time made these instrumental disturbances a serious burden. It is clear that they disrupted a longstanding pattern in the allocation of work and home responsibilities.

The episodic nature of instrumental role failure, excessive drinking, and emotional lability demonstrate a critical systemic problem of deviance tied to psychiatric disturbances: *unpredictability.* A basic function of role specification is to introduce predictable behavior. It is an equilibrating mechanism. Unpredictability is thus tantamount to social disorganization.

Expressive role failure. Mrs. Nelson's moodiness, argumentativeness, and withdrawal directly violated expressive role expectations. She was also keenly aware that other deviance, such as excessive drinking and the conflict and argumentation associated with it, resulted in the breach of her relationship with her husband and daughter.

The systemic character of roles is also reflected in the fact that her deviance resulted in *a loss of authority* and *prestige* vis-à-vis her daughter. Feeling that she should be a companion, an advisor, and an influence over her daughter's behavior, she experienced this loss with considerable concern.

Representational role failure. Certain role expectations in every group are essentially symbolic. Individuals are expected to behave in ways which appropriately *represent* their position in the group and the group itself. Stephanie's embarrassment over her mother's drinking, which had been a matter of public knowledge and social gossip, may be understood partly in these terms. Mrs. Nelson's improper drinking at business conventions and Mr. Nelson's cancellation of various social engagements may be similarly understood. These representational roles were also possibly attached to maintaining social status in the community and their particular social class. It is clear that Mrs. Nelson regarded her daughter's concern about her drinking as symbolic of her failure as a mother. She once stated, "Let me tell you that not to be admired by your daughter is a very crushing thing."

These observations dramatize the fact that deviant behavior has a social psychological impact not only on other individuals in the family but on the deviant himself. Under *what conditions* might this stimulate secondary deviance or illness? Most research on mental illness and the family tends to focus on the impact on other members of the family and neglects this aspect.

What is labeled as "inappropriate drinking" is an instructive example of how norms are attached to statuses, rules, and social situations. Cross-culturally, there are intriguing examples of how groups regulate whether people can drink at all, what, when, why, how, and with what *resulting behavior.*[7] Typically, these norms are attached to status characteristics—age, sex, race, religion, social class—and to specific social situations. Drinking in this family was a highly valued activity associated with sociability and business relationships. It was when the patient's drinking was regarded as intruding on role performances that her husband defined it as socially inappropriate and "out of control."

Processes and Problems of Reequilibration

The interdependence of individuals in the group and the systemic character of the group are revealed in a variety of attempts to restore role functioning and repair relationships. The family's attempt to reequilibrate, and its difficulties in doing so, should be of central concern to the clinician because they may provide the generic motivation which prompts treatment contacts.

One way of reequilibrating a social system is to restore the pattern which existed prior to crisis. Another way is to change the system along some idealized or preferred lines. In either case, of course, the system must be acceptable to the principal parties in the conflict. Attempts at both alternatives were exhibited in this family, but they were conflictual and unstable. Mrs. Nelson vacillated between efforts to resume her usual roles and relationships (as nearly as possible) and an attempt to change substantially her relationship with her husband. For the most part Mr. Nelson attempted to restore the status quo ante and to resist any changes which might imply any serious revision in his usual occupational role. The nature and basis of this untoward situation, and the mechanisms which reflected these variant reequilibrating strivings, require examination.

Sanctioning is the most widely recognized technique of social persuasion. As such, it is also a mechanism of social control and reequilibration. Conflict and tension typically arise in a social system when deviance occurs. These may be quite simply "natural" responses on the part of the frustrated or threatened party. They may also be deliberate attempts to communicate the unacceptability of particular behaviors and to pursuade conformity. In either event, conflict, tension, and avoidance serve as punitive sanctions. Mrs. Nelson experienced many such responses from her husband, daughter, and son.

Conflict and rejection are ways of delivering the message, "You are deviant." If the message is successfully delivered, the individual is assigned a new identity, status, and role. It is his responsibility to do what is necessary to "correct" his behavior.[8] The deviant role and the sick role [9] are both examples of corrective roles. Both imply a loss of status. One question, of course, is whether the individual can be persuaded that his behavior is deviant. This was not the issue in this case, as Mrs. Nelson agreed that her behavior was inappropriate, but she and her husband differed remarkably on why she behaved as she did.

That deviance and conflict may be functional, however problematic, requires special emphasis.[10] Conceptions of the nature and significance of conflict may be culturally patterned. The romanticization of the American family may have implied that "conflict should not occur in a good marriage," and that its occurrence is foreboding. However, it is true that when deviance, conflict, and dissensus persist, the results are destructive.

The loss of status and authority associated with being labeled "deviant" reveals that sanctioning is not only a reactive process, but is built into social structure. When an individual performs according to role expectations, he validates his position and is legitimately entitled to the prestige, power, rights, and privileges attached to this position. Mrs. Nelson desperately sought the interpersonal gratifications exchanged with membership in good standing, but she was at once also unable and unwilling to do so.

Perceptual distortions reveal a desperate attempt to restore the status quo ante in the face of severe threats. The denial of mental illness and deviance has been well documented.[11] While regarded as intrapsychic defense mechanisms, however, they have not generally been examined as *preferred social definitions* with persuasive intent.[12]

Despite an extraordinary series of personal losses, for example, Mrs. Nelson was unable to account for her acute depression and anxiety. Describing this as "the what's-the-matter-with-me stage," she said, "I guess I would say to myself, I'll bet nine million times, you have no reason in the world to feel like this!" Subsequent to her mother's death, her compulsion to give gifts to old ladies apparently was not recognized as a transparent sign of her grief reaction. Despite her initiative in seeking psychiatric help, she focused on her symptoms of depression and anxiety and denied any problems that might be related to her drinking. She was resistant to psychotherapy and broke off treatment relationships.

The conflictual *social functions* of perceptual distortions were exemplified in the *alcoholism versus mental illness controversy*. Mr. Nelson reported that his wife only got depressed and anxious *as a result of excessive drinking.* He claimed that she had adjusted well to family losses, minimized any problems between them, and claimed that she had "no particular worries." Mr. Nelson stated that his wife, generally speaking, was optimistic, even-tempered, and not moody: "It seems that the little bad habits of her family irritate her more than anything else. She may feel a little neglected because I have to spend many nights on the road and work a lot when I'm at home."

While he recognized that she would drink only after he left home, he attached no significance to this fact. He attributed her new-found inability to drink in a controlled manner to "some biochemical change in her body." "Why can't they [psychiatrists] tell people they have a drinking problem instead of insisting they have other problems?" he asked, with thinly disguised contempt.

Later Mrs. Nelson regarded her drinking, depression, and nervousness as related to other problems. Unlike her husband, she did not believe that "everything would be okay if I just stop drinking." This struggle was also reflected in Mrs. Nelson's recourse to psychiatrists, while he pressed her to go to an alcoholic treatment center. She obliged him when he told her "we can't go on like this." Mrs. Nelson certainly communicated the "need for change" in direct as well as oblique ways, but she recognized the difficulty in effecting change and feared being totally rejected. She also realized that her behavior was "driving people away rather than making them closer." Further illustrating these issues, Mrs. Nelson stated: "If I discuss too much the kinds of things I wanted to change, it would be overpowering for him. On the other hand, if I keep sneaking them in, it won't make any impression. Do you think it would jolt him into thinking if I said I decided if I quit drinking it would neither make him or myself happy unless other things were changed? I can destroy what I have by wanting so much more than what I have. I realize all these things aren't silly, but I don't want him to think they're all-powerful. I feel if I went into these things I can't help but feel he couldn't help feeling I didn't love him."

On the occasion of one hospitalization, it was noted: "She constantly remarks that she knows what is best for her, but isn't able to go through with it and the reason she can't is what bothers her."

Faced with the failure of remedially oriented efforts on one hand, and the prospect of "dissolving" the family on the other, accommodation may result. Accommodation refers to the revision of expectations and reallocation of functions. It is a compromise or stalemate (no pun intended). Accommodation is a means of "living with" deviance and reducing its impact. Like other attempts at equilibration, it may require perceptual distortion and socially shared "myths."

Probably all groups exhibit patterns of accommodation; the issue is, at what "cost-benefit"? As in *Who's Afraid of Virginia Woolf?*, if myth-maintained accommodations become extensive, or are challenged by some special event, they will break down. Several researchers have noted that hospitalization may be precipitated by the breakdown of accommodative patterns.[13] Either the incentives for accommodation may change, or the threshhold of tolerance may be exceeded. That families often accommodate to chronic and severe deviance which is broken by dangerous behavior has been noted. Sociocultural factors affect the family's *capacity for accommodation*. For example, whether the family is nuclear or extended, rural or urban influences its capacity for accommodation.

All Nelson family members made some accommodations to perceived deviance. Neither sanctioning, pressures for treatment, nor deviance was unremitting. However, when Mrs. Nelson withdrew to her bed for several weeks—described by Mr. Nelson as "her longest binge" —he advised her that he was reaching the end of his rope, and persuaded her to seek treatment for alcoholism.

Limitations of Treatment

Mrs. Nelson's history of disturbance and treatment is not encouraging. Having documented a five-year span of progressive disturbance at the time of my study, I was to learn, some two years later, that she was continuing to exhibit serious difficulties. During her history she had been treated by numerous professionals: psychiatrists, physicians, social workers, psychologists, and others. She was able to purchase quality care by well-trained professionals.

It is thus tempting to conclude that her problem was intractable —inherently poor in prognosis, or unlikely to respond to current knowledge and treatment techniques. It might be argued that she was resistant to treatment, or a poor candidate for therapy. Without dismissing these considerations, and without impugning the professional treatment she received, it is possible to identify some important limitations to the conceptualization of her disturbances and treatment efforts. It is, of course, impossible to establish that a broader appreciation of social dimensions would have led to more effective results, although one may argue for the plausibility of this thesis. In any event, our concern here is instructional, and the reader can draw his own conclusions about the record of intervention and the critical judgments which our perspective inclines us to suggest.

Psychological reductionism. There was a conspicuous tendency for clinicians to reduce her problem to an intrapsychic personality problem of developmental origin. The following notes are illustrative:

The impression is that this is a woman who has been somewhat of a mixed neurotic most of her life who is showing considerable depression, probably associated with early involutional changes—or rather her feelings about these changes. . . .

The patient was sent here for psychiatric treatment. It was apparent that she had a basic personality disturbance and in an attempt to control the point that it was beginning to disturb her normal social and family life. She was in the involutional age. She had some depression, some anxiety and was a rather hostile, outspoken individual. Electric shock treatment was considered initially; however, after she was placed on Deprol, her depression subsided sufficiently so it was felt that convulsive therapy was not warranted at this particular time. . . . FINAL DIAGNOSIS: Psychoneurotic reaction, anxiety, and depression.[14]

While it may be assumed that Mrs. Nelson's reactions to menopause would be influenced by her personality (as would anyone else's), the view that this was a neurotic crisis has qualities of prejudgment and encapsulation. No developmental information is offered in support of that conclusion, and no reference is made to external events or her life situation, which might be weighed against or integrated into that conclusion. Why did she become grossly symptomatic at this particular time? Why did she show her specific symptoms of anxiety, depression, and drinking? Within *any* conceptual model, what was she depressed *about*, anxious *about*, or nervous *about*?

Solipsism refers to the philosophical view that only the self exists and that only the self is an object of verifiable knowledge. It is apparently the implicit perspective with which clinicians regarded Mrs. Nelson's case. There is little evidence of any effort to document or analyze the remarkable external realities of her life situation and their possible impact on a relatively "healthy personality"—not to mention one judged as having a *persistent neurotic conflict*.

Taking a life-situational approach to this case as part of the research method revealed a number of important facts. The onset of Mrs. Nelson's depression was associated in time with the death of a sister. Her symptoms subsequently waxed and waned in conjunction with a number of personal "crises," broken by intervals. After her sister's untimely death, her son went off to college. She began to experience an intensive need for affection from her husband. On one occasion, shortly after he left home, she flew several hundred miles to tell him, "You forgot to kiss me good-bye." Subsequently Mrs. Nelson's elderly and ailing mother came to live with her and became an expensive and difficult management problem. Her mother suffered a stroke and was placed in an institution. Mrs. Nelson again experienced acute nervousness and depression. A gynecologist informed her that she was going through menopause. Due to her persistent symptoms she saw a local psychiatrist. After her mother's death Mrs. Nelson displayed increasing nervousness, depression, and alcohol abuse. These symptoms abated periodically—to be exacerbated by other family deaths.

Beyond personality. To be sure, not all clinicians were unmindful of the various meanings of menopause. Yet apparently no one looked far beyond the boundaries of personality to environmental events. There were no formulations or inquiries, for example of the family, even as a system of interacting personalities. There was no substantial exploration of the family as a sociocultural system in change, disorganization, and reorganization. The husband, to the extent that he was consulted at all, was treated as a source of diagnostic information regarding his *wife's problem*.

The personal and system problems implicated in this case—and the definitions elicited in response to them—may be conceived as basic problems in the sociology and social psychology of the life cycle. With reference to the concepts of the family life cycle and developmental tasks, the reallocation of expressive and instrumental functions in conjunction with changes in family composition implicates both personal problems of adaptation and system problems of accommodation.[15] It may be expected that when Mr. Nelson confronts a de facto change in his relationships to work—for example, retirement—he may incur a profound personal crisis. A number of sociological papers have suggested that role changes associated with the life cycle may constitute crises contributory to illness.[16]

Treatment Contacts

Contact with "outside" professional sources of help is probably generally a reluctant and tardy response. It may be usefully viewed as socially motivated in many guises. As such, it is a special effort at reequilibration.

Perhaps most typically, recourse to professional help reflects the limiting conditions of tolerance being exceeded by cumulative stress, dangerous behavior, unpredictability, or the capacity for accommodation. That treatment contacts occur despite denial, uncertainty, and conflicting definitions of the existence of illness reflects their social control functions.

For some patients treatment is an act of reluctant compliance, an effort to regain entry into the family, job, or community. For others it is a voluntary effort to change themselves and the social systems of which they are a part. Too often, as in this case, there are conflicting social motives in seeking or failing to seek professional help. And perhaps too often, clinicians are insufficiently aware of the social struggle that prologues treatment contacts; wittingly or unwittingly clinicians may ally themselves with the patient or family members or otherwise neglect the social foundations of treatment contacts.

The Clinician and the Social System

In keeping with the spirit of this book, I hope various clinicians will make independent judgments of the clinical implications of these observations and concepts. I shall attempt to suggest briefly some of my own.

First, I believe that they offer extensions and alternatives to the personality and biological models which still dominate mental health approaches. While American psychiatry has always recognized the importance of social factors, sociological data and concepts have not been as systematically incorporated into the field's mainstream perspectives and practices. Whatever validity and utility there might be in conceptualizing Mrs. Nelson's disturbances in terms of personality or biology, it is clear that preoccupation with such concepts would result in reductionistic errors of omission and commission. Similarly, intervention in this case implies a family-centered approach. The particular concepts considered are specifically useful to the social diagnosis and social therapy of families confronted with severe psychiatric disturbances. These families require special attention to the social processes of deviance, conflict, and social control. However, these types of data and concepts have broad application to the full variety of psychiatric disturbances; to primary, secondary, and tertiary intervention; and to individual or group therapy.

The concept of equilibrium in social systems not only specifically increases our understanding of social processes, but provides an important bridge among biologic, sociologic, and psychologic systems. The concept of equilibrium moves us beyond the static confines of "structure" (whether it be biologic, psychologic, or social) and into the areas of *process* and *change.*

Beyond their informational and conceptual implications, these studies imply the need for a reexamination of therapeutic roles. Clinicians are faced with "presenting problems" which imply not only the "treatment" of some special class of problems, but the restoration of equilibrium in these multiple systems. This does not mean that the clinician's client shifts from the patient to the family (which is one possibility); it does mean that his treatment of the patient must have reference to the family system.

Sometimes, it seems to me, there is a curious bias in psychoanalytic psychotherapy. It tends to view the patient's group as a source of his problem, as a context which thwarts his growth, development, and autonomy. To this must be added a corrective which recognizes human groups—particularly primary groups—as a setting in which the individual inevitably strives to fulfill some of his most important needs, and which, indeed, enables him to do so.

Some studies have indicated that the best predictor of the post-hospital performances of severely disturbed patients is a relatively high level of family expectations.[17] A possible implication of this finding is that despite the deviance and symptomatology which these patients had exhibited, the family still regarded them as important members; were important sources of support; and provided the patients with motivation to restore their health and social functioning.

The progressive attrition of roles assigned to the patient—due to accommodation—may thus be antitherapeutic. Paradoxically, as the individual is charged with fewer roles, his deviance has less impact, and he may function at lower levels without risk of sanctioning or treatment efforts. This is exemplified in the "downward spiral" of chronic alcoholics. Family ties are broken, and they slide into less demanding occupational roles which will tolerate their deviance. This may have a double-edged result: It may prompt the disturbed person to make an extraordinary effort to regain important relationships and roles, or it may encourage him to slip into increasingly lower levels of adaptation. The efficacy of "artificial" helping groups, such as Alcoholics Anonymous, may be that they function as surrogate primary groups. Similarly, family-centered and other group therapies may gain unique therapeutic properties by simulating natural groups.

The reequilibrating role of the therapist may oblige him to re-examine the confines of the doctor-patient relationship and the problems and prospects of its extension to other family members. There is substantial evidence that clinicians generally hold rather limited, specialized role conceptions. Efforts at "comprehensive" care are still plagued with the problem of differentiating and coordinating the roles of the *team*.

It is clear that the functions of defining the nature and implications of illness and deviance to patients and family members, of social diagnosis and social therapy, are not being adequately addressed.[18] The application of social science requires not only incorporation of a body of knowledge, but its integration into a system of professional roles. But that is another story.

NOTES

1. Homeostasis: a relatively stable state of equilibrium or tendency toward such a state between the different but interdependent elements or groups of elements of an organism or group. *Webster's Seventh New Collegiate Dictionary*, p. 398.

2. See, for example, Shirley S. Angrist, Mark Lefton, Simon Dinitz, and Benjamin Pasamanick, *Women After Treatment* (New York: Appleton-Century-Crofts, 1968); John Clausen and Marian Radke Yarrow, issue eds., "The Impact of Mental Illness on the Family," *Journal of Social Issues* 11, no. 4 (Spring 1955); Alfred Dean, "Alcoholism and Social Structure: A Sociological Study of Illness, Deviance and Social Response" (Ph.D. diss., University of North Carolina, Chapel Hill, 1965); Howard E. Freeman and Ozzie G. Simmons, *The Mental Patient Comes Home* (New York: Wiley, 1963); Joan K. Jackson and Kate L. Kogan, "The Search for Solutions: Help-seeking Patterns of Families of Active and Inactive Alcoholics," *Quarterly Journal of Studies on Alcohol* 24 (September 1963): 449–472; Marjorie Fiske Lowenthal, *Lives in Distress: The Paths of the Elderly to the Psychiatric Ward* (New York: Basic Books, 1964); Benjamin Pasamanick, Frank R. Scarpitti, and Simon Dinitz, *Schizophrenics in the Community: An Experimental Study in the Prevention of Hospitalization* (New York: Appleton-Century-Crofts, 1967); Harold Sampson, Sheldon L. Messinger, and Robert D. Towne, "Family Processes and Becoming a Mental Patient," *American Journal of Sociology* 68 (July 1962): 88–96; Charlotte Green Schwartz, "Perspectives on Deviance—Wives' Definitions of Their Husbands' Mental Illness," *Psychiatry* 20 (August 1957): 275–291; Carroll A. Whitmer and Glen C. Conover, "A Study of Critical Incidents in the Hospitalization of Mentally Ill," *Journal of the National Association of Social Work* 4 (January 1959): 89–94; and Edwin C. Wood, John M. Rakusin, and Emanuel Morse, "Interpersonal Aspects of Psychiatric Hospitalization," *Archives of General Psychiatry* 3 (December 1960): 443–454.

3. For a review of our prior examination of the family, see Chapters 4, 7, and 10. There is a wide range of literature on the family in sociology. See, for example,

Harold T. Christensen, ed., *Handbook of Marriage and the Family* (Chicago: Rand McNally, 1964); Robert O. Blood, Jr., *Marriage,* 2nd ed. (New York: Free Press, 1969); Gerald R. Leslie, *The Family in Social Context* (New York: Oxford University Press, 1967); and Robert F. Winch and Louis W. Goodman, *Selected Studies in Marriage and the Family,* 3rd ed. (New York: Holt, Rinehart, 1968).

4. Jessie R. Pitts, "The Structural-Functional Approach," in *Handbook of Marriage,* ed. Christensen, p. 71. This article (pp. 51–124) also offers a further discussion of instrumental and expressive functions.

5. For a further appreciation of central trends and variant patterns in the family in American culture, see Ruth S. Cavan, "Subcultural Variations and Mobility," in *Handbook of Marriage,* ed. Christensen, pp. 535–585; Leslie, *Family in Social Context,* pp. 255–312; Lee Rainwater, "Crucible of Identity: The Negro Lower-Class Family," in *The Negro American,* ed. Talcott Parsons and Kenneth B. Clark (Boston: Houghton Mifflin, 1966), pp. 172–196; and Florence Kluckhohn, "Variations in the Basic Values of Family Systems," in *A Modern Introduction to the Family,* ed. Norman Bell and Ezra Vogel, rev. ed. (New York: Free Press, 1958), pp. 319–330.

6. For a more extensive examination of mental illness as deviant behavior, see Alfred Dean, "The Social System, Deviance, and Treatment Efforts," in *Further Explorations in Social Psychiatry,* ed. Berton H. Kaplan, Alexander Leighton, and Robert N. Wilson (New York: Basic Books, 1976), pp. 75–93.

7. See, for example, David J. Pittman and Charles R. Snyder, eds., *Alcohol, Culture and Drinking Patterns* (New York: Wiley, 1962).

8. For a further discussion of corrective roles, see Dean, "Social System."

9. For an analysis of the sick role, see Talcott Parsons, "Illness and the Role of the Physician: A Sociological Perspective," in *Personality in Nature, Society and Culture,* ed. Clyde Kluckhohn and Henry A. Murray, 2nd ed. (New York: Knopf, 1954), pp. 609–617, and Talcott Parsons and Renee C. Fox, "Illness, Therapy and the Urban American Family," in *Modern Introduction to the Family,* ed. Bell and Vogel, pp. 347–360.

10. There has been an unfortunate tendency in sociology to focus upon the *negative* consequences of deviance and conflict. While pointing to some of the problematics of deviance, I do not wish to imply that it is entirely, or even necessarily, dysfunctional. Deviance and conflict may signal an individual's inability or unwillingness to accept certain roles—and lead to changes which improve the gratifications of group members and the social system as a whole. On the other hand, suppression of deviance and conflict may lead to perpetuation of hidden dissatisfactions and oblique expressions of deviance, which become complex and destructive. In many respects this was the situation in the Nelson case, as is partly shown later in this paper. Thus the *clear identification* of role disturbances and conflict—and their *solution*—may *increase* group functioning and solidarity. See Lewis Coser, *The Functions of Social Conflict* (New York: Free Press, 1956).

11. See, for example, Clausen and Yarrow, "Impact of Mental Illness."

12. I have found that patients and family members *prefer* to define the nature of their problem in certain ways. They show an emotional investment in certain "definitions of the situation." In this case the patient regarded her drinking as the symptom of a problem, while her husband defined it as the source of the problem. Preferred definitions attempt to serve social and social psychological functions. See Dean, "Alcoholism and Social Structure," 517–533.

13. The concept of accommodation and its empirical referents, however, are developed differently by researchers. See Antonio J. Ferreira, "Family Myth and Homeostasis," *Archives of General Psychiatry* 9 (November 1963): 55–61; Dean, "Alcoholism and Social Structure"; and Sampson, Messinger, and Towne, "Family Processes."

14. Howard Psychiatric Hospital, *Admission and Discharge Report,* 4. Cited in Dean, "Alcoholism and Social Structure," p. 301.

15. Like the individual, the family goes through a life cycle which includes, for example, pre–child bearing, child rearing, and so on. Given the social psychological significance of the primary group, it is important to link our understanding of the individual and family life cycles. See Leslie, *Family in Social Context,* pp. 262–265 and passim.

16. Note, for example, Ruth Benedict's hypothesis about adolescent turmoil in American society (Chapter 8). See also Thomas H. Holmes and Richard Rahe, "The Social Readjustment Rating Scale," *Journal of Psychosomatic Research* 11 (1967): 213–218; J. Tyhurst, "The Role of Transition States—Including Disasters—in Mental Illness," *Symposium on Preventive and Social Psychiatry* (Washington, D.C.: Walter Reed Army Medical Center, 1957), pp. 149–167; and Robert N. Wilson, *The Sociology of Health: An Introduction* (New York: Random House, 1970), pp. 95–98.

17. See, for example, Freeman and Simmons, *Mental Patient Comes Home,* pp. 139 ff. and passim.

18. See Dean, "Social System."

COMMENTARY

Dean uses the case of the Nelson family to illustrate the complementarity of the social science perspective with the biological and psychological. The case demonstrates that the clinical problems of the identified patient, Mrs. Nelson, may be understood in three very different ways. The biological: She was undergoing a major endocrinologic dysfunction associated with the menopause and characterized by depression, anxiety, and alcoholism. The psychological: Given the "premorbid personality structure" of a passive dependent character type, Mrs. Nelson decompensated under the stress of losing several important love subjects. Unable to express her anger adequately and appropriately, she turned it on herself, becoming depressed, and through her alcoholism expressing helplessness, anger, and a plea for help. The social: After thirty years of marriage the Nelson family structure and therefore its functions were undergoing some radical changes. The children were growing more independent, no longer requiring of Mrs. Nelson the same kind of mothering functions. The parents and older siblings of Mr. and Mrs. Nelson were of an age where their health and survival were in jeopardy. The independence of the children left the marital couple increasingly alone with each other and required the further evolution of their relationship, a task the Nelsons had not yet accomplished.

These three alternative viewpoints, while capable of articulation independent of each other, are each incomplete. Each offers important but partial insights. Without diminishing the relevance of biological or psychoanalytic concepts, Dean identifies sociological elements of this case which appear to require further development and integration into a comprehensive perspective.

Dean's analysis demonstrates that concepts and theories serve not only to organize data, but to direct observation. The following further illustrate clinically relevant inquiries suggested by sociological concepts.

What of the deaths of significant persons following in tragic succession? What import can be attached to the apparent coincidence of the initial loss of her sister with the onset of depression? What of the patterned association between the loss of significant persons—primary relationships—and the vicissitudes of symptomatic behavior? Of what significance is her son's going off to college and the same prospect arising for her daughter? Even if Mrs. Nelson had not become grossly symptomatic and deviant, was not the prior social system already substantially disequilibrated? Can her compulsion to give gifts to old ladies (subsequent to her mother's death), and her hostile behavior toward family members, be reduced to "neurotic fears and doubts stirred up by the involutional period"?

What is the objective and subjective significance of menopause? Is it simply a biochemical upheaval marked by demonstrable periods of nervousness and depression? Is it an upheaval of the id, marked by primitive reveries and regression? Is it a symbol of aging, decline, social change, and death? How do individuals deal with these universal experiences—and with what chemistries of personality, culture, and social networks? What is the function of religion here? Did anyone record: Religious Background: Catholic; Current Religious Affiliation: Episcopalian? *And what might be made of it? What is the role of religious belief in the experience of aging, death, and other crises? What is the role of primary relationships in the communication, ventilation, working through, and interpersonal support for emotional crises? Are these sociocultural and social-psychological processes mere* epiphenomena compared to the massive realities of unconscious, neurotic phenomena? *Is their understanding and manipulation so feebly significant compared to the remedies of medication and insight psychotherapy?*

This paper also moves beyond a view of a patient with problems to a social system faced with stress, deviance, disorganization, conflict, and change. A number of questions are also stimulated by this perspective. Have the clinicians' perspectives of Mrs. Nelson's "intrapsychic disturbances" unwittingly aligned them with Mr. Nelson and preservation of the status quo? Does therapy imply an effort to assist family members to new social relationships and a reorganization of roles? Are the conflicting views of Mr. and Mrs. Nelson regarding the nature and causes of her disturbance a matter for redefinition by the clinician? Do the conflicting interests of Mr. and Mrs. Nelson in stability versus change serve to undermine psychotherapy? Does Szasz' argument with the "myth" of "mental illness" apply here?

These are among the difficult but inviting questions which reward our efforts to obtain and integrate multiple perspectives. The reward is a broader and deeper understanding of the adaptive and adjustive processes implicated in the lives of patients.

PART IV

THE MENTAL HEALTH SYSTEM IN SOCIETY

CHAPTER 22

The Mental Health System in Society

Bert Pepper

The editors have designed this book to lead along a twisted but continuous path: from the fertile plains of basic social science definitions and concepts, through the canyons of the conceptual bases of treatment for individuals and for groups, into and beyond the thicket of challenges to the medical model, and now into the crowded cosmopolitan environment of our contemporary society, where all of these ideas and forces play upon each other.

Whether a tree falling in the forest causes a sound in the absence of a listener is a fascinating philosophical question which is of little concern to pragmatists. Similarly, whether mental disorder can exist in an individual in the absence of a society to help create and observe it is interesting, but irrelevant for all practical purposes. The editors believe that it has been demonstrated that the elements of each kind of mental disorder and sociocultural structures are inexorably interdependent with regard to causation, labeling, classification, and response. Even a nutritional deficiency psychosis is in part dependent on the food-raising and feeding habits of both the culture and the individual. Chemically produced psychoses are dependent on others in the community for at least one of several elements: laboratory synthesis; cultivation and gathering of mushroom, poppy, or hemp; or the distribution and sale arrangements of the "drug *culture*."

The eternal interdependence of psychological, biological, and social factors has been noted in earlier chapters. No behavioral expression of a psychological state is properly interpreted in isolation; some consideration of the biological and social context seems essential.

Even before arriving at behavior, one may need to consider a socio-cultural context in order to understand thought and feeling. One of Harry Stack Sullivan's special contributions to psychoanalysis was to demonstrate that even the "unique"—dereistic or autistic—thoughts of the schizophrenic person have an interpersonal basis. He created the term *parataxic distortion* to describe the patient's highly individual-istic interpretation of family of social events.

Who Should Be Treated: The Individual or Society?

Many authoritative mental health professionals recommend that the treatment system limit its activities to direct services to symptomatic individuals, leaving the responsibility for changing society to others. Political scientists, politicians, and interested citizens may be con-sidered as competent as or more competent than health professionals to deal with "treating" or changing society and the world. In a sense, such an attitude eliminates the possibility of effectively preventing mental disorders, since preventive efforts require both better adap-tation of the individual to community demands, and the reverse as well. The family and small social system communities of the patient need assistance in carrying out their tasks if the individual is to retain or regain a normal role and status in society. While the patient may have to give up certain completely unacceptable deviant behaviors, the community in turn may be called upon to redefine some categories of deviance, and thus relabel some behaviors as within normal limits.

Over the last few decades some developing nations have been able to learn from the experiences of countries which developed their mental disorder attitudes and treatment systems some time ago. Ni-geria, for example, has made efforts to minimize the stigmatizing labeling which occurs when mentally ill persons are removed from their home communities and placed in psychiatric hospitals. The Ni-gerian government essentially elected to avoid development of a psy-chiatric hospital system. Instead, a primary focus has been placed upon maintaining psychiatrically ill persons in special communities where they can be brought together for treatment efforts during the day, but return to foster families and normal village life in the evening, so as to prevent community exclusion or extrusion.

Correlations Between Environmental Patterns and Mental Disorders

While many interactions between each person and society are doubt-less individualistic, identifiable patterns exist. Some of these lead to the development of the kinds of thinking and behavior which we have come to call mental illness or mental disorder. These causal and re-sponsive reactions have been studied over the last several decades by numerous psychiatric epidemiologists and social scientists, and a great deal of specific information has been gathered. The next two chapters provide extensive reviews of these studies, coupled with thoughtful analyses from quite different perspectives.

The basic method of epidemiologic studies is to look for correlations between classes of events; in terms of our particular interests, correlations between socioenvironmental conditions and specific psychiatric states. The conditions found to be relevant are diverse and, at first glance, seemingly unrelated. A sample list includes financial status, social mobility, ethnicity, national unemployment and economic conditions, war, the presence of lead or other toxins in the environment of developing children, nutritional opportunities and customs, types of housing, population density, and the incidence of certain mental disorders in blood relatives. Much can be learned by analysis of correlations of such factors with the occurrence of cases of schizophrenia, manic-depressive psychosis, and other mental disorders. But cautious interpretation is required; such broad generalizations as "mental illness is increasing in frequency because of the stress of modern society" or "mental illness is much more common among the poor" have no basis in the data, and are counterproductive to our scientific, professional, and humane goals.

Two consequences flow from epidemiologic research efforts. The first is that some specific socially based etiologic factors of particular psychiatric disorders have been identified. The second is that more focused preventive programs and treatment modalities have been designed. For example, knowledge of increased risk to the bereaved and to immigrants has led to effective preventive efforts directed at the recently widowed and the recently arrived.

Crisis Intervention—From Hypotheses to Modalities

Recent developments in the theory and practice of crisis intervention have created a practical and successful approach to providing effective early intervention by the combined use of all available approaches. Chapter 27 reviews this subject in detail. Briefly, it involves prompt evaluation of the psychological, biological, and social aspects of a state of acute mental disequilibrium in a personal or family system. The first approach is investigative—to identify all known or suspected causes of the loss of homeostasis in the individual-family system. While multifactorial analysis of the causes of disruption is still being worked on, treatment of each identified aspect is undertaken immediately and simultaneously. The primary goal of intervention may be defined as assisting in the development of a new balance point for the individual, family, and personal community as quickly as possible, to prevent the role of deviant from being permanently ascribed. This approach has been so effective that a second goal is set by many practitioners: to assist the individual in arriving at a new balance which is even more productive and satisfying than the one which preceded the crisis.

A cautionary note may be in order when dealing with the subject of prevention and early intervention: It seems possible to go too far in identifying society as the culprit, and weighting efforts at intervention and change exclusively in the direction of the community. All available evidence supports the notion that social labels, categories of deviant behavior, and responses to social deviance are legitimate and essential functions of each culture. Role assignments and limitations on the behavior of the individual are probably as necessary as are positive social reinforcers in the effort to make individual *Homo sapiens* into a social animal who can live, work, and play in groups. These functions are not limited to human societies alone; innumerable studies in animal ethology show that animal groups have cultures with similar rules. Indeed, human ethologists have showed that many of our own social rules are directly derivative of or identical to those of some animal societies.

Cultural Change and Social Balance

After giving full recognition to the points made above—the need for limits on the behavior of the individual; the need for role assignments; the value of both negative and positive rewards for behaviors, as judged by sociocultural values—there still seems to be plenty of room for movement. Interested parties may legitimately seek experimentation and change. The fact that a set of rules of conduct and a structured public order are essential does not assure us that our present structures are either perfect, require their present degree of stringency, or are incapable of being improved upon.

But there are intrinsic problems in altering things, the first being that newness is always frightening. Impending or actual social change invariably causes a fear reaction: "What are we coming to? . . . Our national standards are declining. . . . Our social fabric is being rent asunder!" In fact, analysis of different cultures can give us confidence that the social fabric is quite strong and resilient, rather than fragile and brittle. If we take advantage of its elasticity in a careful way it need not be as confining to the individual as it has been. Of course there are limits to the degree of safe relaxation of social rules and, regrettably, the only way to learn that we have gone beyond the limit of elasticity is by experiment: When the tolerance has been exceeded and a small tear develops, a slight step backward is necessary so that it can be repaired.

There is no need, however, to go back to the starting point of the experiment. For example, in order to deal with the excessive use of psychiatric hospitalization in the United States over the last century—

this matter is reviewed at length in Chapter 29—successful efforts have been mounted in recent years to reduce both the frequency and length of state hospitalization. This change has apparently gone too far in some places and produced a new social problem, straining the social fabric. Large numbers of seriously mentally disordered persons are now living without care or treatment in single-room occupancies in welfare hotels, where they often have substandard living conditions and intermittent or token care and treatment. It would seem appropriate for mental health professionals and civil libertarians to recognize that the movement against hospitalization may have gone too far in some areas. Perhaps they should now provide impetus and direction for a review of care and treatment policies and practices for seriously and chronically mentally disordered persons, aimed at providing them with a socially and professionally acceptable treatment and care system—be it based in hospitals, hospital-like institutions, or adequate congregate living facilities in the community.

Both theory and analysis teach us that all systems in nature try to retain the balance arrived at at any point in time. This is true of the mental health system in society: homeostasis requires the system to stabilize society's expectations of its members, the behavior of individuals, and methods of professional response toward mentally ill persons. Chapter 28 is devoted to some consequences of this last point.

Several techniques are regularly used by mental health and other social systems to maintain homeostatic balance. The first is simply to resist all attempts at change: "Why do we bathe patients this way?" "Why, it's always been done like this, even before I started working here." Or, "Why don't we do it that way?" "We *never* have done it that way!" The second stabilizing technique is to deny that there are any difficulties in the present arrangements; if accepted, this obviates any need for change: "This hospital takes pretty good care of these chronic patients, even if they aren't being actively treated. Even if we had the staff, most of them wouldn't get better anyway. Besides, most of them like it here, and don't even want to leave."

A third technique for stabilization, when it must be admitted that there is a problem and that some change is necessary, is to limit and delay necessary alterations in the system for as long as possible. Many successful governors and other public officials have completed their terms of office reasonably successfully by following this rule: Never do today what you can possibly put off until tomorrow. The director of a large and famous state hospital responded to a staff recommendation that a day treatment program be started by agreeing that it was probably a good idea. But, he argued, he was about to retire, beginning such a new program would require a lot of effort on his part, and he didn't feel up to it. He thereby delayed the change for a decade, for he did not retire for nine more years.

The methods touched upon in the preceding paragraphs are assisted by a fourth, ritualization, which gives an added and special value to elements of the present balance. Even when the efficacy of a present method cannot be supported, it may be continued on the grounds of respect for tradition. Innumerable patients in general hospitals have unsuccessfully railed against the time-honored procedure of waking patients at 5:00 or 6:00 A.M. for a 9:00 A.M. breakfast, only to find that the culture of the nursing department had elevated these procedures above criticism; they had acquired the value of tribal traditions. In a related way, psychiatric methods of organizing staffs into separate inpatient and outpatient clinic departments have gained ritualistic value and meaning, despite the resultant failure to provide necessary continuity of treatment. By becoming part of the historic tradition of psychiatric hospitals and university departments of psychiatry, such structures have become virtually inaccessible to scientific critique. Alternative forms, as recommended in Chapters 15 and 28, can thus be disregarded.

Proposals for change may also be met by a fifth method of maintaining the status quo—requiring an innovation to meet a significantly higher standard of proof of efficacy than present methods: "Maybe that *would* be better than what we do now, but at least our present method does *some* good; it's unwise to switch horses in midstream."

To the extent that mental health professionals wish to make the field more rational and scientific at some necessary sacrifice of tradition, effort is required in order to gain distance from the participant viewpoint. A slightly distant perspective, permitting an observer role, is necessary if a balanced and more objective conception of alternatives is to be gained. Such a goal, while held worthy by most, is rendered difficult by the fact that most *are* direct participants in the mental health system—whether as therapists, planners, or administrators. As such, we are all agents of homeostasis, and this tends to lead the kinds of resistance to change discussed above as challenges—such as are offered throughout this volume—to the present system are proposed.

CHAPTER 23

Patterns: A Key to Causes

INTRODUCTION

Psychiatric epidemiology provides the general mental health field with a set of basic and proven research techniques—an investigative tool kit—essential in attempts to understand causes, effectiveness of treatment, prognosis, and interactions between mentally disordered persons and their social settings. It bridges and interconnects the fields of biological, psychological, and social research. As Gruenberg points out, the apparent dichotomy between medical-biological research and social research is a relatively recent fiction; Hippocrates saw them as two sides of the same coin.

The following reading surveys epidemiologic approaches, techniques, and findings. It brings together several kinds of research which are often thought of separately: clinical study of medical disorders in animal models; studies in animal and human ethology; biostatistical evaluations of mental health service programs; sociological research into the origins of mental disorders; genetic work; psychodynamic studies; identification of iatrogenic syndromes—the list could go on indefinitely.

Mental health professionals have always had an epidemiological perspective on the cases they care for: They have an idea whether the conditions are becoming more common, and ideas about the circumstances under which a particular condition is likely to arise. Such ideas are generally based on their teachers' loosely formulated notions, combined with their own unique background and personal clinical experience.

In the last decade organized epidemiological information about mental disorders has begun to become integrated into the formal training of mental health professionals. Knowledge accumulated in the last thirty years thus becomes the common property of all the mental health professions, and areas of debate and uncertainty are reduced. Of course, what is not yet known remains a vast area for future work.

The group that wrote the following selection was headed by Ernest Gruenberg, a foremost contributor to our epidemiologic knowledge over the past thirty years. The article offers a basic survey of methods and their uses, as well as a broad review of key findings regarding the major mental disorders.

THE EPIDEMIOLOGY OF MENTAL DISORDERS

Ernest M. Gruenberg, Danielle M. Terns, and Bert Pepper

Definition

Psychiatric epidemiology has been defined as "the study of the occurrence of mental disorder within a specified population." [1] It concerns itself with *patterns* of occurrence; with the ecologic and human factors which influence these patterns; and with studying the outcome of attempts to alter these factors. It is both a basic and an applied science which helps to suggest, define, and evaluate strategies to prevent and control mental disorders. By relating the distribution, incidence, and duration of disorders to the physical, biological, and social environment in which people live, epidemiology results in what Gordon [2] calls "medical ecology." Epidemiology is the scientific basis of preventive medicine and preventive psychiatry.

Historical Review

Knowledge of medical epidemiological facts can be found early in the history of mankind, as witnessed by the Mosaic Laws (1200 B.C.) stipulating dietary rules and prescriptions for isolating the lepers and the sick, and for disposing of the dead. Hippocrates (460 B.C.) may be considered the first true epidemiologist. He recognized that disease is a mass phenomenon, as well as one affecting the sick individual; he differentiated between epidemic and endemic distributions, and noted the association of disease with environmental factors.

The first major successful applications of epidemiological methods came in the nineteenth century and resulted in the control of smallpox, cholera, yellow fever, and other infectious diseases. Successes in the early twentieth century led to breakthroughs in noninfectious deficiency conditions such as scurvy, pellagra, and beriberi.

Most early studies concentrated on finding a single, primary cause for a disease, but it became apparent that other matters required consideration: Why do some people escape illness when exposed to the same agent that caused illness in others? What factors determined death for one sufferer and recovery for another? These questions led to a serious consideration of *host factors*—determining the vulnerability of the individual—and *environmental factors*. Such studies led to research into the multifactorial etiology of diseases and paved the way for the sophisticated study of mental disorders.

Incidence and Prevalence Rates

These words distinguish the two most common ways of measuring the frequency of a disorder. The *annual incidence rate* is the number of new cases which develop in a population during a year, divided by the population. This is usually multiplied by 1,000 or 100,000 to produce the annual incidence rate per thousand or per hundred thousand population. On rare occasions the incidence rate is calculated per month, per decade, or for some other time unit.

The *prevalence rate* is the number of cases present in a population. Diseases which occur frequently but which are of short duration, such as measles, have a high incidence rate and a low prevalence rate. A disease which generally lasts longer than a year, such as chronic schizophrenia, has a prevalence which is greater than its incidence. In a general way the prevalence rate of a condition is equal to the annual incidence rate multiplied by the average number of years the cases last, that is, their average duration. "Prevalence" and "incidence" are defined here as generally used today. These technical epidemiological definitions, however, are not used in this precise way by all writers and the reader can expect to find them used in their older, more general meaning—as synonyms for "frequency," and for each other.

Uses of Epidemiology

Morris[3] noted seven uses for epidemiologic studies in medicine: (1) to study historical trends; (2) for community diagnosis; (3) to study the working of health services; (4) to estimate individual risks; (5)

to complete the clinical picture; (6) to identify syndromes; and (7) to search for causes. These categories have been helpful in organizing this article.

Study of Historical Trends

We know that some mental disorders are sources of increasing concern, while others are on the wane. Expert opinion [4] in 1961 agreed that general paresis, pellagra psychosis, and conversion hysteria were occurring with significantly decreased frequency. In the case of general paresis, the decline in incidence can be documented by a review of mental hospital admission data, and can be attributed largely to the use of drug treatment—arsphenamine (Salvarsan) and later, penicillin. Reasons for the decrease in pellagra psychosis are less clear; no specific program of prevention or treatment was introduced, and yet this condition declined in frequency after it was identified as a nutritional deficiency in the 1920s. As with general paresis, we can document a decline of hospital admissions for the treatment of pellagra psychosis. In the case of conversion hysteria, the conclusion that there has been a marked decrease in incidence is based solely on expert opinion, since this was not a condition usually treated by hospitalization.

From the above comments we can surmise that statistical data are helpful, but not absolutely necessary, in making judgments about the changing incidence of certain conditions. Statistical recording of the occurrence of diseases is a relatively recent phenomenon, although we can safely assume that diseases were changing their patterns of occurrence prior to the collection of data. Even when we have data, interpretation requires awareness of changing styles in the use of diagnostic labels and treatment modalities.

We know that some conditions have increased because of medical or technical advances. Prolonging the life of infants with Down's Syndrome (mongolism) by treating their frequent, previously fatal, respiratory infections with new antibiotic drugs has made prevalence rise, as shown by Carter.[5]

New pesticides and pharmacologic substances—cortisone, amphetamines, and LSD are a few examples—have caused new toxic psychoses. Drug addiction has risen in incidence, illustrated by the fact that in New York City the number of deaths from narcotic abuse has quintupled since 1960;[6] the increase has been most notable in persons under age twenty. Simultaneously, the number of subtypes of addiction has increased due to the laboratory development of barbiturates, amphetamines, minor tranquilizers, and methadone. Goldhamer and Marshall [7] demonstrated a striking rise in the admission rates of the elderly to state hospitals over time; this trend, apparently due to an increase in longevity as well as changing social conditions which pressed for removal from community to hospital, continued unabated through the mid-1960s, when new public policies stemmed the tide. Interestingly, the data revealed no major increase in the rate of functional psychosis first admissions for persons *under* age sixty-five.

Community Diagnosis

Community diagnosis estimates the nature and size of a health problem. Since the 1963 Comprehensive Community Mental Health Center legislation, the need to plan centers produced a demand for persons with epidemiological expertise to provide quantified information about service needs.

The first approximation of a community's mental disorder cases can be obtained by counting cases in treatment (by private practitioners and community agencies). Hollingshead and Redlich [8] did this for New Haven, Connecticut, and found that the rate of psychotic conditions in treatment was 139/100,000 in the lowest social class (V) and only 104/100,000 in all other social classes combined. This was not true of the neurosis cases. A picture of this kind is important in understanding how many cases there are and where they are to be found.

But identifying and counting cases in treatment and describing and analyzing their personal characteristics gives only a general picture of the number and kinds of psychiatric disorders and the segments of the community which contain them. Epidemiologists have long known that these cases in treatment are only the tip of an iceberg; several times as many cases are not known to clinicians. Srole and his associates [9] reported that only 5 percent of impaired individuals were in treatment at the time of the "Midtown" survey, and Gruenberg,[10] in the Syracuse Survey of the Elderly, found four untreated "certifiable" cases for each one actually in the hospital.

If we examine all members of a community and sort them into sick and well at the time of examination, we are conducting what is called a morbidity survey. Such a prevalence survey (often done on only a random sample of members of a community) reports rates which depend both on the criteria for labeling used to distinguish a "case" from other people, and on how hard the investigators searched for these cases. These two factors vary so much between surveys that they can account for almost all the variations in the findings of various community surveys.[11]

The relationship often reported between low socioeconomic status (SES) and high rates of severe mental disorders is most striking in studies which deal only with treated cases. This may be because lower-class people tend to be sent for treatment to understaffed state hospitals, where they are treated by the least trained staff for longer periods of time.[12] In studies which have surveyed an entire population intensively, the narrow variation of SES in those test communities has not permitted an adequate study of this relationship. In studies where there are large SES variations in the population, the diagnostic criteria are too soft to relate SES to standard diagnostic terminology. In the Midtown study Srole [13] reported a higher proportion of psychiatrically "impaired" persons in the lower SES groups, but we do not know to what nosologic or diagnostic categories the "impaired" belong.

Factors other than SES influence community rates. In Chicago, Faris and Dunham [14] found that high admission rates for schizophrenia existed in certain census tracts, while other tracts had high rates of manic-depressive psychosis or organic psychosis. The high schizophrenia rate tracts were located in the deteriorating center of the city— the business district and rooming house areas—characterized by social disorganization. It appears that specific community characteristics may affect the occurrence of some specific mental disorders more than others.

There are, in addition, other factors, such as age, sex, and marital status, which affect the risk of mental disorders. For example, Hagnell,[15] Srole and associates,[16] Leighton and associates,[17] and Gruenberg [18] found that increased rates of mental disorders—defined either as "mental illness," "incapacitated," "most certainly psychiatrically impaired," or "certifiable"—were associated with rising age. So the demographic makeup of communities is to be taken into consideration when comparing their overall crude morbidity rates. "Adjusting for" demographic factors is a standard statistical tool in such studies.

Working of Mental Health Services

Studies of how services actually work provide information as to why some patients are in the visible (treated) tip of the iceberg while many others are below the water line, undiagnosed, untreated, and unknown to treatment agencies.

Admission rates to psychiatric services depend on factors other than illnesses. These other factors include: (1) the geographic availability of treatment centers; (2) the acceptability of available facilities to the population; (3) characteristics of the community; and (4) personal characteristics of patients.

Differences in service utilization rates between communities do not necessarily tell us anything about the incidence of disorders. For example, in 1886 Jarvis [19] demonstrated that admission rates to mental hospitals are higher in populations geographically close to the hospital and lower in communities located far away (Jarvis' law of distance). When a facility is well accepted by the community, its residents will be less reluctant to send their sick members for treatment there. This may be an explanation of why Dutchess County, New York, for example, has one of the highest admission rates among New York State counties—Hudson River State Hospital is a major job provider and everybody knows somebody who works there.

Regarding characteristics of a community, controlling for distance, rural areas tend to send fewer people to mental hospitals than urban ones, and small cities in general have lower admission rates than large cities.[20] Admissions within a city may vary according to the types and conditions of housing.[21] Controlling for the effect of economic status, the rate of first admissions of elderly persons to mental hospitals was found to be higher in urban areas with apartment houses, and lower in single-family home areas. Wealthy and poor areas of each type had approximately equal admission rates.

Personal characteristics of patients also affect utilization rates. In general, blacks, the poor, and the unmarried are hospitalized more frequently[22] and remain hospitalized for longer periods of time. Private hospitals tend to treat more patients from the upper SES categories. Outpatient clinics deal with a younger and higher SES population than the state hospitals. Last, but not least, the nature of the psychiatric disorder for which a person is treated determines the kind of facility to which he or she goes. As a general rule, severely mentally ill persons go to public hospitals, while those who are less impaired go to outpatient clinics or general hospital inpatient psychiatric units.

Table 1[23] compares admissions to all United States psychiatric facilities in 1970. The diagnostic distribution discriminates clearly between outpatient and inpatient services and also shows a differential use of hospitals according to their sponsorship. The lower section of the table rank orders admission rates: private hospital admissions are dominated by neuroses, while schizophrenia is the leading diagnosis for state hospitals. When all facilities are combined, it is interesting to note that neuroses are the most commonly treated conditions, followed by schizophrenia and alcoholism, while manic-depressive psychosis contributes very little to the overall pattern.

But any interpretation based on such statistics ought to recognize that utilization rates, particularly those of public inpatient facilities, are highly sensitive to social and administrative policies. In the last twenty years the number of admissions to state hospitals had markedly increased while the number of resident patients had dropped by about 50 percent, facts which do not reflect a change in incidence or prevalence of mental disorders and can be related directly to implementation of new policies.

As an example, let us consider what happened to state hospitals' patterns of hospitalization. From 1945 on, the resident patient population had been growing at a steady rate, reaching an all-time high of 560,000 in 1955.[24] A slow decline which began in 1956 can be credited to the introduction of neuroleptic drugs. However, in 1960 the number was still 535,000. At that time a systematic policy to release patients promptly was initiated, based on the successful results of British hospital reform (reduction of patient census there had preceded the use of neuroleptics). Criteria for both admission and release were liberalized; as a result, the resident patient census dropped as the number of admissions increased, transforming the custodial hospitals into short-term intensive therapy centers. It is useful

TABLE 1

Number, Percent Distribution, Rated per 100,000 Population and Rank Order of Admissions to Psychiatric Faculties by Diagnosis and Type of Facility, United States, 1970

Diagnosis (DSMII Code)	NUMBER					PER CENT DISTRIBUTION				
	All Facilities	State and County Mental Hosp.	Private Mental Hosp.	General Hosp. Inpatient Psych. Unit *	Outpatient Psych. Services †	All Facilities	State and County Mental Hosp.	Private Mental Hosp.	General Hosp. Inpatient Psych. Unit	Outpatient Psych. Services
Total	1,920,120	459,523	87,000	507,904	865,693	100.0	100.0	100.0	100.0	100.0
Mental retardation (310–315)	50,038	12,754	227	4,354	32,703	2.6	2.8	0.3	0.8	3.8
Organic brain syndromes (290–294 and 309 excluding 291, 294.3, 309.13, 309.14)	97,919	42,243	4,052	28,317	23,307	5.1	9.2	4.7	5.6	2.7
Schizophrenia (295)	335,468	135,529	18,791	74,470	106,678	17.5	29.4	21.6	14.7	12.3
Major affective disorders (296)	63,933	15,335	6,099	29,841	12,658	3.3	3.3	7.0	5.9	1.5
Other psychoses (297, 298, 299)	60,161	9,645	6,827	32,360	11,329	3.1	2.1	7.8	6.4	1.3
Neuroses (300)	378,344	34,728	30,282	185,255	128,079	19.7	7.6	34.8	36.4	14.8
Personality disorders (301)	160,995	25,193	4,616	25,202	105,984	8.4	5.5	5.3	5.0	12.2
Alcohol disorders (291, 309.13, 303)	267,999	103,787	8,296	61,387	34,529	10.8	22.6	9.5	12.1	4.0
Drug disorders (294.3, 309.14, 304)	57,020	21,704	2,451	16,674	16,191	3.0	4.7	2.8	3.3	1.9
Transient situational disturbances (307)	163,184	11,283	2,957	19,346	129,598	8.5	2.5	3.4	3.8	15.0
All other (all other codes)	345,059	47,322	2,402	30,698	264,637	18.0	10.3	2.8	6.0	30.5

	RATES PER 100,000 POPULATION †					RANK ORDER (BASED ON RATES PER 100,000 POPULATION)				
Total	951.9	227.8	43.1	251.8	429.1	—	—	—	—	—
Mental retardation (310–315)	24.8	6.3	0.1	2.2	16.2	10	8	10	10	6
Organic brain syndromes (290–294 and 304 excluding 291, 294.3, 309.13, 309.14)	48.5	20.9	2.0	14.0	11.5	6	3	7	7	7
Schizophrenia (295)	166.3	67.2	9.3	36.9	52.9	2	1	2	2	3
Major affective disorders (296)	31.7	7.6	3.0	14.8	6.3	7	7	5	5	9
Other psychoses (297, 298, 299)	29.8	4.8	3.4	16.0	5.6	8	10	4	4	10
Neuroses (300)	187.6	17.2	15.0	91.8	63.5	1	4	1	1	2
Personality disorders (301)	79.8	12.5	2.3	12.5	52.5	5	5	6	6	4
Alcohol disorders (291, 309.13, 303)	103.1	51.5	4.1	30.4	17.1	3	2	3	3	5
Drug disorders (294.3, 309.14, 304)	28.3	10.8	1.2	8.3	8.0	9	6	9	9	8
Transient situational disturbances (307)	80.9	5.6	1.5	9.6	64.2	4	9	8	8	1
All other (all other codes)	171.1	23.5	1.2	15.2	131.2	—	—	—	—	—

* Numbers shown are discharges.
† Numbers shown are terminations. Data shown *exclude* the outpatient services at community mental health centers because the diagnostic breakdown of admissions to these centers was not comparable.
‡ Estimated July 1, 1970; United States civilian population (201,722,000) was used as base population.

when studying a hospital or a state hospital system to note the year in which the number of admissions first exceeded the census; this helps to indicate which systems were in advance of others. In 1969, for the first time, the number of resident patients in the United States (375,000) became equal to the number of admissions. In areas where the new policy had first been implemented, such as Dutchess County, the crossing took place four years earlier. In New York State as a whole this crossing has not taken place as yet. Sponsors of the "re-volving door" policy were acutely aware of the need for continuous com-munity treatment, preferably by a unified clinical team taking re-sponsibility for in- and outpatient care, and the need for an "easy in—easy out" policy. Facilitating return to the hospital in time of crisis was what made early releases possible. Unfortunately, this kind of service was not provided everywhere and too many chronic patients were sent out of hospitals to fend for themselves in a world neither prepared for them nor willing to afford the supportive services they needed.[25] This not only gave the revolving-door policy a bad name, it also created unnecessary suffering for the patients and, as the consequence of their bizarre and sometimes frightening behavior, in-creased rejection by the community. Failure to understand that previous successes had been based on the principle that early release requires easy readmission led to chaos and reaction rather than progress.[26] Some results of this backlash in public opinion are already visible with the reappearance of locked doors in some previously open institutions.

Another example of policy affecting utilization rates is the de-crease in admission rates of the elderly in New York State hospitals. In 1968 the New York State Department of Mental Hygiene restricted the admission of people over sixty-five to those clearly needing hospital-ization for a severe psychiatric disorder. This was done because too many of the admissions were felt to be unnecessary, with communities "dumping" elderly persons for whom less than inpatient hospital care would have been more appropriate. As a result, first admissions dropped from about 7,000 a year in 1967 to 2,000 in 1972.

In sum, the census of state hospitals was reduced by the decision to facilitate admissions and releases for the population under sixty-five, and in New York State, to restrict admissions of the elderly. Need-less to say, this only means that the visible portion of the iceberg has been reduced by policy decision; the iceberg itself has not changed.

Epidemiology also contributes to the evaluation of health services. This implies that the services have a definite goal, such as decreasing the incidence of groups of disorders in a population. Epidemiological methods are needed to determine whether the goal is being achieved. An interesting example of evaluation research was carried out by Bagley [27] in England and Wales to assess the impact of suicide preven-tion centers. Bagley compared the suicide rate of some fifteen towns where Samaritan groups had been in operation for two years or more to two groups of control towns in which there were no such services. He found that there had been only a slight decline in the Samaritan cities' suicide rate (– 6 percent). But in the control towns during the same period of time, the suicide rate had increased significantly (+ 20 percent for one group, + 7 percent for the other). In this case the services' impact was not reflected by a major decrease in suicide, but they had been successful in preventing an unexpected increase.

These examples of epidemiologic studies of how well health services are working show how the abstract theorists and passionate advocates can be forced to face reality.

Individual Risks and Chances

"The actual arithmetic of the individual risk of suffering a disease is for practical purposes the simple addition of annual age specific incidence rates." [28] Because of the accumulation of new cases over time, the individual risk of developing mental disorder or of being hospitalized increases with life expectancy.

Assessment of individual risk is relevant to the physician and to the planners and providers of prevention and treatment services. The more clearly we identify a population at risk, the better our chances of organizing useful screening services and applying effective primary prevention efforts. Hagnell [29] examined an entire population to determine the proportion who would develop mental disorders before age sixty. For ten years he followed the Lundby population first studied by Essen-Moller [30] in 1947. Hagnell was able to gather information on 99.6 percent of the original population of 2,550, ten years after Essen-Moller and colleagues did their prevalence survey. Hagnell estimated the accumulated risk of developing at least one mental disorder at least one time between the ages of ten and sixty as being 43.4 percent for men and 73 percent for women.

By the technique of summing the new cases occurring in each age group, Hagnell estimated that 13.7 percent of women and 5.5 percent of men would, by age sixty, develop a mental disorder lasting more than three years. Only a small number of these disorders were found to be of psychotic type or proportion. Despite the higher overall incidence of disorder in women, men ran a slightly higher risk of psychotic disorder.

Men had a 2 percent risk of schizophrenia, a 1 percent risk of other psychoses, and a 5.4 percent risk of organic syndrome. Women had a 0.7 percent risk for schizophrenia, 2.8 percent for other psychoses, 1.4 percent for organic syndromes. Hagnell's much higher probability that men would develop schizophrenic or organic syndromes is in sharp contrast to other studies which depend on age-specific incidence and prevalence rates of *treated* disorder. Hagnell further calculated the risk of first admission to a mental hospital at 4.1 percent for men and 5.5 percent for women up to age sixty.

Completing the Clinical Picture and Identifying New Syndromes

When we broaden our search beyond cases already in treatment we may markedly alter the clinical descriptions and prognoses of an illness or condition. This may be done by seeking out cases that have not come to clinical attention through referral to treatment—community surveys and studies of individual risks attempt to do this. Alternatively, patients may be followed after conclusion of treatment to learn more about the natural course of their condition. Such studies have provided more optimistic predictions about the long-term prognosis for many schizophrenics,[31] and informed us of the high medical morbidity and death rates associated with severe psychiatric illnesses.

Expert opinion in the United States often states that 3 percent of the population suffer from some degree of mental retardation—mild, moderate, severe, or profound. Most cases fall into the mild category. However, it has been noted that the age-specific prevalence drops markedly from adolescence onward.[32] The rate drop is too large to be accounted for by death, and it therefore appears likely that significant numbers of individuals who were labeled "mildly retarded" during childhood improved their functioning and lost their label during their adolescent or adult years. Investigations have revealed that mild intellectual deficit is particularly evident during childhood years in school, but is no longer remarkable when the individuals leave school and enter the unskilled manual labor market. The British deal with this situation in a practical way, with good social consequences, by using the term *educationally subnormal* to refer to cases we would classify as mildly retarded. Such individuals escape the retardation label; if they are not included in United States estimates, the frequency of retardation in the population becomes closer to 1 percent, rather than 3 percent, and there is less of a prevalence drop with age.

The long-term prognosis for some schizophrenics was altered by identification of new syndromes. Barton [33] first described the syndrome of *institutional neurosis* in 1961. It is characterized by passive compliance, self-neglect, occasional outbursts of aggressive behavior, indifference, and apathy. Barton reported this as developing after many years of living in a total institution, such as described by Goffman,[34] which had deprived the person of a sense of self, dignity, and opportunities for indivdual initiative. Barton's success in rehabilitating chronic mental patients in such hospitals showed that some of their disability was of sociogenic origin. Efforts to prevent secondary chronic deterioration led to recognition of a more severe syndrome, only some cases of which are institutional neurosis: *social breakdown syndrome* [35] is characterized by a variety of psychological and social decompensations, including lack of self-care, episodes of aggressive or self-destructive behavior, and failure to initiate recreational, vocational, or conversational activities. Most episodes of the syndrome were found to be short-lived, beginning in the community and ending not long after admission to a mental hospital. However, some cases were noted to last for many years and had been thought, prior to identification of the syndrome, to be due to chronic deterioration brought about by the primary diagnosis—schizophrenia in half the cases, but a wide variety of different disorders in the other half.

People who have been psychiatric patients die faster than the rest of the population. Babigian and Odoroff [36] monitored death certificates of people on the psychiatric case register in Monroe County, New York, and reported that the risk of death (adjusted for age, sex, marital status, and SES) was two- to threefold higher than for the rest of the population. When they removed psychiatric patients who were also chronically medically ill, the aged, and alcoholics (high-risk groups) from their data, the relative risk of dying was still 1.5 to 2 times that of the general population. Munoz and associates [37] showed that of 314 patients who reported to a psychiatric emergency service, 6 percent died within two years of the initial visit. The expected death rate for a population of similar age, race, and sex was only 1.6 percent.

The brief examples cited above are illustrative of the notion that longitudinal studies of specific disorders or of whole populations can teach us a great deal about the outcome and nature of various mental disorders. Such studies have revealed that the deterioration which was long thought an inevitable consequence of schizophrenia may be a largely preventable iatrogenic or sociogenic complication of treatment. In contrast to this optimistic finding, other data derived from studies designed to complete the clinical picture support the hypothesis that mental disorders may be components within a broad constellation of illnesses suffered by at-risk individuals in society; medical and social morbidity of all sorts, as well as early death, are the consequences.

In Search of Causes

The most valuable use of epidemiology is to discover preventable causes of illnesses and disabilities. Epidemiology is part of a joint enterprise in the search for causes. New understanding about the origins of mental disorder emerges when clinical research, laboratory studies, sociological inquiries, and epidemiology interact with one another. Epidemiological studies are stimulated by clinical and laboratory observations which by themselves cannot provide the information needed for generalizations. Population studies are required to amplify new ideas about disease prevention. Field studies are needed to validate etiologic and treatment hypotheses, and to test whether a specific method actually reduces the rate at which a particular disorder occurs. Such *preventive trials* may sometimes be done early, before the primary etiology of the disorder is known. For example, Pasamanick, Scarpitti, and Dinitz [38] conducted a preventive trial of institutionalization of schizophrenic patients.

An experimental group, constituting 70 percent of the total study cohort, was quickly released from the hospital for continued treatment at home. Treatment for this entire group consisted of home care by specifically trained public health nurses. Of this experimental group, 40 percent received clinically indicated active psychopharmacologic drug treatment, while the other 30 percent treated at home received a placebo. The remaining 30 percent of the patients in the cohort were a control group and were provided the usual, relatively longer hospital stay, as well as other treatment generally afforded hospitalized schizophrenics. During the follow-up period of six to thirty months the group which received drug treatment plus home treatment spent 90 percent of their time out of the hospital; the group treated with placebos at home spent 80 percent of their time out of the hospital; the control group spent 75 percent of their time out of the hospital. Pasamanick thus identified two preventable causes of institutionalization: relatively lengthy initial hospitalizations and absence of active psychopharmacologic treatment.

Sometimes a preventive trial does not permit proper research design, including use of a control group. This may happen because of reorganization or reform of the delivery of mental health services involving an entire community. For example, the mental health services provided to the residents of Dutchess County, New York, were reorganized in 1960 [39] to provide unified clinical teams to care for patients during both inpatient stay and community treatment. The goal of reorganization was to reduce the incidence of chronic social breakdown syndrome. A research survey showed that the annual incidence of the syndrome in persons aged sixteen to sixty-five declined by more than 50 percent during the first years after reorganization. As a consequence of epidemiologic study of the new service pattern, it was possible to document the dozens of person-years of severe disability prevented annually.

The kinds of studies just discussed are obviously useful as evaluation research, but beyond that they also add to our fund of knowledge supporting the hypothesis that many forms of chronic deterioration of psychiatric patients are sociogenic or iatrogenic, preventable complications of various mental disorders.

Genetic and Familial Factors

Mental health workers have long been impressed with the high frequency of mental disorders among relatives of their patients. The family history has long been a used and abused part of the standard psychiatric workup. It was assumed that when family histories of a particular disorder were being studied, one was studying the transmission of genetic material. However, genetic-epidemiologic studies have partially supported but greatly complicated this simple theory. Book [40] noted that early morbidity surveys of mental disorders showed the existence of definite familial aggregations of cases of both schizophrenia and manic-depressive psychosis. While the risk of schizophrenia in a general population is about 1 percent, the risk in the relatives of schizophrenic probands is higher (siblings, 7–15 percent; children, 7–15 percent; parents, 5–10 percent). In manic-depressive psychosis the estimated risk is approximately equal for first-degree relatives (10–15 percent for parents, children, and siblings).

Book noted that while each of these conditions occurs in family aggregations, they do not tend to overlap. That is, families of manic-depressives show no higher frequency of schizophrenia than the general population, nor do families of schizophrenic patients show an excess of manic-depressive disorders. This segregation of two sets of families implies that the two conditions are the results of different causes. He theorized that perhaps family clusters of schizophrenia can be explained by the existence of a single very *low penetrance* recessive gene. *Low penetrance* means that the phenotype occurs in only a small proportion of people with the genotype. Gene disorders only become manifest when the appropirate environmental conditions are present—in some conditions the environmental conditions are rare (low penetrance), and in others they are common (high penetrance).[41]

Further support for a genetic etiology for schizophrenia was provided by Kety, as reviewed by Wender and associates.[42] He studied children of schizophrenic parents who had been adopted by others, and found an incidence of schizophrenia similar to that which would have been expected if the children had been raised by their natural parents. Yet these schizophrenic children had been raised by adoptive parents who were not schizophrenic.

Some who were unconvinced by the early genetic evidence looked to psychodynamic theories to explain the development of schizophrenia. Manfred Bleuler [43] suggested that data on secondary cases provided evidence for the psychological transmission of the disorder. Bateson and associates [44] described schizophrenogenic patterns of mothering and family life, including the *double bind*, to explain the influence of child-rearing patterns on later development of schizophrenic syndromes. Lidz [45] and Wynne and Singer [46] also argued for a psychogenic etiology of schizophrenia. The eugenicists tended to think that families share only a common set of genes, ignoring the social inheritance of money, language, and culture. The psychogeneticists think only of the latter and ignore the former.

Eugen Bleuler [47] referred to the *group of schizophrenias*, rather than to a single schizophrenic condition with a single cause. Wender and associates [48] studied children of schizophrenics who had been adopted and showed that a broad range of conditions, the "schizophrenic spectrum," appeared to be genetically determined. Contemporary community treatment of schizophrenics may tend to increase the genetic pool for this condition, as well as for other psychiatric disorders. This potential problem, as well as the sociogenic risk to children being reared by intermittently psychotic parents who are now hospitalized for briefer periods than was the case even a few years ago, may also be important.

Fear of contaminated or inferior gene pools leading to great increases of mental disorders has not been supported by research. The United States was once regarded as being at great risk because some European countries were alleged to be subsidizing migration of mentally ill persons. Studies by Malzberg [49] and Ödegaard [50] showed this fear to be unfounded, because the immigrants had no more mental disorder than the native-born.

Sociopsychological Theories

In 1897 Durkheim [51] introduced the concept of "anomie," that is, disruption of traditional societies with their unquestioned value systems. He related anomie, created by industrialization and increasing rationalism and secularism, to suicide rates. Durkheim also verified the fact that social characteristics and forces were reflected in the behavior of individuals. Shaw and McKay,[52] following a similar approach, related patterns of social disorganization in one city (Chicago) to delinquency rates, and opened the way for Faris and Dunham's study [53] of first admission rates for mental disorders Their key finding, commented on earlier in the section on community diagnosis, was that social isolation and disorganization caused the behavioral and psychological characteristics of schizophrenia. Alternate hypotheses were subsequently advanced. Ödegaard [54] cited *self-selection*, which holds that persons with certain characteristics drift to certain areas, social classes, or even professions; Myerson [55] suggested that the concentration of schizophrenia in the high-rate areas was due to *downward drift*, and not caused by the characteristics of the areas. A variation of the drift hypothesis, the *segregation hypothesis*, explains the downward drift of the schizophrenic not as a passive phenomenon but as an active search by the individual for areas where isolation and anonymity protect him against the demands—for him unbearable—of conventional society.

The hypothesis of *differential tolerance* holds that differences between communities in rate of admission are determined by familial and cultural attitudes, their tolerance of deviant behavior, and their reluctance or willingness to resort to public agencies for treatment. A case in point would be the Eaton and Weil [56] survey of the Hutterites in 1958: This small sect in the Midwest had never had one of its members hospitalized for mental disorders. Some had assumed that in this tightly knit, highly religious community, living patterns prevented mental disorders. Eaton and Weil found that, in fact, mental disorders were as prevalent in this society as in others, but all of the sick members were cared for at home.

None of the subsequent studies dealing with sociocultural indices settled the issue definitely. Some did support the drift hypothesis; [57] some did not.[58] A recent book by Levy Rowitz,[59] which repeated the Faris and Dunham study with some variations, had some findings supporting the drift hypothesis and others supporting the differential tolerance hypothesis (renamed here as extrusion or antiextrusion bias).

Srole and Leighton [60] had linked social disintegration with increases in the prevalence of mental disorders in their community surveys. Recently Leighton [61] summarized much of the work testing the anomie hypothesis. He recommended that community mental health centers employ a new kind of mental health professional—the community catalyst—to address community needs for reintegrative efforts which can, by supporting individual needs, prevent psychiatric disorder. Caplan [62] made a similar recommendation, urging that nonprofessional self-help support groups be encouraged in the community to assist individuals judged to be at high risk of psychiatric decompensation.

Stress-Related Etiologic Factors

Hans Selye [63] emphasized the *diseases of adaptation;* he popularized the concept of stress and its impact on the health of the individual. Unfortunately, there is as yet no general agreement of a definition of stress; this leads to difficulties in comparing the hypotheses and outcomes of various studies. Levine and Scotch [64] in 1970 provided a valuable summary of recent contributions to the study of social stress and its consequences.

Holmes and Rahe [65] focused attention on the impact of life events on the health of individuals. Their social readjustment scale includes forty-three types of events, such as marriage, leaving school, losing or getting a job, and death of a significant other. Each event is given a weight according to a judgment as to the amount of adjustment required to deal with it. Adding up the point values of the events occurring for an individual during a given period of time gives the life change units score. Individuals whose score exceeded 300 points were found to have an increased morbidity as compared with those with low score. Other workers [66] have related the number of life events experienced to the frequency of episodes of psychiatric disorder. A recent volume edited by B. and B. Dohrenwend [67] summarizes new findings and developments in life events research.

Crowding, and the disturbance of interpersonal relations it entails, has been reviewed recently by Cassel.[68] There is evidence, much of it from animal studies, suggesting that "one of the more important aspects of the environment for man (from a disease etiology point of

view) may be the presence of other members of the same species."
However, Cassel adds that attempts to demonstrate that increased population density and crowding per se are related to poorer health status
in humans have led to confusing and often conflicting results.[69] Cassel
has refined the crowding hypothesis and offers several more specific
theorems.

1. When population density in human groups leads to *disordered
interpersonal relationships,* the specific cause may be:

> failure to elicit anticipated responses to what were previously appropriate
> cues and an increasing disregard of traditional obligations and rights. . . .
> The failure of behavior patterns to accomplish their intended results
> (that is, lead to predictable responses on the part of others) leads fre-
> quently to repetition of these behaviors with, presumably, concomitant
> chronic alterations in the autonomic nervous system activity and hormo-
> nal secretions associated with such activity. These, in turn, alter the
> homeostatic mechanisms of the organisms, leading to increased suscepti-
> bility to disease . . . [when] individuals are not receiving any evidence
> (feedback) that their actions are leading to desirable and/or anticipated
> consequences. In particular this would be true when these actions are
> designed to modify the individual's relationships to the important social
> groups with whom he interacts.[70]

2. Animal studies suggest that not all members of a population
may be equally susceptible to noxious social processes. The more
dominant animals in a group tend to show the least effects, while the
submissive members show the most extreme consequeneces.[71]

3. Cassel suggests that available protective factors may include
both biologic and social mechanisms. In addition to the biological
adaptive capacities which are usually considered, he suggests that social processes have also been shown to be protective. Conger and associates [72] demonstrated that rats may develop peptic ulcers when
given unexpected electric shocks. Social support seems able to provide
a measure of protection from the biopsychologic stress of the shocks;
fewer rats developed ulcers if they were shocked in the company of
their littermates. Crowding will produce hypertension in mice only
when the crowd consists of strangers.[73] Studies of small human
groups have shown that insoluble dilemmas produce higher states of
autonomic nervous system excitement when the group is made up of
strangers than when it consists of friends.[74]

Cassel has developed a summary formulation based on the above
data and hypothesis which holds that:

> . . . The health consequences of disordered social relationships will not
> be universal, affecting all people in the same manner. A more adequate
> formulation would hold that such consequences will depend on (1) the
> importance or salience of the relationships that become disordered; (2)
> the position of the individuals experiencing such disordered relationships
> in the status hierarchy; (3) the degree to which the population under
> study has been unprepared by previous experience for this particular situ-
> ation (that is, has had insufficient time to adapt); and (4) the nature
> and strength of the available group supports.[75]

Summary

Social changes and new techniques can be expected to produce alterations in the patterns of occurrence of mental disorders; our state of knowledge is changing as well. The actual picture of mental health services that exists today differs from that of twenty-five years ago. What we knew twenty-five years ago did not permit us to predict today's situation; we still do not know enough to predict the psychiatric situation of the year 2000, in spite of important advances in our knowledge. Nevertheless, while the specifics may change, this principle will remain true: Epidemiology is the basic science of preventive psychiatry and treatment evaluation.

Some mental health professionals may be "turned off" by the epidemiological approach, which tries to amass relevant facts and reason cautiously from them. Some may prefer simpler polemical debates about whether *mental illness* is a medical or a political term. Whether or not *mental illness* exists, there is a powerful body of evidence which indicates that there are many separately identifiable mental illnesses or disorders. Sufferers from these serious conditions deserve treatment efforts based on thorough study of available knowledge of their specific illness. That is the responsibility of every treating mental health professional. We have presented this primer on epidemiology in the hope that the reader will become interested enough to become a student of the field and pursue some of the references cited in the notes.

NOTES

1. L. E. Hinsie and R. J. Campbell, *Psychiatric Dictionary*, 4th ed. (New York: Oxford University Press, 1970).

2. J. E. Gordon, "The Twentieth Century: Yesterday, Today, and Tomorrow," in *The History of American Epidemiology*, ed. F. H. Top (St. Louis: C.V. Mosby, 1952), p. 114.

3. J. N. Morris, *Uses of Epidemiology*, 2nd ed. (London: Livingston, 1970).

4. Group for the Advancement of Psychiatry, Committee on Preventive Psychiatry, *Problems of Estimating Changes in Frequency of Mental Disorders. Report 50* (New York: Group for the Advancement of Psychiatry, 1961).

5. C. O. Carter, "A Life-table for Mongols with the Causes of Death," *Journal of Mental Deficiency Research* 2, no. 64 (1958).

6. Milton Helpern, "Fatalities from Narcotic Addiction in New York City," *Human Pathology* 3 (March 1972): 13–21.

7. H. Goldhamer and A. W. Marshall, *Psychosis and Civilization* (New York: Free Press, 1949).

8. August B. Hollingshead and Frederick C. Redlich, *Social Class and Mental Illness: A Community Study* (New York: Wiley, 1958).

9. Leo Srole et al., *Mental Health in the Metropolis*, vol. 1, *The Midtown Manhattan Study*, Thomas A. C. Rennie Series in Social Psychiatry (New York: McGraw-Hill, 1962).

10. E. M. Gruenberg and staff of the Mental Health Research Unit, *A Mental Health Survey of Older People* (Utica, N.Y.: State Hospitals Press, 1960).

11. Srole et al., *Mental Health;* Gruenberg, *Mental Health Survey;* Dorothea C. Leighton et al., *Psychiatric Symptoms in Selected Communities*, vol. 3, *The Character*

of Danger (New York: Basic Books, 1963); Paul Lemkau, Christopher Tietze, and Marcia Cooper, "Mental Hygiene Problems in an Urban District," *Mental Hygiene* 25, no. 4 (1941): 624–646; and Robert E. L. Faris and H. Warren Dunham, *Mental Disorders in Urban Areas: An Ecological Study of Schizophrenia and Other Psychoses* (Chicago: University of Chicago Press, 1939).

12. Hollingshead and Redlich, *Social Class.*
13. Srole et al., *Mental Health.*
14. Faris and Dunham, *Mental Disorders.*
15. Olle Hagnell, *A Prospective Study of the Incidence of Mental Disorder* (Stockholm: Scandinavian University Books, 1966).
16. Srole et al., *Mental Health.*
17. Leighton et al., *Psychiatric Symptoms.*
18. Gruenberg, *Mental Health Survey.*
19. Edward P. Jarvis, "Influence of Distance From and Nearness to an Insane Hospital on its Use by the People," *American Journal of Insanity* 22 (1866):361–406.
20. B. P. Dohrenwend and B. S. Dohrenwend, "Psychiatric Disorders in Urban Settings," in *American Handbook of Psychiatry,* ed. G. Caplan (New York: Basic Books, 1974), pp. 424–447.
21. E. M. Gruenberg, "An Isolation of Social from Economic Concomitants of Mental Hospital Admission Rates" (Ph.D. diss., Yale University, 1955).
22. M. Kramer et al., *Mental Disorders—Suicide,* Vital and Health Statistics Monographs, APHA (Cambridge, Mass.: Harvard University Press, 1972).
23. M. Kramer and R. Redick, unpublished data.
24. Kramer et al., *Mental Disorders—Suicide.*
25. Robert Reich, "The Chronically Mentally Ill: Their Fate in New York City," *The Bulletin* (New York State District Branches, APA) 15, no. 4 (1972): 6.
26. Gruenberg, "Benefits of Short-term Hospitalization," in *Strategic Intervention in Schizophrenia: Currenut Developments in Treatment,* ed. Robert Cancro, Norma Fox, and Lester E. Shapiro (New York: Behavioral Publications, 1974), pp. 251–257.
27. C. Bagley, "The Evaluation of a Suicide Prevention Scheme by an Ecological Method," *Social Science and Medicine* 2, no. 1 (1968): 1–14.
28. Morris, *Uses of Epidemiology.*
29. Hagnell, *A Prospective Study.*
30. Erick Essen-Moller, "Individual Traits and Morbidity in a Swedish Population," *Acta Psychiatria Neurologica Scandinavia* 100 (1956).
31. Manfred Bleuler, "Research and Changes in Concepts on the Study of Schizophrenia 1941–50," *Bulletin of the Isaac Ray Medical Library* (Butler Hospital, Providence, R.I.) 3, nos. 1 and 2 (1955): 1–132, and E. M. Gruenberg, "Epidemiology of Schizophrenia," in *American Handbook of Psychiatry,* ed. Caplan, pp. 448–463.
32. E. M. Gruenberg and A. Kiev, "The Age Distribution of Mental Retardation," in *Psychopathology of Mental Development,* ed. J. Zubin and G. A. Jervis (New York: Grune & Stratton, 1967), p. 233.
33. R. Barton, "Consideration, Clinical Features and Differential Diagnosis of Institutional Neurosis," *Proceedings of the Third World Congress of Psychiatry* 2 (June 1961): 890–895.
34. E. Goffman, *Asylums* (Garden City, N.Y.: Doubleday-Anchor, 1961).
35. E. M. Gruenberg, R. V. Kasius, and M. Huxley, "Objective Appraisal of Deterioration in a Group of Long-stay Hospital Patients," *Milbank Memorial Fund Quarterly* 40, no. 90 (1962).
36. Haroutun M. Babigian and Charles L. Odoroff, "The Mortality Experience of a Population with Psychiatric Illness," *American Journal of Psychiatry* 126, no. 4 (1969): 470–480.
37. Rodrigo A. Munoz et al., "Mortality Following a Psychiatric Emergency Room Visit: An 18-Month Follow-Up Study," *American Journal of Psychiatry* 128, no. 2 (1971): 112–116.
38. Benjamin Pasamanick, Frank P. Scarpitti, and Simon Dinitz, *Schizophrenics in the Community: An Experimental Study in the Prevention of Hospitalization* (New York: Appleton-Century-Crofts, 1967).
39. E. M. Gruenberg, "Can the Reorganization of Psychiatric Services Prevent Some Cases of Social Breakdown?" in *Psychiatry in Transition 1966–67,* ed. A. B. Stokes (Toronto: Clark Institute of Psychiatry, University of Toronto Press, 1967): 95–109.
40. J. A. Book, "Genetical Etiology in Mental Illness," in *Causes of Mental Disorders: A Review of Epidemiological Knowledge, 1959* (New York: Milbank Memorial Fund, 1961): 14–33.

41. B. McMahon, "Gene-Environment Interaction in Human Disease," in *The Transmission of Schizophrenia*, ed. D. Rosenthal and S. Kety (London: Pergamon Press, 1968), pp. 393–402.

42. P. H. Wender et al., "The Psychiatric Adjustment of the Adopting Parents of Schizophrenics," *American Journal of Psychiatry* 127 (1971): 1013–1018.

43. Bleuler, "Research and Changes."

44. G. Bateson et al., "Toward a Theory of Schizophrenia," *Behavioral Science* 1 (1956): 251–264.

45. T. Lidz, *The Family and Human Adaptation* (New York: International Universities Press, 1963).

46. L. C. Wynne and M. T. Singer, "Thought Disorder and Family Relations of Schizophrenics: I. A Research Strategy; II. A Classification of Form of Thinking," *Archives of General Psychiatry* 9 (1963): 191–206.

47. E. Bleuler, *Dementia Praecox or the Group of Schizophrenias* (New York: International Universities Press, 1950).

48. Wender et al., "Psychiatric Adjustment."

49. Benjamin Malzberg, "Mental Disease Among the Native and Foreign-born White Populations of New York State, 1939–1941," *Mental Hygiene* 39, no. 4 (1955): 545–563.

50. O. Ödegaard, "Emigration and Insanity: A Study of Mental Disease Among the Norwegian-born Population of Minnesota," *Acta Psychiatria Neurologica Scandinavica*, supp. 4 (1932).

51. Emile Durkheim, *Suicide: A Study in Sociology*, ed. George Simpson (New York: Free Press, 1951).

52. C. R. Shaw and H. D. McKay, "Social Factors in Juvenile Delinquency: A Study of the Community, the Family, and the Gang, in Relation to Delinquent Behavior," in *Report on the Causes of Crime*, National Commission on Law Observance and Enforcement, vol. 2, no. 13 (Washington, D.C.: Government Printing Office, 1931), pp. i–xv, 3–401.

53. Faris and Dunham, *Mental Disorders*.

54. O. Ödegaard, "The Incidence of Psychoses in Various Occupations," *International Journal of Social Psychiatry* 2, no. 2 (Autumn 1956): 85–104.

55. A. Myerson, "A Review of Mental Disorders in Urban Areas," *American Journal of Psychiatry* 96 (1940): 995–997.

56. J. W. Eaton and R. J. Weil, *Culture and Mental Disorders* (New York: Free Press, 1955).

57. E. M. Goldberg and E. S. Morrison, "Schizophrenia and Social Class," *British Journal of Psychiatry* 109 (1963): 785, and P. H. Wender et al., "Social Class and Psychopathology in Adoptees," *Archives of General Psychiatry* 28 (1973): 318.

58. J. A. Clausen and M. I. Kohn, "Relation of Schizophrenia to the Social Structure of a Small City," in *Epidemiology of Mental Disorder*, ed. B. Pasamanick (Washington, D.C.: American Association for the Advancement of Science, 1959), p. 69, and R. J. Turner and M. D. Wagnefeld, "Occupational Mobility and Schizophrenia: An Assessment of Social Causation and Social Selection Hypothesis," *American Sociological Review* 32 (1967): 104–113.

59. L. Levy and L. Rowitz, *The Ecology of Mental Disorders* (New York: Behavioral Publications, 1973).

60. Srole et al., *Mental Health;* Leighton et al., *Psychiatric Symptoms.*

61. A. H. Leighton, "Social Disintegration and Mental Disorder," in *American Handbook of Psychiatry*, ed. Caplan, pp. 411–423.

62. G. Caplan, *Support Systems and Community Mental Health* (New York: Behavioral Publications, 1974). (Ms. p. 24:28)

63. H. Selye, *The Stress of Life* (New York: McGraw-Hill, 1956).

64. S. Levine and N. A. Scotch, *Social Stress* (Chicago: Aldine, 1970).

65. T. Holmes and R. H. Rahe, "The Social Readjustment Rating Scale," *Journal of Psychosomatic Research* 11 (1967): 213.

66. J. K. Myers, J. J. Lindenthal, and M. P. Pepper, "Life Events and Psychiatric Impairment," *Journal of Nervous and Mental Diseases* 152 (1971): 149–157; G. W. Brown and J. L. T. Birley, "Crises and Life Changes and the Onset of Schizophrenia," *Journal of Health and Social Behavior* 9, no. 3 (1968): 203–214; and E. S. Paykel et al., "Life Events and Depression. A Controlled Study," *Archives of General Psychiatry* 21 (1969): 753.

67. B. S. Dohrenwend and B. P. Dohrenwend, eds., *Stressful Life Events: Their Nature and Effects* (New York: Wiley, 1974).

68. J. C. Cassel, "Psychiatric Epidemiology," in *American Handbook of Psychiatry*, ed. Silvano Arieti (New York: Basic Books, 1974), 2: 401–411.

69. J. C. Cassel, "Health Consequences of Population Density and Crowding," in *Rapid Population Growth,* prepared by a Study of the Office of the Foreign Secretary, National Academy of Science (Baltimore: The John Hopkins Press, 1971), pp. 462–478.

70. Cassel, "Psychiatric Epidemiology," p. 405.

71. J. J. Christian, "The Potential Role of the Adrenal Cortex as Affected by Social Rank and Population Density in Experimental Epidemics," *American Journal of Epidemiology* 87 (1968): 255–264.

72. J. J. Conger et al., "The Role of Social Experience in the Production of Gastric Ulcers in Hooded Rats Placed in a Conflict Situation," *Journal of Abnormal and Social Psychology* 57 (1958): 216.

73. J. P. Henry. J. P. Meehan, and P. M. Stephens, "The Use of Psychosocial Stimuli to Induce Prolonged Hypertension in Mice," *Psychosomatic Medicine* 29 (1967): 408–432.

74. N. D. Bogdanoff et al., "The Physiologic Response to Conformity Pressure in Man," *Annals of Internal Medicine* 57 (1962).

75. Cassel, "Health Consequences," p. 407.

COMMENTARY

The preceding paper has noted that both the pattern of occurrence of mental disorders, and our state of knowledge about them, are changing. However, basic epidemiologic thinking and concepts are unlikely to be altered greatly, even as the problems we face change and new investigatory methods are developed.

Mental illness and mental disorder are broad terms which sweep within their embrace a multitude of events, concepts, issues, scientific concerns, ethical values, and moral dilemmas. Such umbrella terms cannot be dealt with meaningfully without first specifying our particular interest in some detail; epidemiology provides us with the tools we need to do so.

The important uses of epidemiology have been explained and demonstrated: to understand historical trends, amplify and clarify diagnostic issues, probe etiology, plan and evaluate mental health services, assist in community diagnosis, and evaluate treatment. Do you agree that the method can be used, regardless of one's primary discipline or professional orientation, to evaluate hypotheses and test concepts derived from biology, sociology, social psychology, or psychoanalysis?

The editors have placed this chapter at the beginning of the last part of this book to assist in the transition from theory to application. As theoreticians and consumers of research we are keenly aware of how little we know definitively and quantitatively. Nevertheless, whether in the courtroom or the consulting room, the mental health professional is the best expert available on questions of mental disorder. Finding yourself in that uncomfortably responsible position, do you feel capable of handling questions put to you on the basis of your objective scientific knowledge? To what extent do you feel your re-

sponses and therapeutic actions are the result of judgments based on "soft" data, such as unquantified clinical experience and learning? How far will epidemiologic research into mental disorders have to go before you might feel yourself a scientist, rather than something of an artist? Many clinicians, we suspect, believe that that day will never come, and are glad of it.

CHAPTER 24

Intrapsychic versus Environmental Determinism: Psychosocial Complementarity

INTRODUCTION

The following article represents an ambitious venture into difficult conceptual areas. The editors feel that the expedition has been successful, and that the paper merits thoughtful reading and analysis despite its length and complexity. Its rich nutrition can best be assimilated by a careful reading, a second reading, and discussion of its many intriguing points with others.

Marc Fried has really written two papers in one. The first begins with a closely reasoned analysis of the basic psychoanalytic (Freudian) and sociological (Durkheimian) theoretical models. Fried points to the value and limitations of both of these models for the understanding of human behavior in general, and psychopathology in particular. Noting that it is essential that we develop conceptual schemes which bridge the psychological system, Fried indicates that not only are linking concepts lacking in the Freudian and Durkheimian frameworks, but the two widely variant perspectives appear to be unbridgeable. However, Fried offers a conceptual scheme which provides for their integration: the complementarity model of psychosocial relationships.

Fried proposes that the ego structures of individuals must be adapted to the types of role expectations that exist in their particular societies. Societies which encourage the pursuit of a wide range of roles demand more individuation and impose upon the individual the burden of a high degree of ego differentiation and integration. This type of ego structure, however, would not be adaptive in a society which had a rigidly defined role structure and few role alternatives. Psychopathology develops when the individual's ego resources, differentiation, and integration are noncomplementary to the social system. This is the principle of psychosocial complementarity.

In the second part of his paper, Fried reviews some compelling epidemiological data suggestive of associations between psychopathology and social class, black-white differences, marital status, migration, and other variables. He considers the merits of the data and carefully weighs various interpretations of them. Finally, he shows how these data may be analyzed within the framework of psychosocial complementarity.

SOCIAL PROBLEMS AND PSYCHOPATHOLOGY

Marc Fried

The Principle of Psychosocial Complementarity

Conceptual advances in the behavioral sciences have led to wide appreciation of the fact that all forms of human behavior involve both intrapsychic and environmental determinants. But this formulation is of little help in understanding any single instance or form of behavior as a manifestation of the interaction between individual and social variables. The problem requires explicit and detailed conceptual models and propositions that can clarify the patterns of interplay among a range of individual and social resources and conflicts, and their consequences for ordered and disordered functioning. Yet, there remains an apparently insuperable gulf in models, concepts, and methods between those fields that stress the primacy of individual variables and those that emphasize the primacy of culture and social structure.

The conceptual dilemma becomes particularly pointed, and our failures to resolve it become particularly unfortunate, when we consider the mutual influences that affect the development and persistence of social pathology and psychopathology. This polarity of views is apparent in comparing those two major figures who provided the most

Marc Fried, "Social Problems and Psychopathology," in *Urban America and the Planning of Mental Health Services*, edited by Leonard J. Duhl. (Revised.) Copyright © 1964, Group for the Advancement of Psychiatry. Reprinted by permission of author and Group for the Advancement of Psychiatry.

basic general models for contemporary investigations of disordered functioning, Freud and Durkheim. Both Freud and Durkheim were concerned with the relationship between stimulation and motivation, between individual and group, between personal and social variables. Yet, despite many similarities in interest, each of them selected a path that led to diametrically opposed conceptualizations.

Freud's Model for Psychopathology.   In his earliest effort at elaborating a fairly comprehensive theory of psychopathology, "The Neuro-Psychoses of Defence," [1] Freud delineated his focus on the internal mechanisms involved in the transposition of a previous social experience into a current symptom or syndrome. Despite his awareness that factors apart from these internal mechanisms might affect the course of subsequent events, his attention remained in the realm of these internal mechanisms themselves.[2] Moreover, Freud repeatedly faced the question of the distinction between those individuals who succumbed to neurosis and those who did not, despite similar prior histories. He employed a number of types of explanation but, as Hartmann and Kris [3] have pointed out, he often resorted to ad hoc support from constitutional factors even when developmental psychoanalytic concepts were at hand to clarify the issue.[4] At no point, however, did he consider the possibility that differences in *external* resources of either a situational or structural nature might account for the differences in subsequent "internal" fate of an event or experience.

In spite of his several great studies of social psychological phenomena, Freud's model [5] implies a number of propositions that are antithetical to Durkheim's views. Briefly, we may summarize several central components of Freud's model: (1) all behavior is motivated and any act can be fully (or almost fully) accounted for by the motives involved in the action and their sources in personal history; (2) the psychological significance of external events can be viewed wholly from the vantage point of the reality principle as one of the guiding forces in the development and functioning of the ego; and (3) the personal history of the individual and the unresolved conflicts that are maintained provide the necessary and sufficient conditions for neurosis or, at the very least, create a predisposition that may readily be precipitated by unfavorable environmental circumstances. Thus, the model of psychopathology can be stated in these terms: *Unresolved conflicts determine both the impulses and the defenses against impulse that result in psychopathology when the ego is incapable of adapting the behavior to the demands of reality.*

Freud was certainly aware that social relationships and social resources could facilitate (or impede) the adaptation of the ego to the demands of reality, but he did not formulate any systematic propositions that took account of this fact.[6] As a consequence, the psychoanalytic model could only treat the external world and its effects on motivation, conflict resolution, and ego structure as an array of random and discrete events and situations. In these terms, individual differences are due primarily to differences in *selection* on the part of the individual rather than to *systematic* differences in social roles, positions, and cultural patterns. Social relationships might influence the development of the individual in critical ways, but differences in socially structured resources and controls could have no consistent and widely observable effects on current behavior or psychopathology.[7]

Contrasting Views of Durkheim. Durkheim presents several striking contrasts to Freud. He was, perhaps, even more aware of the operation of psychological forces than Freud was of social forces and never rejected their empirical importance. However, Durkheim self-consciously set himself the task of developing a field of sociology and rejected the fundamental *theoretical* importance of psychological factors as basic, explanatory variables. The work in which he most explicitly addressed himself to the clarification of this problem was *Suicide*.[8] In his analysis of suicide, Durkheim recognized that particular psychological states are frequently associated with suicide but maintained that these are sufficiently diverse and result from a wide enough variety of actual experiences that they cannot provide a general explanation for suicide. Durkheim realized that consciousness did not represent the most critical aspect of human motivation. But he did not explore the underlying commonalities among apparently diverse psychological states. For Durkheim, psychological events were, thus, random and discrete factors determined by highly idiosyncratic personal histories. Despite the fact that individual psychological experiences might account for individual instances of suicide, they could provide no basis for generalizations regarding the common factors that caused suicidal behavior.

> Sometimes men who kill themselves have had family sorrows or disappointments to their pride, sometimes they have had to suffer poverty or sickness, at others they have had some moral fault with which to reproach themselves. But . . . these individual peculiarities could not explain the social suicide-rate; for the latter varies in considerable proportions, whereas the different combinations of circumstances which constitute the immediate antecedents of individual cases of suicide retain approximately the same relative frequency. They are therefore not the determining cause of the act which they precede. Their occasionally important role in the premeditation of suicide is no proof of being a causal one.[9]

In effect, Durkheim points out that individual behavior is the individualized expression of socially determined tendencies. Certainly he admits that selective factors operate to produce individual instances of suicide. But he rejects the idea that these selective factors can be formulated as the causal factors. The differences in suicide rate are associated with differences in social organization and, thus, an "individual yields to the slightest shock of circumstances because the state of society has made him a ready prey to suicide."

Durkheim developed neither a model nor a theory as fully as did Freud. However, certain fundamental propositions stand out as components of a model and of a theory. In contrast to Freud's emphasis on individual motivation to action, Durkheim stressed the social regulation of behavior inherent in the cohesiveness and stability of the society and in the individual's commitment to social relationships. His analysis of suicide distinguishes several types of suicide: those which are due to decreased social organization and heightened individualism (egoistic suicide); those in which suicide represents a societal ideal or expectation (altruistic suicide); and those in which the disruption of familiar patterns of social organization and of the bases for social behavior lead to suicide (anomic suicide). Although Durkheim did not examine motivation closely, he clearly conceived of the motivation itself as social in origin. The social origin of suicidal motivation might be of three different types, related to the three forms of suicide: (1) it might involve a sense of *emptiness* (as in egoistic suicide) resulting from the absence of that social cohesiveness which alone makes living meaningful and worthwhile; (2) it might be a sense of *courageous self-sacrifice* or social fulfillment (as in altruistic suicide) because the individual participates in the social good through suicide; or (3) it would be a gesture of *anger and bitterness* (as in anomic suicide) when social instability and crisis disrupt the patterns of experience that are the foundation for the individual's entire set of expectations. In this formulation, Durkheim comes close, indeed, to a statement of mutual influences but maintains that the individual state is largely a reflection of the social condition which produces the particular type and rate of suicide.

These conceptualizations of Durkheim imply a more general conception of man and society than do Freud's views. For Freud, the individual can achieve gratification only *despite* society; the reality principle determines the price he must pay in the reorganization and delay of impulse expression. Neurosis, in fact, can be conceived as the result of excessive conformity in which the more personal aspects of impulse life can be given only symptomatic expression. For Durkheim, on the other hand, the individual can achieve gratification and meaning only *through* social commitment. Complex and highly differentiated modern societies involve a high degree of individuation and individualism that place an enormous burden on the individual. If there is a lack of cohesiveness within smaller segments of the individual's systems of social relationship due to marital disruption, to economic crises, or to the absence of a religious community, there is ready and widespread disenchantment with life.

In stating the formulations of Freud and of Durkheim in this way, it is apparent that although there is a sharp contrast in the models, they are not truly disjunctive. Freud [10] was well aware of the importance of social cohesiveness and saw clearly that social commitment was the central feature guiding the fate of libidinal and aggressive drives. Similarly, Durkheim was well aware of the importance of individualism and the meaning inherent in fulfillment of individual desires and goals. His analysis of the development of industrial societies in *On the Division of Labor in Society* [11] introduces a distinction between two modes of social organization that lead to differences in the tolerance for individualism in personality. The first of these bases for social organization is *mechanic* solidarity. It presupposes a relatively simple society in which commitments are to the larger group with a common set of values and sentiments; there is little opportunity for the development of individuality since cohesiveness depends upon the fact that each person is an embodiment of the collectivity. The second basis for social organization he calls *organic* solidarity. It is characteristic of industrial societies with a highly developed division of labor; there is a high degree of social differentiation, and the primary foci of social commitment are in the reciprocities among individuals in small groups (family, neighborhood, friendships, work groups). Opportunities for individuality and for the development and expression of individual personality are at a maximum in societies with organic solidarity.

When Freud and Durkheim address a common problem, such as the increased complexity and potential for disorder in highly civilized societies, they appear to be speaking in opposite terms. Freud stresses the greater need for self-denial and repression of impulses; Durkheim talks of the narrower framework for social solidarity and the conditions of social disorganization in which individuality becomes a burden. Yet both of these views are tenable, and it requires only a slight shift in perspective to see them as formulations of a *complementary relationship between the individual and his society.*

The greater the difficulty of establishing social solidarity, the more the individual must rely upon himself and his own resources and regulatory mechanisms. The more he must rely upon himself, the less can he develop facility in anticipating common desires and sentiments or the degree of self-subordination necessary for maintaining reciprocity in the regulation of impulse and desire. To this extent in the absence of social resources for regulation and fulfillment, the burden of repression is in greater degree an individual expectation and a personal necessity. We come, thus, to the apparent paradox that the most civilized populations are those in which individual freedom and personality regulation replace communal resources and social control to a considerable extent; and social solidarity involves a greater degree of independently achieved and developed reciprocity, commitment, and social affiliation. But while there is heightened emphasis on individuality and increased opportunity for the personal fulfillment of sublimated goals in highly differentiated, industrial societies, the individual pays a price in decreased security, in an increased need for the inhibition of impulses, and in greater danger of isolation and estrangement under conditions of social disruption.

Psychosocial Relationships: The Congruence Model. The opposition between individual and social regulatory mechanisms, the fact that extensive development of internal and, thus, individual regulatory mechanisms precludes a high degree of responsiveness to external and, thus, social regulatory mechanisms and, conversely, that extensive organization of external and, thus, social regulatory mechanisms precludes a high degree of internal regulation, provides the basis for one form of interactional model of behavior. This model implies that social and psychological mechanisms of regulation, which we shall categorize as resources and controls, are virtually interchangeable phenomena in establishing and insuring ordered, adaptive, goal-oriented behavior. However, there are many aspects of development and functioning for which this is not the case, which require concurrence or compliance between social stimuli and psychological motives. Social development rests upon the socialization of a biological organism dependent on the environment for growth and development to different degrees.

Effective socialization involves learning to modify and channelize impulses, desires, affects, and actions to accord more closely with the individual's actual or anticipated statuses and roles or, under certain conditions, to modify these statuses and roles to accord more closely with impulses, desires, and goals. Integrated development and effective performance require considerable congruence among psychological dispositions, among social roles, and between psychological dispositions and social roles. The content of social expectations must be sufficiently similar to individual desires, strivings, and plans to allow at least a moderate degree of personal meaning or fulfillment in social commitments and in social action. We may speak of these social expectations and norms, in a highly condensed way, as the content of roles; the individual, inner (conscious or unconscious) desires and strivings may be referred to, in equally condensed fashion, as the content of *goals*. Thus, effective functioning necessitates a moderately high degree of congruence between the content of roles and the content of goals, sufficient so that some degree of pleasure in goal achievement is commensurate with socially acceptable role performance and so that the pursuit of individual goals is compatible with the limits of actual or potential role performance.[12]

To the extent that theories of behavior have made any attempt to explain the interaction of psychological and social processes, they have almost invariably devoted primary attention to the similarity between individual strivings and sociocultural expectations. This emphasis on the parallelism between the individual and his society we may say is based upon an implicit or explicit *congruence* model.[13] It is clear that the existence of such congruence between psychological motives and social expectations is quite fundamental. However, the congruence model has serious limitations in accounting for specific behaviors, in permitting us to distinguish deviance from conformity, and in separating pathological from normal functioning except under highly restricted conditions. These are several reasons for these difficulties in modeling all relationships between the individual and his society on the basis of congruence, and their explication helps to point up some of the central problems that have characterized psychosocial explanations of behavior.

The transformation of drives and impulses in the course of social development and their effects on the structure of a relatively autonomous ego organization never dispose wholly of the potential conflict between personal wishes and social expectations. There can be little doubt that relatively primitive and undifferentiated impulses persist in adulthood and are accessible to consciousness (or even direct action) under conditions which are only moderately disruptive of familiar, socialized ego patterns. Thus, despite the enormous impact of socialization, congruence can be maintained only with persisting environmental regulation (stimulation and control) and with constant adjudication between roles and goals.

Certainly this is a dimension of individual variability, and the more effective the ego resources and controls, the more extreme must the disruptive factors be to facilitate the primitivization of goals. It is also, however, a dimension of societal variability; the more varied the roles an individual fulfills, the more complex the roles and role relationships involved, the less can any simple set of principles guarantee congruence between motives and expectations. In a highly differentiated "open" society such as those in urban, industrial countries, it is manifestly impossible for socialization to guarantee a high degree of congruence, and it becomes essential that the demands and expectations most fundamental for the integration of the society be represented *internally* in the goals and organizational principles of the ego.

The social environment is not only a source of demands and constraints. It also provides rewards, gratifications in role performance (role satisfaction) that do not depend entirely upon the satisfaction of impulses, and pleasures in social relationship and social experience that only secondarily become associated with personal motives. The fact of environmental reward implies that it is possible for individuals to develop patterns of social conformity without an initial investment in and desire for the particular behaviors and roles required by such conformity. The extent to which "reinforced" behaviors are dependent on environmental stimuli and can occur or develop only under conditions that forcibly restrict individuality and freedom accounts for the regularities obtained by reinforcement in the laboratory. Moreover, conformity that derives from social rewards need not be as constricted or narrowly defined as conformity that operates primarily under threat of punishment. Conformity based on efforts to obtain better pay, to receive group support and even group control, or to establish reciprocal and meaningful obligations may become quite generalized in behavior and in social orientations. Asch's study [14] of the effects of "rigged" group unanimity on individual judgments of a stimulus reveals that, even under the limited conditions of a laboratory experiment, it is possible to obtain great variability in the extent to which individuals make quite "unrealistic" judgments in order to maintain conformity with the group.[15] Prior congruence between roles and goals is, clearly, not a necessary condition for social conformity.

Beyond constraints and rewards, the social environment is a source of opportunities, stimulation, and challenge, which can lead to changes in behavior and to changes in ego structure that alter the balance of intraphysic forces. In conditions of social change, a most pervasive characteristic of industrial societies, opportunity and challenge are multiplied. Even in relatively restricted situations, as for the more deprived groups in industrial societies or for the tradition-bound peasant, the roles for which an individual was prepared during growth have generally altered sufficiently to require new adjustments and adaptations for which no socialization experience could have prepared him. As a consequence, any equilibrium between role expectations and goal aspirations toward which socialization is directed is likely to be constantly disrupted by changes from both societal and individual forces. The very concept of adaptation implies the readiness to alter familiar modes of orientation in the face of internal or external changes; in the extreme, it implies the ability to alter or modify internal goals in the presence of changing environmental potentials and to redefine external roles under the direction of changing personality potentials. Thus, congruence between roles and goals can only represent a rudimentary base that delimits the range of behavior and serves as a gross orientation for anticipation and planning.

We have already indicated that there is both individual and societal variability in the socialization of primitive impulses and desires; in the variety and complexity of roles that allow more differentiated motivational fulfillment; in the degree to which immediate social (group) rewards are meaningful and can generate attitudinal conformity; and in abilities to utilize environmental opportunities and challenges for realizing personal goals in adaptive achievements. We are familiar with all of these patterns as important differences between people (e.g., Riesman's "inner-directed" and "other-directed" patterns), as differences which can only synoptically be described as the primacy of personal goal aspirations as determinants of behavior. The actual ways in which different people equilibrate roles and goals to avoid disruptive conflict are infinitely varied and idiosyncratic. But the fact of the dominance of commitments to roles or to goals, and, by extension, the primacy of group-oriented or of ego-oriented behavior, is neither so varied, so flexible, nor so completely individual. It is, rather, a dimension of variability from one society to another and from one subgroup in society to other subgroups.

Some societies allow little room for independent goal definition and individuality and, through tradition and group observability, maintain relatively clear and specific role definitions and minimal-maximal performance expectations.[16] Socialization is directed to conformity, to compliance with group expectations, to the rewards of consensus, to the comforts of being like others. As a consequence, there is little opportunity for the development of independence and initiative and little encouragement to the differentiation of ego resources and ego controls. Under these conditions, a highly developed ego organization is maladaptive, except in circumstances that provide extensive opportunities for mobility out of the group or which require leadership roles.

Those societies or societal subgroups that emphasize the importance of autonomous behavior, of independent choices among alternative courses of action, and of initiative in changing external circumstances to meet inner desires, must allow wide latitude for the exercise of personal goals and of internal controls. All efforts of socialization are directed to the development of the ego even if, in immediate behavior, it involves nonconformity and strain. The expression of personal goals and the manifestation of inner resources for goal achievement, anticipation, planning, mastery, and ambition are necessarily rewarded and often can justify a wide range of otherwise deviant behaviors. The proliferation of external restrictions or rewards is viewed as potentially dangerous for, in fact, they tend to undermine the functional significance of internal mechanisms as sources of constraints or esteem.

Psychosocial Relationships: The Complementarity Model. We arrive by this route at a principle of psychosocial complementarity: *Adaptive behavior is based on the central regulative function of internal resources and controls when mechanisms of social regulation are relatively undifferentiated and role definitions are diffuse and flexible; it is based on the central regulative function of external resources and controls when mechanisms of ego regulation are relatively undifferentiated and goal directions are ambiguous and limited.* The distinction between these types can be made at the level of personality (e.g., ego differentiation and ego diffusion) or at the level of the social system (e.g., organic or contractual solidarity). The principle of complementarity implies that the modal pattern will always involve the predominance of *either* personal *or* societal regulation. At the extremes, of course, all societies must have institutionalized mechanisms for insuring a modicum of conformity and for minimizing severely disruptive forms of deviance. Similarly, human behavior requires some minimal commitment to societal expectations and some minimal demand for personal satisfaction. Within these extremes, however, an emphasis on the priority of role expectations and social conformity virtually precludes the extensive development or functioning of an ego organization capable of supplying internal resources or maintaining internal controls. The widespread development of individuality, of personal strivings for mastery, of personal desires for achievement can only arise in a relatively "open" society and, in turn, is likely to encourage the attrition of laws, regulations, ascribed statuses, and rigidly defined roles that too drastically limit the exercise of independence and initiative. Even the bureaucratization of industrial societies only modifies the degree to which and the roles within which such independence and initiative are desirable and is incomparably more flexible than the monolithic organization of preindustrial communities.

Although we may describe the modal patterns of effective adaptation in terms of the complementary relationships between individual and group mechanisms of regulation, it is evident that such complementarity does not obtain for all individuals in a society. Complementary patterns have considerable stability, but they are by no means static. An individual may move out of these relatively stable situations for many reasons of internal or external change. Under ordinary circumstances, individuals move into and out of complementary arrangements throughout the course of growth. In fact, the major transitions of human development may be seen as the disruption of temporarily stable and complementary states, disruption due to changes in internal desire or social demand, and their transformation into noncomplementary patterns. In turn, the noncomplementary patterns lead to subsequent efforts and expectations to achieve new forms of complementarity.

These movements away from the "ideal type" of complementary relationship between ego structure and social organization can be designated as noncomplementary patterns because they represent either the *simultaneous* force of individual goals and social expectation or the *simultaneous* absence of individual goals and of social resources.

Thus, the noncomplementary situation of a struggle for freedom from the family on the basis of intensified individuality during adolescence is often associated with the development of increased complementarity in the somewhat less binding expectations of peers; phases of apathy or indifference toward goal achievement coupled with the lack of adequate supportive or interactive social relationships is a typically unstable non-complementary pattern in adolescence. Noncomplementary patterns are as varied in type and in consequence as are complementary patterns. They differ, however, from complementary patterns by virtue of their intrinsic instability. Noncomplementary patterns in which *both* social and psychological regulatory mechanisms are powerful or in which *neither* type of regulation is notably available are the primary sources of change either in the direction of more satisfying and social effective arrangements or of dysfunction and pathology. The dynamic forces involved in developing noncomplementary relationships and in reestablishing complementarity are complex, and it is possible only to delineate several major sources and directions of these patterns.[17]

In modern industrial societies, it is primarily in working-class communities that one finds the basic conditions for that complementary pattern which involves the subordination of personal goals to social roles and the modest development of ego resources and controls in the presence of highly cohesive and omnipresent group relationships. This pattern is relatively stable despite the manifest pressures toward and opportunities for social and residential mobility into higher status positions.[18] Data from a working-class community in the West End of Boston reveal how frequently individuals are reluctant to relinquish their close-knit network ties despite the development of ego resources and of competence for independent activity. At the same time, such noncomplementary patterns are unstable, and those individuals with high ego resources *and* available social resources most frequently plan to move out of the area.

Although we cannot trace the full early history of these people, they tend to be distinguished from those in the same community who show a complementary pattern in a number of ways: (1) they often maintain close contact with parents but are not as often embedded in highly obligatory local kinship or network ties; (2) they are relatively content with the dependability and "encapsulating" presence of long-term ties to others but show an ability to establish new ties *de novo* outside the framework of the residential community; (3) they are frequently "central persons" in neighborhood groups and manifest many forms of initiative in small ways that do not obtrude themselves in their social role behavior; (4) clearly they show more highly developed ego functions and superego orientations that tend, however, to be inhibited by a "common man" ideology; and (5) there is a relatively high degree of "role articulation" in the marital relationship, indicating the greater capacity of the nuclear family to serve as a residual resource in the absence of the neighborhood peer group. All of these attributes define them as "transitional types" between the characteristics typical of the working class and those of the middle class.

This noncomplementary pattern is, par excellence, the basis for social mobility. With social mobility, implying mobility out of the socially cohesive group, a new pattern of complementarity is established, one which involves increased opportunity for goal-directed behavior without a constant requirement to fit these goals to already defined roles and social expectations. The transition is not an easy one, and undoubtedly many people experience it as a severe deprivation.[19] In fact, if ego resources are not commensurate with the task of freeing oneself from the constant availability of group resources and controls, familiar patterns of psychopathology may develop. An even more frequent source of psychopathological development would appear to arise from another direction of movement out of the working-class pattern of complementarity. This is the pattern that results from movement out of communally oriented group resources under the impact of psychological or social deprivation and results in the absence of *either* effective ego organization *or* effective social organization.

The principle of psychosocial complementarity implies that group resources provide alternative bases to ego resources in encouraging effective adaptation. Under conditions of intensified social deprivation, whether due to loss of employment, marital disruption, lack of familiarity with the group, ill health, or any other of the many potential factors, there is simultaneously an intensified need for group resources and a more perceptible inability of the group to meet these needs. In working-class communities there are many mechanisms of mutual assistance in emergency, but these are insufficiently based in a stable collectivity to maintain unrelated individuals through long-term deprivations.

On the basis of the data from the West End before and after relocation,[20] several factors stand out as common characteristics of this particularly problem-prone group: (1) quite frequently, they are discrepant in cultural background from the major population groups in the community; (2) they tend either to have fewer group contacts or do not utilize the group as compensation for deficits in other relationships (e.g., distance from the husband); (3) far more often do they have significant reservations about various "slummy" features of the environment (rats, buildings, space, amenities); (4) despite frequent complaints about the West End they often show an *increase* in positive feelings and longing after leaving; and (5) both in the past and the present, they more frequently seem beset with deprivations and disruptions, with past neglect, loss, and trauma, and with current unemployment, alcoholic spouses, illnesses, and problems with children.

For those with few ego resources and few group resources, it is evident that difficulties in establishing close-knit relationships have generally been quite extensive over long periods of time, and that with the move from the West End and its ever-present "friendliness," the precarious balance that many of these people maintained was totally disrupted. Although the crisis of transition was quite global and affected a majority of this working-class population, those who were least integrated into the socially cohesive patterns and who suffered less pure "grief" also could least cope with the added (and not wholly expected) deprivation. Thus, this noncomplementary pattern involved a set of circular reinforcements in which social resources and controls do not as readily become available and, when present cannot as easily be utilized to supplement the lack or inadequacy of psychological resources and controls.

From a psychological viewpoint, we often conceive only of the presence or absence of differentiated ego regulation (in the form of "ego strength") as a source of pathological behavior. From a sociological viewpoint, deviance is often attributed only to the absence of differentiated mechanisms of social regulation and of social integration. Despite their larger understanding of many concrete situations, Freud and Durkheim represent these opposing viewpoints. In the light of a principle of psychosocial complementarity, it is apparent that the analysis of both ego organization and of social organization is essential for an adequate explanation of normal or pathological functioning. The absence of a differentiated ego structure with effective regulatory mechanisms is not, in itself, an indication of adaptive failure or of psychopathology. In the presence of meaningful social networks that define role expectations and demand little in self-definition of goals, it may result in a most effective pattern of stable adaptation. Only when this organization of ego functions is coupled with ineffective mechanisms of social regulation or in crises that cause the loss or disruption of familiar patterns of group organization [21] do problems arise that lead to increasing maladaptation and the development of social pathology and psychopathology.

The many forms of social deprivation that occur in our society result in an intensified need for these external social resources. In the extreme, they involve a need that goes beyond the resources of any available natural group structure. The failure of community groups to meet these needs is likely to increase the degree of social isolation. Here we can visualize one primary function of professional health and welfare services, including psychiatric hospitalization, as virtually the only forms of organization that can supply external resources and controls adequate for establishing a more stable and complementary base for the emergence of more effective patterns of individual adaptation. With an understanding of the fundamental nature of complementary relationships, it may be possible to delineate these functions more precisely or to appreciate the potentials of alternative social resources in meeting the need for social regulatory mechanisms under conditions of psychological disorganization.

Psychiatric Epidemiology of Social Problems

Epidemiological Studies and Psychosocial Analysis. Ideally, a rigorous test of the hypotheses and derivations from the principle of psychosocial complementarity requires some form of highly controlled experimental or quasi-experimental design. In the absence of more adequate materials, however, it is useful to examine a readily available source of data in order to consider the more general implications of the principle of psychosocial complementarity. Such a source of data lies in the epidemiological literature on psychiatric hospitalization and the different conditions which reveal increases or decreases in rates of psychiatric hospitalization for an entire segment of the population or for some subgroup. The use of epidemiological data for such analytic purposes has not become widespread but offers considerable possibility for the examination of theoretical questions that require large population studies. For present purposes, however, these data can only be used to exemplify two components of the complementarity theses: (1) the rather general proposition that there is a close link (and, often, an arbitrary distinction) between psychological and social determinants; and (2) the more specific proposition that crises and transitions are particularly disruptive for lower status people. It does not, clearly, permit us to test the feature of the complementarity thesis that is more specific to this principle, that these disruptive effects are selectively important among those people with relatively few internal resources who are thereby more vulnerable to changes in the availability of situational resources.

In considering the theoretical issue of the interaction between psychological and social processes through the relationship between social problems and psychopathology, we have an opportunity to study relatively extreme instances. The most evident bases of social problems lie in that realm which we may describe as deprivation. In its simplest and starkest forms, it may include deprivation of material resources for daily living, such as food, shelter, and clothing. In more elaborate or subtle ways, it can involve deprivation of security or freedom, of opportunities and access, of social relationships and social esteem, or of skills, abilities, and privileges.

The use of epidemiological data for purposes of psychosocial analysis presents a number of problems and, in attempting to organize these data according to their implications for the effects of social deprivation, we shall rely more heavily on epidemiological findings than the solidity of the data warrants. Thus, it is essential to note certain important limitations. There is an excellent discussion of the utility of data on the first admissions to psychiatric hospitals as evidence for the incidence of psychiatric disorders by Kramer and his coworkers.[22] This provides sufficient caution against any interpretation of these data that does not, at the very least, understand these findings as indices of complex social phenomena. There is no path to treatment, no diagnostic procedure, and, consequently, no rate of psychiatric disorder that is not influenced, at every point in the process of being counted, by various social phenomena which literally create the rates of observed illness. In principle, this is neither more nor less true for psychiatric disorders than for any form of behavior or performance that must be evaluated by various human beings in different social contexts, by individuals who have specific value orientations and stable commitments to a relatively narrow range of functioning.

On the other hand, the development of institutionalized facilities for dealing with specific types of disturbed behavior and the education of communities to the use of these facilities necessarily results in some degree of uniformity. In most communities this means that those individuals who are least able to deal with the normal range of roles and role expectations, and whose failure appears to be associated with marked affective or cognitive deviation from community norms, will be defined as mentally ill. When there are similarities in the social structure of communities, common expectations for role performance within these communities, and common criteria among a body of professional "experts," we can anticipate some minimal common core of psychological and social malfunctioning among people who are classified as psychiatrically ill. These facts preclude a meaningful comparison of rates in different societies unless the comparison takes such variability into account. However, given such general similarity in "mental health" values, the analysis of internal relationships between rates of hospitalized or treated disorders and other variables is a legitimate basis for the interpretation of results.[23]

In comparing the effects of different conditions of social deprivation on rates of psychiatric hospitalization, we shall use data based on first hospitalization or those that approximate first hospitalizations almost exclusively. Technically, these are closest to the epidemiological category of "incidence" studies in which the first occurrence of a particular symptom or disease is the datum to be aggregated. The reason for this limitation is that, whatever the variations in designating a person as mentally ill or in hospitalizing people for psychiatric disorders, it is almost certain that there is even greater variability in the conditions and evaluations that determine whether or not a person remains in the hospital, having been once hospitalized, or returns to the psychiatric hospital after prior discharge.

Social Class Status.   Numerous studies suggest that the form of adult deprivation implied by lower social class position is a significant determinant of severely disordered psychological functioning. This issue has received widespread attention in recent years as a result of the work of Hollingshead and Redlich,[24] although the relationship between social class and psychiatric hospitalization has been observed and reported over many years. In a recent and extensive review, Mishler and Scotch [25] have carefully considered the most substantial studies of social class and hospitalization for schizophrenia and other psychoses. They point out that eight of the nine studies reviewed show that the highest incidence of psychiatric hospitalization occurs in the lowest social class groupings used in each study. Similarly, and almost as consistently, the lowest rates occur among the managerial group. Between these extremes of social class position, however, relationships are less clear and consistent.

If we consider the entire range of social class statuses, there is no warrant for the proposition that a simple, inverse relationship obtains between social class position and the incidence of psychiatric hospitalization. However, the lowest status groups do show the highest rates of hospitalized (or treated) psychiatric disorders. In addition to those studies selected for review by Mishler and Scotch, numerous other findings provide further evidence for this conclusion with few contrary results.[26]

Although the data appear relatively clear and consistent, the meaning of this association is more ambiguous. Many hypotheses have been suggested to account for the relationship: differences in community tolerance, class influences on psychiatric diagnosis, downward social mobility as an expression of early psychiatric disorder, and the cumulative stress most readily engendered among lower status groups.[27] The influence of differences in community tolerance for psychiatric disturbance is difficult to assess. The one study specifically directed to this problem [28] indicates fewer instances of nonhospitalized psychosis in a lower-middle-class area. Freeman and Simmons [29] show that the lower the social class, the less the feeling of stigma concerning patients who had been hospitalized. Jaco's data [30] indicate that if we consider only public treatment for psychosis, the incidence rates more nearly approximate a linear distribution of greater frequency with decreasing social class position (with the exception of the professional and semi-professional group). Although these results suggest higher extrusion rates among lower status people, they do not offer much promise of explaining the larger findings so simply.

There can be little doubt that the cultural patterns associated with social class status influence diagnostic judgments, and the lower the status, the more severe the diagnoses are likely to be.[31] But if this factor were to account for the relationship between social class position and psychiatric hospitalization, we would expect consistently linear associations for all status levels, and least of all would we anticipate high rates among professional groups. Thus, although the influence of diagnostic bias leading to higher rates of psychiatric hospitalization for low status groups cannot be dismissed, it would not appear to be sufficiently powerful or consistent to provide the single most general explanation.

The effect of predispositions to psychosis on downward social mobility has frequently been hypothesized as an explanation for the relationship between social class and psychiatric hospitalization. On logical grounds, the effect of predispositional factors on downward mobility should produce roughly equivalent effects at all status levels and lead to a linear association between social class status and psychiatric disorder. We have already indicated that such linearity does not obtain. Moreover, although the various efforts to examine the relationship between downward mobility and psychiatric hospitalization do not adequately dispose of this hypothesis, they lend little substantial support to this proposition as a general explanation.[32] We may also note that higher rates of psychiatric disorder are observed at the lowest educational levels as well as at the lowest occupational levels.[33] Since the finding is most notable for extreme educational deprivation, one could account for the causal influence of predispositions to psychosis only by maintaining that there is a widespread effect of such predispositions on educational attainment prior to adolescence. This proposition cannot be documented, nor can it explain the high rates among people with high educational achievements. Thus, it must remain an hypothesis that requires more systematic study and, in any case, is unlikely to be the predominant source of the social class relationship.[34]

The final hypothesis to be considered is that higher rates of psychiatric disorder appear among the lowest status groups because low status is itself stressful or because the limited resources available to people of low status result in greater impact and/or cumulation of other stresses and crises. One of the findings in Jaco's study [35] of psychiatric disorders in Texas offers some suggestions. In contrast to most other studies on social class and psychiatric disorder, Jaco distinguishes the unemployed from all other occupational categories and finds that the rates of treated psychiatric disorder are disproportionately high in this group. Among the employed manual laborers and service workers, the rates are high, but this is not so marked as in other studies. To what extent, one may legitimately wonder, are the very high rates of psychiatric disorder found in the lowest status groups a function of an association between *unemployment* and psychiatric hospitalization? The lowest status groups, by occupational or educational criteria, have by far the highest rates of unemployment.[36] Thus, the strong association of low socioeconomic status and treated psychiatric disorders could result largely from the fact that unemployment is higher in the lowest status levels and is also markedly associated with psychiatric hospitalization or treatment.

Such a relationship in which the higher rates of psychiatric hospitalization among lower status people are largely accounted for by the higher rates of unemployment might provide a basis for a more dynamic explanation of the perplexing social class finding but, for the time being, must remain a promising conjecture. In any case, it would hardly soften the conclusion that extreme, overt deprivation is a prominent source of manifest psychiatric disorder.[37] However, it would tend to contradict the proposition that low social class status per se is a form of deprivation leading to increased psychiatric impairment. It would suggest rather some more complex hypotheses: either (1) a greater variety of deprivations and/or stresses occur at lower status levels, leading to a cumulative effect on impairment; or (2) there is greater likelihood that the characteristic deprivations among lower status groups will be more severe and incapacitating crises; or (3) because of less adequate internal resources among lower status people, the same frequency and same severity of deprivation and/or stress will produce more severe impairments.[38]

Up to this point we have considered each possible explanation of the relationship between extreme status deprivation and psychiatric hospitalization as if it were a unitary factor that had to account for all or most of the association. Such singular explanations, whether directly revealed by the data or based on a more comprehensive conceptual formulation, are particularly satisfying to the aesthetic of science. Clearly, however, it is possible that all of the factors considered (and others as well) might account for these findings. Certainly it is possible that higher rates of hospitalization among the lowest socioeconomic status groups could result from a conjunction of: (1) differences in the frequency or severity of, or the resources for handling, deprivation in different social class groups; (2) the downward mobility potential of psychologically disturbed, relatively low status people; and (3) their frequent "extrusion" from the community and readier diagnosis of psychosis. Even if we assume that for any moderate proportion of the cases the disturbed psychological state is antecedent to the situation of social deprivation, it is evident that the greater frequency of, greater severity of, or less effective mechanisms for dealing with deprivation engendered by very low status necessarily means a far greater likelihood that disturbing and disruptive situations will occur. The larger number of factors that, alone or in concert, might produce disproportionate rates of psychiatric hospitalization among the lowest status group tends, thus, to highlight the ways in which the simple form of deprivation indicated by lower social class position may have complex and varied ramifications. We shall turn, therefore, to further areas in which social deprivation or social disruption may play significant parts in the observed rate differentials for severe psychiatric disorders.

Negro-White Differences. Although it is possible to regard Negro-white differences as one aspect of social stratification, the situation of the Negro is sufficiently different from that of the white at equivalent educational or occupational levels to warrant special consideration. At every level of social class status, the Negro suffers a greater range and more intense forms of overt deprivation (and implicit threat) than do whites. If extreme deprivation is a causal factor in hospitalization for psychiatric disorder, then Negro rates of psychiatric hospitalization lend considerable support to its importance. *At the present time, Negro rates of first admission to psychiatric hospitalization are consistently and overwhelmingly higher than white rates for both sexes and for virtually every age group.*

The full extent of this finding has only emerged in data for relatively recent periods. Pugh and MacMahon [39] point out that by 1922 the rates for Negroes had risen to parity with white rates and by 1933 "the non-white population was entering mental hospitals at higher rates than the native white in all except nine of the states. . . ." However, as Malzberg [40] had previously shown, even in the 1922 statistics the rates for the white population exceeded that for the Negroes only in several of the southern regions of the United States in which there were inadequate psychiatric hospital facilities for Negroes. Most studies show that current rates are at least twice as high for Negroes as for whites with the greatest differentials in the younger age groups and greater for males than for females.[41] Moreover, the same indices of deprivation or disruption that lead to increased rates for whites also cause increments to the Negro rates: low education, low occupation, migration, divorce, and separation.[42]

Unfortunately, the available data do not allow us to go much beyond this descriptive statement about the extremely high rates of first admission to psychiatric hospitals among Negroes. Nonetheless, more clearly than in any other situation, it is essential to conclude from these data that being Negro is of basic causal significance in producing higher rates of severe psychiatric disorder. The extreme versions of a selection hypothesis are rather evidently ruled out. There can be no question that being a Negro is *not* the result of predispositions to psychosis. Moreover, although psychological deprivation and disorganizing experiences of personal history may occur more frequently among Negroes than among whites, social deprivation and disruption, systematically related to many features of social structure that affect the Negro at all phases of development and functioning, are considerably more frequent and more severe among Negroes than among whites. If we consider the numerous other spheres in which malfunctioning is manifest, in unemployment and underemployment, in delinquency and crime, in poor health and high mortality rates, in dependence on social agency assistance, it is evident that overall rates of deviance and disorder are so great among Negroes that few alternative hypotheses are reasonable. We are bound to conclude that *severe social deprivation of the type so widely experienced among Negroes is of fundamental causal significance for psychological impairment.*

We have pointed to evidence that extremes of status deprivation, manifest among the lowest socioeconomic groups and among Negroes, are rather powerful components of the causal network leading to increased rates of first admission to psychiatric hospitals. In the absence of contrary data, the evidence is quite convincing that the extreme social deprivation implicit in these status positions, either directly or in conjunction with the frequent and relatively severe associated threats, disruptions, and crises, must be placed at a relatively early point in the causal chain that accounts for psychiatric disorder and hospitalization. At the same time, it becomes increasingly apparent that social deprivation is hardly ever *simply* deprivation. Extreme deprivation, at the least, implies frequent threat, likely frustration of many desires and impulses, widespread experiences of helplessness and futility, and the lack of inner or outer resources to serve as equilibrating mechanisms in a crisis, thereby intensifying the disruptive significance of modest frustrations and stresses. At an unconscious level, it is likely that more primitive impulses and fantasies are engendered by the same "objective" threat, deprivation, stress, or crisis and thus make the adaptive task more difficult. *Deprivation is the focal point in extremes of low status, but it is most often associated with a manifold of other social and psychological sources of disruption.*

Schematically, we can diagram the immediate sequences leading to psychiatric hospitalization as in Figure 1. The scheme is not meant as an inclusive substantive statement; it attempts only to diagram major points in the sequences and in the interactions. The middle column is labeled *Descriptive Clinical Sequence* because, without implying any specific causal theory, it takes account of precipitating circumstances

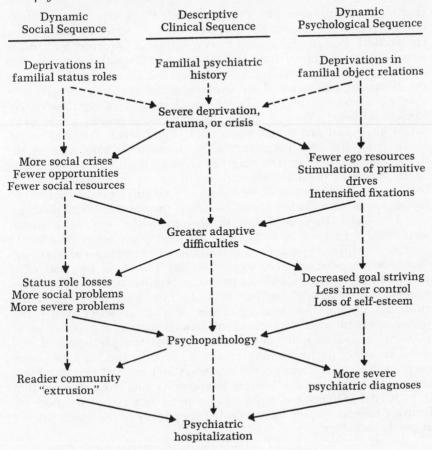

FIGURE 1
Causal Sequences Leading to Psychiatric Hospitalization

and the downhill course that so often appear to characterize the emergence of psychopathology prior to hospitalization. The first column, labeled *Dynamic Social Sequence*, indicates that with deprivations at the level of familial status and familial roles, two major directions may be traced: (1) a series of further deprivations, disruptions, crises, lacks, and losses are more likely to arise given the initial deprivations; and (2) at any point in the sequence those social deprivations may lead to intermediate "clinical" manifestations and, more significantly, can result in psychological changes that may be traced through the levels of "inner" psychological malfunctioning. Similarly, the *Dynamic Psychological Sequence* implies that deprivation at the level of familial object relations, on the one hand, leads to increased likelihood of additional forms of psychological deficit and, on the other, can result in both "clinical" manifestations and in social deprivations and disruptions at any point in the sequence.

This chart is, thus, a synopsis of many possible paths to psychiatric hospitalization. For any given individual, the primary direction of "regressive" movement may be seen as a series of shifts along the vertical axis of the Dynamic Psychological Sequence with occasional, diagonal forays into the Descriptive Clinical Sequence. For another person, the most appropriate characterization may be through the increasing difficulties of the Dynamic Social Sequence, occasionally showing up as one of the clinical manifestations in the Descriptive Clinical Sequence. We may suspect that, for most people, a very careful psychological and social assessment would reveal frequent movements from Dynamic Psychological Sequence to Dynamic Social Sequence and the reverse. The diagonal arrows, which stress these shifts in the sphere of manifest difficulty, point up the interaction of forces that are easily overlooked if we follow any singular psychodynamic or sociodynamic formulation of the causes of psychiatric hospitalization.

The chart, thus, is drawn in this particular way, with multidirectional sequences, to emphasize this one point: *It is possible to treat one of these sequences as systematic and everything else as random, idiosyncratic, or situational, but this is only a function of a particular perspective which understands psychological or social phenomena systematically, but not both.* In fact, both represent distinguishable systems that bear upon one another at select points and with respect to specific problems of human action. But problems of pathological behavior are precisely issues that are psychological *and* social in origin, in intervening processes, in definition, and in consequences. The more clearly we can understand the independent functioning of each sequence *and* its interactions with other factors that form partial systems and sequences in their own right, the more effectively may we be able to explain the complexity of observed patterns of psychopathology.

Social Deprivation and Situational Crises. We have pointed to the fact that at the lowest levels of status, socioeconomic deprivation is accompanied by many other problems of living and that for any given level of "objective" stress the absence of inner or outer resources to facilitate adaptation means a greater degree of *relative* deprivation or experienced stress. Although there is little evidence concerning the effects of cumulative difficulties on psychiatric disorder, there is some suggestion in the data that an increase in overt psychiatric pathology occurs with an increased number of deprivations and stresses.[43] Moreover, as we have suggested, even if there is no greater likelihood that a particular form of deprivation or disruption will occur among the lowest status groups, it is likely that when these do occur in any form they will be more seriously incapacitating. There are no available data that allow us to assess this problem directly. However, a number of situational crises for which data exist do permit us to evaluate more fully the effects of social problems more generally on psychiatric hospitalizations. We shall turn to a brief consideration of some of these data on economic disruption, marital disruption, and residential disruption before evaluating the larger problem posed.

ECONOMIC DISRUPTION. We have already indicated that unemployment may well be a particularly significant intervening variable accounting for high rates of psychiatric disorder. There is also evidence, although not unambiguous, that serious economic depressions, which produce high rates of unemployment and drastic alterations in economic and social status, produce high rates of disordered functioning. The data are most clear for suicide and appear to be consistently confirmed. There is a direct statistical relationship between indices of economic depression and rates of suicide.[44]

For psychiatric hospitalization, the data are more difficult to evaluate. If we consider all first admissions to psychiatric hospitals, there is evidence for a relationship between the economic depression of the 1930s and psychiatric disorders.[45] The issue, however, is complicated by two factors: (1) From Dayton's data [46] it would appear that the critical period of rising rates for psychiatric hospitalization occurred during the onset of unemployment before the depression was in full evidence, and a similar pattern holds for suicide.[47] But there are few series of data available for the relevant periods which permit replicating Dayton's findings. (2) The increase in psychiatric hospitalization during the depression period was considerably greater for persons without mental disorder than for those with mental disorder. It is unclear whether the criteria for hospitalization or those for diagnosing mental disorder were more drastically affected by the widespread evidence of realistic deprivation during the crisis. In any case, Dayton does show that the effect holds for cases with mental disorder, albeit less strongly, and there is also a subsequent rise during the onset phase of the recession which occurred in 1937.[48] Thus, we are led to conclude, tentatively, that the type of crisis manifested in an economic depression increases the likelihood of psychiatric disorders.

MARITAL DISRUPTION. The data on marital status and psychiatric hospitalization are virtually as clear and unambiguous as one could desire. Despite minor variations within subcategories, *first admission rates for psychiatric hospitalization are consistently higher for the divorced than for any other group.*[49] Moreover, the rank position of first admission rates is generally the same for different marital status groups. The divorced, single, widowed, and married represent a decreasing order of rates. A similar pattern exists for suicides and lends further support to the general significance for malfunctioning of these different marital situations.[50]

More clearly than any other set of findings, the data on marital status and psychiatric hospitalization necessitate a model of multiple causation. In the higher rates for the widowed than for the married there is evidence for the importance of deprivation or disruption rather than selective factors. Selection might account for some unknown proportion of the high rates among both the single and the divorced, although the components of deprivation among the single and of disruption among the divorced are too apparent to require comment. However, since there is every reason to believe that selective factors should affect rates among the single to a considerably greater extent than among those who did marry but were later divorced, and yet the rates for the latter are the highest of all, we must grant a good deal of importance to the crisis of divorce or separation as one determinant of subsequent psychiatric hospitalization. Finally, the differential between the married, at one extreme, and the divorced, at the other, tends to be dramatic; first admission ratios of psychiatric hospitalization are of the order of three to five times higher for the divorced than for the married. The rate differences according to marital status are strong, and the factors involved do not lend themselves readily to any simple explanation. Rather the combinations of predispositional selective factors and of the stabilizing effects of cohesive marital relationships stand out as forces that reinforce one another in producing the observed effects on rates of psychiatric hospitalization.

RESIDENTIAL DISRUPTION.   Differences in rates of psychiatric hospitalization for mental disorder between the native-born and foreignborn had become a public issue of considerable importance in the United States after World War I, when legislation was pending for more restricted immigration.[51] A frequent thesis in this argument was that these higher rates were due to the inherent inferiority of the immigrant nationalities. Ødegaard's famous study of Norwegians [52] showed that the immigrants to the United States from Norway had higher rates than did those Norwegians who remained in Norway. These data could be interpreted in several ways—but Ødegaard chose to make a case for the selection hypothesis. Subsequent work clarified the fact that it was migration (whether due to selection or to the process of migrating) rather than nativity which bore the responsibility for these higher rates.[53]

Increasing evidence has given greater credence to the central importance of the disruptive experience of migration, although the selection hypothesis has not been ruled out as a general explanation or as a way of accounting for some proportion of cases.[54] Several recent studies introduce either new ways of ordering the data or new ways of accounting for them. Recent rates of psychiatric hospitalization for mental disorder show the persistence of a relatively small difference between the foreign-born and native white rates,[55] with several negative findings.[56] Of striking interest in these studies is the new evidence that *migrants from one state to another have even higher rates than do the foreign-born, and that this differential holds for both Negroes and whites.*

An important hypothesis to account for migration ratio differentials in psychiatric disorder has been suggested by Murphy.[57] He points out that there are differences in migrant rates that correspond to differences in the situation of the migrant in the specific host society. A wide range of migration situations require that the immigrant adapt to a wholly unfamiliar situation without adequate support or resources for making the transition, and it is in these societies that high migrant rates of psychiatric hospitalization appear. Migration from rural to urban areas and from preindustrial to industrial societies produces a crisis of transition in which, for a relatively long time, the migrant is deprived of the educational and cultural background necessary for effective functioning, of the occupational and prestige opportunities fundamental in urban life, and of the social resources of familiar and dependable ties and relationships to other people.[58] Crises have an inherent potential for creating disorder although they may also lead to higher levels of functioning.[59] But the potential for change intrinsic to such crises of transition requires meaningful resources to maximize the opportunities and to minimize the dangers. Since the rural or peasant migrant rarely has commensurate internal resources for dealing independently with these unfamiliar challenges at the outset, he must find equivalent external resources. For many former peasants, these were available in the urban, ethnic, working-class slums.[60] For the migrant who moves from one state to another, few such communities exist, and under these circumstances, without adequate internal or external resources, psychiatric disorder and hospitalization appear to be one of a number of manifestations of a high frequency of failures in adaptation.

Social Problems and Psychopathology: A Causal Matrix. In reviewing data on the relationships among social deprivation, social disruption, and differential rates of psychiatric hospitalization, we have come to several conclusions. Some of these are quite unambiguous, others less clear, and some remain as tentative hypotheses. In summarizing these results, it is possible to see the main lines of interpretation and their implications.

1. Extreme overt deprivation of economic and social resources and opportunities associated with the lowest status positions in our society is a serious impediment to effective functioning and is statistically associated with higher rates of first admission to psychiatric hospitalization. Although no simple causal explanation accounts either for all the cases or for the fact that other persons in similar status positions show less marked (if any) evidence of psychological disorder, severe deprivation appears to have a very significant determining influence at numerous points in the complex sequences that result in psychopathology.

2. Overt social and economic deprivation, both in its most extreme form and in more modest degree, is very often related to various types of psychological disruption and deprivation. There are undoubtedly conditions in which *psychological* deprivation is a primary causal factor leading to *psychological* disorganization and resulting in *social* deprivation. With equal certainty, however, *social* deprivation may lead to *social* disruption and, in turn, may result in *psychological* disorganization.

3. There is no adequate evidence that overt social deprivation and rates of observed psychiatric disorder are related in a simple, linear pattern. In trying to account for the distinctiveness of the pattern among the most severely deprived groups, we suggested that available social resources can often counteract the more severe consequences of social or psychological deprivation. By implication, it is the effect of social deprivation on social disruption that potentiates the relationship between social deprivation and severe psychopathology.

Their cumulative impact and consequences for psychological disorganization give dynamic meaning to the sequences that start with social deprivation and end with psychiatric hospitalization.

4. Crises of transition, manifest in such disruptions as economic depression, divorce, and migration, also produce marked increases in rates of psychiatric hospitalization. There is presumptive evidence that a social principle equivalent to Freud's concept of "over determination," elaborated in Waelder's principle of multiple function,[61] holds for multiple external deprivations and disruptions. Moreover, any single deprivation or disruption increases the likelihood that other deprivations and disruptions will occur. It is also possible that when disruptions are experienced as severe deprivations and losses, their consequences for psychopathology are most serious.[62]

5. If we try to understand the great importance of extreme deprivation for psychopathology in relation to the disproportionate reduction of potentials for psychiatric disorder with less severe conditions of social deprivation, we come upon the considerable importance of the resources, social *or* psychological, that seem to modify the impact of deprivation or disruption. There are several factors that appear to be involved in this relationship: (1) the sense of security in the availability of resources during crises of transition; (2) actual assistance (economic aid, advice, homemaker service) of various types to compensate for deficits in temporary crises of deprivation or disruption; (3) implicit and explicit encouragement to reorganize psychological resources either through group denial of hopelessness or through ego support by clarifying alternatives. These appear only to be effective in relatively close-knit community relationships in which there is a sense of common "cultural identity" with widespread knowledge of deprivation.[63]

6. Finally, these results provide provisional support for the general view that numerous transitional states and situations are the most specific proximal causes of high rates of psychopathology. It is not so much the prior status of deprived groups (e.g., as lower class of Negro) but rather the particular vulnerability of these populations to conditions of internal or external change which appear to be associated with the incidence of psychiatric hospitalization. On theoretical grounds, we would anticipate that these transitions would represent noncomplementary conditions in which there is a simultaneous deprivation of internal and external regulatory mechanisms or a simultaneous convergence of internal and external regulatory mechanisms. While it is not altogether possible to draw from these findings a more precise conclusion than that these are, in fact and most fundamentally, noncomplementary conditions, the data indicate that this is one of the more plausible explanations for differences in rates of psychiatric hospitalization.

NOTES

1. Sigmund Freud, "The Neuro-psychoses of Defence (1894)," in *Complete Psychological Works of Sigmund Freud,* vol. 3 (London: Hogarth, 1962): 43–68.

2. In referring to his formulation of the primary defensive act, Freud stated: "I cannot, of course, maintain that an effort of will to thrust things of this kind out of one's thoughts is a pathological act; nor do I know whether and in what way intentional forgetting succeeds in those people who, under the same psychical influences, remain healthy. I only know that this kind of 'forgetting' did not succeed with the patients I analyzed, but led to various pathological actions." Freud, "A Reply to Criticisms of My Paper on Anxiety Neurosis (1895)" in *Complete Psychological Works of Sigmund Freud,* pp. 121–139; Marc Fried, "Social Problems and Psychopathology," in *Social Psychology and Mental Health,* ed. Wechsler et al. (New York: Holt, Rinehart and Winston, 1970), p. 627.

3. Heinz Hartmann and Ernest Kris, "The Genetic Approach in Psychoanalysis," in *Psychoanalytical Study of the Child* 1 (1945): 11–30.

4. This is particularly striking in view of his own earlier efforts to stress "acquired" factors in neurosis in contrast to the predominant view. In fact, he was highly critical of the fact that "others may declare the case to be determined by heredity even when there is no heredity, so that they overlook the whole category of acquired neuroses." Freud, "A Reply"; Fried, "Social Problems," p. 426.

5. Freud, "Totem and Taboo (1913)," in *Complete Psychological Works of Sigmund Freud,* vol. 13, 1–162; "Group Psychology and the Analysis of the Ego (1921)," in *Complete Psychological Works of Sigmund Freud,* vol. 18, 67–143; "The Future of an Illusion (1927)," in *Complete Psychological Works of Sigmund Freud,* vol. 21, 3–63; "Civilization and Its Discontents (1930)," in *Complete Psychological Works of Sigmund Freud,* vol. 21, 59–157.

6. It is worth noting that Freud, like other great thinkers, was aware of many more issues and complexities than he was ever able to formulate systematically in the framework of his model. In this sense, Freud left a heritage that goes beyond the model or the theory he formulated or even implied. Unfortunately, the very force of the model and of the theory makes it that much more difficult to utilize these profoundly insightful but passing observations more systematically than he did since, almost inevitably, it would mean altering the model and the theory. Even in those instances in which he went further and delineated the fundamental components of a new model and a new theory, as with ego psychology, there appears to be considerable reluctance to carry its implications to their logical conclusions.

7. Freud realized the potential influence of differences in social organization (social class, religious affiliation) on adult personality and behavior. However, this did not alter his basic model. This is particularly evident in *Civilization and Its Discontents,* in which he discusses social cohesiveness. Clearly, he regards the pressures for stable social organization as impediments to the free expression of impulses and therefore as limitations on happiness. He never conceives of social relationships as intrinsically rewarding but conceptualizes only the limitations they impose on impulse gratification. This is partly due to his equating impulse gratification and happiness, a formulation that is untenable in the light of psychoanalytic ego psychology. In effect, the developmental primacy and partial persistence into adulthood of primitive sexual and aggressive wishes played an inordinate part in his formulation of their *theoretical* primacy. The issue is, in part, taken into account in Hartmann's formulation of the primary and secondary autonomy of the ego. As in Allport's statement of the principle of functional autonomy, developmental changes in the vicissitudes of drives and of their objects lead to a total change in the structure of the ego and, therefore, of the relative significance one may attribute to any single motivating factor. This conceptualization is, in a sense, already implicit in Freud's distinctions between primary and secondary processes or of pleasure and reality principles. But Freud did not carry to its logical conclusions his own dictum that the reality principle involved the postponement of immediate pleasure for the sake of greater future rewards, since he was, generally speaking, more strongly influenced by problems of pain and their diminution than of rewards and their maximization. N. A. Dayton, *New Facts on Mental Disorders* (Springfield, Ill.: Charles C Thomas, 1940); Freud, "Civilization and Its Discontents"; Heinz Hartmann, "Notes on the Reality Principle," *Psychoanalytical Study of the Child* 11 (1956): 31–53; Hartmann, *The Ego and the Problem of Adaptation* (New York: International Universities Press, 1958); Gordon W. Allport, "The Open System in Personality Theory," in *Journal of Abnormal Social Psychology* 61 (1960): 301–310; Allport, "Personality: Normal and Abnormal," in *Personality and Social Encounter,* ed. Allport (Boston: Beacon, 1964), pp. 155–168.

8. Emile Durkheim, *Le Suicide* (Paris: F. Alcan, 1897); English translation. New York: Free Press, 1951.

9. Ibid.

10. Freud, "Civilization and Its Discontents."

11. Durkheim, *On the Division of Labor in Society* (New York: Macmillan, 1933).

12. Erikson and Parsons have contributed particularly to our understanding of the mechanisms involved in developing this form of congruence. In a recent essay, Inkeles has generalized and further clarified an integrated approach to this problem for the study of adult behavior. Hartmann's concept of social compliance refers to a related phenomenon. E. H. Erikson, "Growth and Crises of the Healthy Personality," in *Symposium on the Health Personality*, ed. M. J. E. Senn (New York: Josiah Macy, Jr. Foundation, 1950); Talcott Parsons, *The Social System* (New York: Free Press, 1951); Alex Inkeles, "Sociology and Psychology," in *Psychology: A Study of Science*, ed. S. Koch, vol. 6 (New York: McGraw-Hill, 1963): 317–387; Fried, "Social Problems," p. 430; Hartmann, "Notes on the Reality Principle."

13. A number of studies fall outside this predominant trend and try to link significant propositions concerning individual impulse and social regulation or control in empirical analysis. These, in addition to the work of Freud and, especially, of Durkheim, form the literature for the complementarity model. One of the most systematic and successful of these studies is in Henry and Short's analysis of *Suicide and Homicide*. A number of other fine examples are Riesman's *The Lonely Crowd*, Aronfreed's study of morality in children, Miller and Swanson's analysis of entrepreneurial and bureaucratic systems, Gouldner and Peterson's provocative study of preliterate social organization, and Fromm's earlier but still important and stimulating work. A. E. Henry and J. F. Short, Jr., *Suicide and Homicide* (New York: Free Press, 1954); David Riesman, *The Lonely Crowd* (New Haven: Yale University Press, 1950); J. Aronfreed, "The Nature, Variety, and Social Patterning of Moral Responses to Transgression," *Journal of Abnormal Social Psychology* 63 (1961): 223–240; D. R. Miller and G. E. Swanson, *The Changing American Parent* (New York: Wiley, 1958); Alvin W. Gouldner and R. A. Peterson, *Notes on Technology and the Moral Order* (Indianapolis: Bobbs-Merrill, 1962); Erich Fromm, *Escape from Freedom* (New York: Farrar and Rinehart, 1941); Fried, "Social Problems," p. 430.

14. Solomon E. Asch, "Studies of Independence and Conformity: I. A Minority of One Against a Unanimous Majority," *Psychology Monographs* 70 (1956): 1–70.

15. In Merton's typology we may refer to the alteration in perception as attitudinal conformity and the alteration in response only as behavioral conformity. It is particularly striking that *attitudinal* conformity could be attained simply through persistent group pressure. Robert K. Merton, "Conformity, Deviation, and Opportunity Structures," *American Sociological Review* 24 (1959): 177–188.

16. The post-feudal European peasantry of the eighteenth and nineteenth centuries are among the best examples of this type, although the contemporary urban, industrial working class approximates it in many ways. The alternative "ideal type" is particularly evident among the elites of expanding empires and in the large middle- and upper middle-class groups of highly developed industrial societies.

17. These refer only to the forms of complementarity involving individual stability and change. The same principle is applicable at a societal level but requires a different level of anlysis in dealing in the large-scale evolutionary or revolutionary social change.

18. Fried, "Transitional Functions of Working-Class Communities: Implications for Forced Relocation," in *Mobility and Mental Health*, ed. M. Kantor (Springfield, Ill.: Charles C Thomas, 1965), pp. 123–165.

19. Fried, "Grieving for a Lost Home," in *The Urban Condition*, ed. L. J. Duhl (New York: Basic Books, 1963), pp. 151–171.

20. Ibid.; Fried, "Effects of Social Change on Mental Health," in *American Journal of Orthopsychiatry* 34 (1964): 3–28.

21. E. Lindemann, "Psycho-social Factors as Stressor Agents," in *Stress and Psychiatric Disorders*, ed. J. M. Tanner (Oxford: Blackwell Scientific Publications, 1960), pp. 13–16.

22. M. Kramer et al., "Studies of the Incidence and Prevalence of Hospitalized Mental Disorders in the United States: Current Status and Future Goals," in *Comparative Epidemiology of the Mental Disorders*, ed. Pauls Hoch and Joseph Zubin (New York: Grune and Stratton, 1961), pp. 56–100.

23. This is one way of stating a more general principle in the analysis of data based on surveys of populations in which the sources of error and bias are unknown. The raw data are subject to greater error than are the interrelationships between variables, with the exception of those instances in which the error (or bias) happens to be systematically selective with respect to the variables being analyzed. One relevant assumption about the discrepancy between psychiatric hospitalization and the incidence of psychosis which is often made is logically unwarranted. This assumption is that the errors are all or mainly in the direction of false negatives resulting from the failure to count all "true" cases of psychosis in the community. In fact, false positives may be the result of numerous factors: transitory behavior which ap-

pears initially more ominous than it proves to be, low tolerance thresholds in certain families or communities, errors of judgment and evaluation. Moreover, it seems likely that the advance of a field tends to reduce both false negatives and false positives. If this is, in fact, the case, two conclusions follow: (1) discrepancies between observed and "true" rates of psychosis are, from the point of view of the accounting system, truly random errors and are not likely to be the source of consistent associations; and (2) in the language of information theory, this increases the signal-to-noise ratio, and in the presence of considerable random error (noise), relatively minor signals that are consistently produced may signify greater underlying uniformities than are clearly revealed in the data.

24. A. B. Hollingshead and F. C. Redlich, *Social Class and Mental Illness* (New York: Wiley, 1958).

25. Elliot G. Mishler and Norman A. Scotch, "Sociocultural Factors in the Epidemiology of Schizophrenia," *Psychiatry* 26 (1963): 315–343.

26. R. W. Hyde and L. V. Kingsley, "Studies in Medical Sociology, I. The Relation of Mental Disorders to the Community Socio-economic Level," *New England Journal of Medicine* 231 (1944): 543–548; Eva Johanson, "A Study of Schizophrenia in the Male: A Psychiatric and Social Study Based on 138 Cases with Follow up," *Acta Psychiatria et Neurologica Scandinavica* (1958, Supplement 125), Copenhagen: Ejnar Munksgaard; Bert Kaplan, Robert B. Ree, and Wyman Richardson, "A Comparison of the Incidence of Hospitalized and Non-Hospitalized Cases of Psychoses in Two Communities," *American Sociological Review* 21 (1956): 472–479; Robert J. Kleiner and J. Tuchman, "Multiple Group Membership and Schizophrenia," *Behavioral Science* 6 (1961): 292–296; T. S. Langner and S. T. Michael, *Life Stress and Mental Health: The Midtown Manhattan Study*, vol. 2 (London: Free Press, 1963); Everett S. Lee, "Socio-economic and Migration Differentials in Mental Disease," *Milbank Memorial Fund Quarterly* 41 (1963): 249–468; Ben Z. Locke, Morton Kramer, and Benjamin Pasamanick, "Immigration and Insanity," *Public Health Report* 75 (1960): 301–306; L. G. Rowntree, K. H. McGill, and L. P. Hellman, "Mental and Personality Disorders in Selective Service Registrants," *Journal of American Medical Association* 126 (1945): 1084–1087; L. Srole et al., *Mental Health in the Metropolis: The Midtown Manhattan Study*, vol. 1 (New York: McGraw-Hill, 1962); Lilli Stein, " 'Social Class' Gradient in Schizophrenia," *British Journal of Preventive Social Medicine* 11 (1957): 181–195; Dorothy Thomas and Ben B. Locke, "Marital Status, Education and Occupational Differentials in Mental Disease," *Milbank Memorial Fund Quarterly* 41 (1963): 145–160; C. Tietze, P. Lemkau and M. Cooper, "Personality Disorder and Spatial Mobility," *American Journal of Sociology* 48 (1942): 29–39.

27. I shall not consider any of the genetic hypotheses here since they represent one type of specification of predispositional factors and, without far more adequate data, are indistinguishable from other formulations which rest on the significance of selective factors in accounting for rate differentials.

28. Kaplan, Ree, and Richardson, "A Comparison."

29. Howard E. Freeman and D. G. Simmons, *The Mental Patient Comes Home* (New York: Wiley, 1963).

30. E. G. Jaco, *The Social Epidemiology of Mental Disorders* (New York: Russell Sage Foundation, 1960).

31. Howard T. Blane, Willis F. Overton, and Morris E. Chafetz, "Social Factors in the Diagnosis of Alcoholism: I. Characteristics of the Patient," *Quarterly Journal of Studies on Alcohol* 24 (1963): 640–663; S. M. Miller and Elliot G. Mishler, "Social Class, Mental Illness, and American Psychiatry: An Expository Review," *Milbank Memorial Fund Quarterly* 37 (1959): 174–199.

32. Mishler and Scotch, "Sociocultural Factors."

33. Jaco, *Social Epidemiology of Mental Disorders;* Kleiner and Tuckman, "Multiple Group Membership"; Lee, "Differentials in Mental Disease"; Locke, Kramer, and Pasamanick, "Immigration and Insanity"; Thomas and Locke, "Marital Status, Education and Occupational Differentials."

34. It is, of course, possible that downward mobility in occupation or minimal education attainment is more readily produced by psychotic predispositions at lower than at higher status levels. This is not an unreasonable hypothesis in view of the fact that socialization to higher levels of performance may facilitate modest effectiveness in occupational and educational activity in spite of relatively severe psychological or even organic impairments. Some support for this view is provided by the observation that, following psychiatric hospitalization, the lower the initial occupational level, the greater the relative frequency of downward occupational mobility. However, if this proved to be an important factor explaining the social class relationship to psychiatric disorder, it would transpose the sphere in which deprivation functioned to produce impairment and to limit adaptive potentials, without neces-

sarily vitiating the significance of deprivation phenomena. Durkheim, *On the Division of Labor in Society.*

35. Jaco, *Social Epidemiology of Mental Disorders.*

36. U.S. Department of Labor, *Manpower Report to the President* (Washington, D.C.: Government Printing Office, 1963).

37. In this connection we may note that Sainsbury found a significant correlation between unemployment and suicide in a case by case analysis, although there was no "ecological correlation" between rates of unemployment in different areas and suicide rates. In spite of the fact that we cannot automatically classify suicides among severe psychiatric disorders, the many parallel conditions associated with suicide rates and with rates of psychiatric hospitalization lend some further support for the view that crises such as unemployment cause a marked increase in severe psychological disruption. One further piece of evidence supporting this view comes from a study of selective service registrants (Rowntree, McGill, and Hellman) in which a mixed category, which included primarily the unemployed and emergency workers, showed a much higher rate of rejection for "mental and personality disorders excluding psychoneurosis" than did any of the occupational categories. Peter Sainsbury, *Suicide in London: An Ecological Study* (London: Chapman and Hall, 1955); Rowntree, McGill, and Hellman, "Mental and Personality Disorders."

38. The study by Langner and Michael arrived too late to be given adequate consideration in this analysis. It is important, however, to note their finding that the number of stress factors was not significantly greater for lower than for higher status people. Their data indicate that for every unit of stress, there was greater impairment among the lower than among the higher status groups. This led to their explanation of the inverse relationship between social class position and psychiatric impairment on the basis of differences in type of adaptation to stress at different social class levels. Langner and Michael, *Life Stress and Mental Health.*

39. T. F. Pugh and B. MacMahon, *Epidemiologic Findings in United States Mental Hospital Data* (Boston: Little, Brown, 1962).

40. B. Malzberg, *Social and Biological Aspects of Mental Disease* (Utica: New York State Research Council, 1940).

41. Kleiner and Tuckman, "Multiple Group Membership"; Lee, "Differentials in Mental Disease"; Thomas and Locke, "Marital Status, Education and Occupational Differentials"; Malzberg, *Social and Biological Aspects;* Pugh and MacMahon, *Epidemiologic Findings.*

42. Jaco, *Social Epidemiology of Mental Disorders;* Judith Lazarus, Ben Z. Locke, and Dorothy S. Thomas, "Migration Differentials in Mental Disease," *Milbank Memorial Fund Quarterly* 41 (1963): 25–42; Lee, "Differentials in Mental Disease"; Locke, Charles E. Timberlake, and Donald Smeltzer, "Problems of Interpretation of Patterns of First Admissions to Ohio State Public Mental Hospitals for Patients with Schizophrenic Reactions," in *Social Aspects of Psychiatry,* ed. Benjamin Pasamanick and Peter H. Knapp (Washington, D.C.: American Psychiatric Association, Psychiatric Research Reports #10, 1958); Malzberg and Lee, *Migration and Mental Disease, A Study of First Admissions to Hospitals for Mental Disease, New York, 1939–1941* (New York: Social Science Research Council, 1956).

43. Apart from Langner and Michael's data the evidence is indirect, and shows that when different forms of deprivation (education, occupation, racial) or disruption (migration, divorce) are superimposed on one another, in the form of controls or statistical adjustments, rates of first admission to psychiatric hospitals are highest for the group representing multiple deprivations or disruptions. See: Langner and Michael, *Life Stress and Mental Health;* Kleiner and Tuckman, "Multiple Group Membership"; Lee, "Differentials in Mental Disease"; Thomas and Locke, "Marital Status, Education and Occupational Differentials"; Lazarus, Locke, and Thomas, "Migration Differentials"; Malzberg and Lee, *Migration and Mental Disease.*

44. See: L. I. Dublin and B. Bunzel, *To Be Or Not To Be: A Study of Suicide,* (New York: Smith, 1933); Freud, "Civilization and Its Discontents"; Henry and Short, *Suicide and Homicide;* Sainsbury, *Suicide in London;* Douglas Swinscow, "Some Suicide Statistics," *British Medical Journal* 1 (1951): 1417–1423.

45. Dayton, *New Facts on Mental Disorders;* H. Warren Dunham, *Sociological Theory and Mental Disorder* (Detroit: Wayne State University Press, 1959); Pugh and MacMahon, *Epidemiologic Findings.*

46. Dayton, *New Facts on Mental Disorders.*

47. Dublin and Bunzel, *To Be Or Not To Be.*

48. Pugh and MacMahon, *Epidemiologic Findings.*

49. Dayton, *New Facts on Mental Disorders;* Locke, Timberlake, and Smeltzer, "Problems of Interpretation"; Malzberg, *Social and Biological Aspects;* Pugh and

MacMahon, *Epidemiologic Findings;* Srole et al., *Mental Health in the Metropolis;* Thomas and Locke, "Marital Status, Education and Occupational Differentials."

50. Dublin and Bunzel, *To Be Or Not To Be;* Durkheim, *Suicide;* Sainsbury, *Suicide in London.*

51. Malzberg, *Social and Biological Aspects;* Thomas, "Introduction," in Benjamin Malzberg and Everett S. Lee, *Migration and Mental Disease,* pp. 1–42.

52. Ornulv Odegaard, "Emigration and Insanity: A Study of Mental Disease Among the Norwegian-born Population of Minnesota," *Acta Psychiatrica et Neurologica Scandinavica* (Copenhagen: Aarhuus Stiftsboytrykkerie, 1932), Supplement 4, pp. 182–184.

53. Locke, Kramer, and Pasamanick, "Immigration and Insanity"; Malzberg, *Social and Biological Aspects;* Malzberg and Lee, *Migration and Mental Disease;* Thomas, "Introduction."

54. Only a few points may indicate the basis for giving relatively little weight to the selection hypothesis. (1) Most of the historical materials suggest that the large migratory movements to the United States selected the best fit and most able among the peasantry and workers. Although the vast majority came to this country during conditions of adversity, those who came tended to be drawn from the group who had been less severely affected, those who could still pay for the voyage, those who could tolerate the extreme hardship. (2) Malzberg pointed out that the rapid decrease in rates for the second generation did not support any available genetic hypotheses. (3) Rates for the foreign-born are particularly high for the very youngest age groups, who had little part in electing migration and, therefore, could not have best represented the relevant selective factors. Regardless of the form of selection hypothesis, their rates should certainly be no greater than rates for their parents. Oscar Handlin, *The Uprooted* (Boston: Little, Brown, 1952); Handlin, *Boston's Immigrants: A Study in Acculturation,* rev. ed. (Cambridge, Mass.: Harvard University Press, 1959); Marcus Lee Hansen, *The Atlantic Migration, 1607–1860* (New York: Harper & Row, 1961); Malzberg, *Social and Biological Aspects.*

55. Fromm, *Escape from Freedom;* Lee, "Differentials in Mental Disease"; Malzberg and Lee, *Migration and Mental Disease.*

56. Jaco, *Social Epidemiology of Mental Disorders;* Pugh and MacMahon, *Epidemiologic Findings.*

57. H. B. M. Murphy, "Migration and the Major Mental Disorders: A Reappraisal," in *Mobility and Mental Health,* M. Kantor ed. (Princeton: Van Nostrand, 1964), pp. 5–29; H. B. M. Murphy, "Social Change and Mental Health," in Milbank Memorial Fund, *Causes of Mental Disorders: A Review of Epidemiological Knowledge, 1959* (New York: Milbank Memorial Fund, 1961).

58. Cassel, Ralph Patrick, and David Jenkins, "Epidemiological Analysis of Health Implications of Culture Change: A Conceptual Model," in *Annals of the New York Academy of Sciences* 84 (1960): 938–949; Fried, "Effects of Social Change" and "Transitional Functions."

59. Gerald Caplan, "Emotional Crises," in *The Encyclopedia of Mental Health,* ed. A. Deutsch and H. Fishman, vol. 2 (New York: Watts, 1963): 521–532; Leonard J. Duhl, "Crisis, Adaptive Potential and the School," in *Psychology in the Schools* 1 (1964): 263–266; E. Lindemann, "The Use of Psychoanalytic Constructs in Preventive Psychiatry," in *Psychoanalytic Study of the Child* 7 (1952): 429–448.

60. Fried, "Grieving for a Lost Home" and "Transitional Functions."

61. Robert Waelder, "The Principle of Multiple Function: Observations on Overdetermination," *Psychoanalytic Quarterly* 5 (1936): 45–62.

62. Differentials between Negro and white rates of first admissions by differences in marital status provide some data suggesting the importance of the meaning of the particular form of disruption. Negro rates of psychiatric hospitalization are considerably higher than white rates. Negro rates of divorce and separation are also considerably higher than white rates. And the effect of divorce and separation on first admissions to psychiatric hospitals is less marked for Negroes than for whites. The data presented here are from Lee and are based on the detailed breakdown by marital status for all New York hospitals for mental disorder during 1950 in age standardized rates per 100,000 population. The nonwhite rates in these data are predominantly Negro. The relative differences according to marital status can be regarded from either extreme. Marital relationships may be less cohesive among Negroes, and a larger proportion may be listed as married although not living with their spouses. There is much data to suggest this is the case. Alternatively, because divorce, separation, and defacto separation are so widespread among Negroes, they may represent less serious disruptions and may involve less serious deprivation. There is also a good deal to suggest this is so. In either event (and certainly if both are correct ex-

planations), we would expect a less marked difference in first admission rates for married and divorced/separated status among Negroes than among whites. Thus, the difference in *meaning* of the marital state and of its disruption would seem to be a useful hypothetical approach in understanding these and other rate differentials. Fried, "Social Problems and Psychopathology," pp. 448–449; Fried, "Effects of Social Change"; Lee, "Differentials in Mental Disease."

Marital Status	White	Non-White	Ratio
Married	62	154	2.48
Widowed	227	472	2.08
Single	266	508	1.91
Divorced	461	419	.91
Separated	482	555	1.15

63. It is hardly necessary to add that just as social deprivation has conscious and unconscious psychological meaning in addition to its "objective" significance as a realistic lack and potential hazard, so do social resources serve as a realistic bulwark against the more primitive interpretation of lacks and losses; even projected blame is less disorganizing psychologically when supported (and modified) by group consensus.

COMMENTARY

Fried's contention that Freud neglected the role of social systems in health or illness may and should be subjected to debate. Similarly, some will quarrel with the author's depiction of the position of the individual in Durkheim's model. If the contrast between intrapsychic *versus* environmental determinism *is overdrawn, it is—like all caricatures—useful, distinguishing, identifying, not representational. Certainly sociology and psychiatry can profit from more reviews of this kind—including the* biological *facts and assumptions implied or expressed in their respective models. Certainly clinicians may instructively consider how the images of Freud, Durkheim, or Fried conveyed in this paper are reflected in his own observations and inferences about psychopathology.*

We expect that there will be more agreement about the need for concepts and facts which more fully elaborate and specify the links between psychological processes and social processes—between the individual and the group. Appreciation of the "why for" and the "how to" of such an attempt is increased by a review of Fried's effort. This appreciation does not depend, necessarily, upon a complete embrace of the particular conceptual scheme which the author applied. Yet Fried's specific constructs invite evaluation—by the criteria which apply to all conceptual schemes. Are terms clearly defined? Do the concepts have clear empirical referents? Do the concepts suggest new facts that need to be gathered? Do the concepts serve to organize and explain existing facts? Do the constructs lead to testable hypotheses? What implications do existing facts have for the further clarification, specification, and qualification of concepts? Certainly these questions do not lend themselves to "yes" or "no" answers, but rather to "in this manner . . ." and "to this extent . . . ."

As Fried himself indicates, the value of his scheme may be measured by the extent to which it illuminates the epidemiological data which he examines. His collation and cool, discriminating analysis of these data are an important contribution to the literature. For example, Fried identifies a number of factors which influence the association between psychiatric hospitalization mates and social class. After due consideration, he meticulously identifies the data and logic which lead him to conclude that there is a causal relationship between social class and psychopathology—"though not a simple, direct or unilinear one." All mental health professionals should be familiar with these provocative, controversial and often clouded arguments and evidence.

CHAPTER 25

Primary Prevention— A Negative View

INTRODUCTION

If we consider the range of attitudes about the usefulness of primary prevention efforts in psychiatry, Elaine Cumming is near the negative pole while the National Institute of Mental Health, Gerald Caplan, and Alexander Leighton approach the positive pole. Leighton's position is presented in Chapter 26. Arguments for investing psychiatric resources in preventive efforts are well summarized by Caplan: "Primary prevention involves studying the provision of resources in a population and attempting to improve the situation when necessary—usually by modifying community-wide practices through changing laws, regulations, administrative patterns, or widespread values and attitudes." [1] *Caplan agrees with Cumming about the lack of a hard, objective analysis of preventive efforts to date: "The efficacy of preventive efforts has been assessed in too few of the programs discussed in this review." Their basic disagreement is over priorities—how much effort should the mental health system make in the area of preventive versus direct treatment efforts. They also disagree about who should be involved in community development. Caplan urges: "Clearly community planning, organization and coordination are fundamental elements in effecting preventive psychiatry. Thus, the key factors which influence mental health in the community must be delineated in the areas of economics, politics, public health, religion, welfare and education, to name a few. It will be obvious that the lines between the roles of psychiatrist, social planner, social activist will often not be clear."* [2]

In contrast, Dr. Cumming's concern is that primary prevention efforts remove needed manpower from treatment; she recommends against the deployment of service-oriented mental health manpower into crisis intervention, community consultation, and community development programs.

Dr. Cumming's arguments are put in a provocative and challenging manner; they merit thoughtful and substantive consideration.

NOTES

1. Gerald Caplan, "Perspectives on Primary Prevention: A Review," *Archives of General Psychiatry* 17 (September 1967): 333.

2. Ibid, p. 332.

PRIMARY PREVENTION—
MORE COST THAN BENEFIT

Elaine Cumming

A history of primary prevention of mental illness might pass for a thumbnail sketch of the changing value preoccupations of an age. The story moves from the evils of proscribed sex to the virtues of efficiency; from there to the importance of the inner man and finally to the moral value of "the community." If the Victorians did not teach their children that self-control and dutifulness would prevent mental illness, perhaps it was because they did not think in those terms, but the notion of primary prevention had crept in by the time of Bleuler's *fin de siècle* prescription "the avoidance of masturbation, of disappointments in love, of strains or fright are recommendations which can be made with a clear conscience because these are things which should be avoided in all circumstances." [1]

By the twenties we were discovering that self-hypnosis, *à la Coué*, for adults and rigorous habit training for children would maintain good mental health. Such optimistic efficiency not surprisingly started to break up during the depression, and by the end of World War II the inner man was paramount and mental health education designed to encourage his expression had taken hold. This stream of activity, together with a preoccupation with permissiveness in child raising, characterized the silent, individualistic, inturned fifties. As approaches to primary prevention, both mental health education and the special emphasis on child raising crested during this period and have since receded, so I will refer to them only briefly before going on to what appear to be the two current strategies, crisis intervention and consultation.

Earlier Strategies

Education was the basis of the prevention programs of the recent past, and this education was centered on both child raising and personal practices. Child-raising practices have always been a vehicle for value statements about the good life. It is important to notice, however, that although beliefs about child raising change, and child-raising practices themselves may change, the rates of mental illness do not appear to change with them.[2] Davis[3] summarizes the child-raising lore of the 1940s and 1950s as "thermodynamic," being centered on the faith that a warm, loving parent will produce a mentally healthy child, but he also points out that there is little evidence for that faith.[4]

In the same monograph, Davis reviewed the many attempts to modify personal attitudes and practices through various kinds of exhortations. He concluded that "the important problem, in mental hygiene campaigns concerned with techniques of personal adjustment and prevention of mental illness, is not the appropriate means of communication and persuasion but the fact that mental health educators have nothing concrete and practical to tell the public." Whether or not this little book delivered the *coup de grâce* to that kind of mental health education, we will never know, but the tide has certainly ebbed since it appeared. In spite of that, education as a strategy should not be lightly abandoned just because trivial content has rendered it futile in the past. I will return to this later.

Newer Strategies

The good life has shifted from the self-realization of individuals and is all tied up with the need for community development, community involvement, the redistribution of power,[5] and saving the world from the violence, corruption, and decay of modern urban life, as well as the fear of a generation that seems actually to be less materialistic than its parents. It is not surprising to find that the prevention of mental illness has draped itself in these more modern garments.

Crisis Intervention. We experience the world as in crisis, and it is easy to blame many of our discomforts upon the atmosphere of crisis that is generated by each day's news. Somehow the idea of crisis as an inherent, but undesirable, aspect of living has seized us.

The conviction that psychological health is dependent in part upon the successful weathering of life's crises is modern; it seems to have grown from a number of sources, among them ideas of vulnerability at times of change [6] and ideas of developmental stages.[7] It seems likely from a variety of evidence that rapid treatment of the crisis of acute mental illness is an essential part of the good practice of psychiatry,[8] and I explicitly exclude from this discussion consideration of crisis intervention as a therapeutic technique.

Caplan [9] appears to have given the first impetus to crisis intervention as a *preventive technique among normal people.* It is worth noting, however, before discussing this strategy that most of the changes of status that punctuate an ordinary life span, except perhaps bereavement, would not have been called crises as little as a generation ago. Now, in an age of crises, entering school, puberty, going to college, marriage, parenthood, and retirement all have this label.

A number of descriptions of crisis intervention programs designed to prevent mental illness among normal people who are undergoing such expectable life crises as adolescence, childbirth, marriage, and bereavement can be found in the literature. These programs are lent a certain *prima facie* validity by retrospective clinical reports of psychologically impaired people who have been found not to have resolved such crises. A classical example of this kind of evidence is Lindemann's 1944 report [10] of unresolved grief among bereaved families. Unfortunately, no study was found that had both a baseline measure and evidence that people who did not adequately resolve their grief were later inclined to a variety of psychological disabilities. It is, therefore, not possible to tell whether or not these same people had been psychologically healthy before the bereavement. While useful therapies have been based upon such post hoc clinical evidence, it is a doubtful basis indeed for a program of prevention that would in its nature require resources sufficient to serve the enormous populations at risk, very few of whom would be expected to be affected. Even if only "high risk groups" were included, such as widows under sixty years of age,[11] the ratio of service delivered to illness prevented would be enormous. Similar criticisms of preventive interventions with the parents of premature infants can be made. Although Caplan's group found that they could predict which parents would meet their criteria of good adaptation by examining patterns of "grappling behavior" during the crisis of having a premature infant,[12] the ability of these people to cope with this crisis is not, of course, independent of their general competence before the crisis.[13] Services routinely supplied to the parents of premature children would be expected to have a very low yield. (Perhaps if obstetricians had more confidence in psychiatrists they would refer to them those patients who were not grappling well.) No studies could be found that showed that intervention at the time of normal crisis had any effect upon subsequent mental illness.

There are two further problems to be raised about the use of this kind of intervention as primary prevention in a society in which every individual can expect to pass through a number of changes from one status to another. First, since there are institutional supports for these transitions in a stable society, there does not seem to be any obvious reason why intervention by psychiatrists should be needed, especially since psychiatrists are needed for treating the mentally ill. If society is in such a condition of change that these crises become difficult for a large number of people, a good argument can be made for trying to strengthen the social fabric rather than the population. This is a task that more and more psychiatrists are in fact willing to undertake, and I will return to this new role later when I discuss consultation. My point here is that primary prevention through crisis intervention is in theory unnecessary in a stable society, and in an unstable one the usefulness of deploying scarce resources for this purpose should have to be demonstrated.

The final objection to crisis intervention as a preventive strategy is perhaps the most important one: In spite of the assumption that in this crisis-ridden world crises are inevitably experienced as strains,[14] such evidence as is available about the relationship of stress to psychiatric breakdown suggests that it is not crisis that leads to personality disorganization and psychiatric casualty, but exposure to continued, unremitting stress.[15] The literature on this matter might be summed up as, "All that stresses is not strain."

When individuals are under long-continued stress, however, there is an implication of a stressful environment and therefore the implication that psychiatric casualties might be more easily avoided by changing the environment than by strengthening the individual. In a brilliant and influential report on the need for a preventive program in the army, Apple and Beebe [16] pointed out that only a change in the structure of the environment of infantrymen could reduce psychiatric casualties. In the army, changes in environment can be made by fiat. In civilian life, not only is major change by executive order impossible, but the stresses are more complex.

We take for granted that slums, poverty, deprivation, and humiliation are stresses that are felt as strains whether or not they generate the surplus of mental illness with which they are associated. It is the core of my argument that the urgent moral imperatives of the day arise in revulsion from and fear of the vile conditions in urban slums, and that these morally debasing conditions are therefore assumed to be causing mental illness, just as yesterday strict child-raising practices and repression of hostile impulses were assumed to cause it then.[17] My guess is that our prevention strategies would be exactly the same even if the statistical associations between slums and rates of schizophrenia were unknown to us. No one knows whether or not vile living conditions actually cause mental illness, but in a civilized society they should be found intolerable just because they are vile. All citizens, not just psychiatrists, should be appalled at them.

If it does turn out to be true that adverse conditions of life cause mental illness, such knowledge will not necessarily help. It is already known that they cause physical illness and mental retardation and are associated with crime, delinquency, despair, suicide, and numbers of other unwanted effects, and always have been. It is clearly not the mandate of any one discipline to remove itself from its central specialty and attend to the moral dilemmas of the nation. We would not be happy if the obstetrician left the ward aide to deliver the babies while he was busy organizing the community to fight the conditions that lead to foetal wastage. The world will change, but it will be changed by socio-political processes, as it has been in the past. There is a certain arrogance in someone who has been trained to heal the sick imagining that he therefore has an expertise beyond that of any other thoughtful citizen in patching up the cracks in society. Indeed, the naiveté of some of the literature in this field must be attributed to this arrogance. When we read that the world can be changed by "altering social arrangements to insure that those who have done the right things are indeed rewarded," and that "a congress on ethics and conduct should be convened to . . . dispel the present confusion about sex and to change society . . . ," [18] we can only wonder whether members of the psychiatric fraternity and their paraprofessional brothers do not have a trained incapacity to understand the history and the structure of American society.

None of this is prejudicial to the so-called storefront movement. Experiments with new forms are needed. Perhaps psychiatric care ought to be delivered to people close to where they are, certainly in terms that they can understand and under conditions that do not humiliate and alienate them. Perhaps this means that treatment must sometimes be delivered in the fronts of stores, church basements, and other unorthodox places, and especially that it be given in the evenings and on weekends, but it is my contention that this should be done in the name of giving humane and efficient care to the mentally ill and that pretensions about it preventing mental illness should be abandoned. They should be abandoned not only because the psychiatrist is unlikely to be particularly effective at such preventive tactics but also, and more importantly, because too often in the excitement the patient, especially the chronically ill patient, is forgotten, "merely clinical" activities are discarded, and the psychiatrist is off on one of his moon journeys doctoring society. These journeys are sometimes called consultation.

Consultation. The literature on consultation makes depressing reading for anyone interested in evidence. Program descriptions abound, but evaluations of these are lacking, perhaps because it is so difficult to conceive of a method of showing that any mental illness is prevented by consultations of any kind. The reason for this difficulty is that both the method of prevention and the implied etiology of the disease are so diffuse. We seem to have adopted a kind of moral miasma theory of causation [19] and we are attacking the disease with a general program of uplift. (At one time the word "uplift" must have had the same with-it modernity that "outreach" had a decade ago. They are equally moral terms.) Mental illness is often so mysterious, unpredictable, and threatening to the moral order that until we know more about it, these diffuse moral attitudes may be inevitable.

CASE CONSULTATION. Some of the hundreds of descriptions of

consultation programs that fill the journals include interesting typologies, most of which reveal that not all consultation is preventive in intent, and the most interesting of which is fourfold. The first type, case consultation, is an absolutely orthodox component of every branch of medicine and an essential part of good practice. When the target of intervention is someone already impaired, consultation must be considered treatment and not prevention. Even so, there is evidence that agencies can be frustrated by consultation. By the time they call for a consultant they really want to make a referral. Often, they have already used all the techniques of which they are capable, and the psychiatrist cannot add anything to their armamentarium of skills in his consulting capacity. Rabiner [20] has suggested that psychiatric consultation will be accepted only when direct services are already in effect, and when there is an active demand for the consulting service. Brodsky,[21] in an interesting intersystem analysis, cautions the psychiatrist to respect the roles of other specialists when he offers his services. In passing, no descriptions of consultation programs being developed in response to a spontaneous community demand could be found. Consultation does not appear to be as good a mousetrap as a treatment program.

CONSULTEE-ORIENTED CONSULTATION. "Consultee-oriented" consultation seems to consist of the psychiatrist somehow making the consultee a better and more mature person. Kiyoshi,[22] describing a consultee-oriented consultation, says, "When the team meets these people in their offices it adopts an attitude of consultee-oriented consultation rather than patient-oriented consultation. This means that the members of the team will not have any direct contact with the agencies' patients. . . . The consultant is concerned primarily with the growth of the skills of the agency workers and *not with the workers' effectiveness*." (Italics mine.) Sometimes it is hard to believe that psychiatrists are not actually fleeing from their patients.[23]

Occasionally, somebody describes a consultation program that had unpleasant and unintended consequences, but such authors, though thoughtful and honest, seem never to question the basic utility of their programs. It is difficult, however, for an outsider to know exactly why a psychiatrist is better at improving the skills of a policeman or a school teacher than a school teacher or a policeman is at improving his.

EDUCATIONAL CONSULTATION. The third kind of consultation is basically education. The psychiatrist lectures at PTA meetings and any other organizations that invite him in the hope that this will change their practices. As Davis [24] concluded from his review of the literature, however, "It appears that there is a continuum in degrees of change from beliefs to attitudes to subjective states to practices. Almost all studies of change in information show positive results while . . . studies of change in practice show negative outcomes." Nevertheless, as Davis says, the possession of information is itself valuable because it reassures people,[25] sets up realistic standards against which people can measure their own performances, and tends to innoculate against overreaction to stress.[26] More research into the long-term effects of specific factual education programs is much needed. The intellect should never be sold too short.

Whether education can ever be specific and rational and still achieve this purpose is perhaps the question. It may be that until we know something more specific about the mental illnesses that remain so hard to control, their implicit threat to society will always evoke moral responses and these will always color educational programs. Perhaps we will never be able to prevent these illnesses until we can cure them.

COMMUNITY CONSULTATION. Finally, in a decade of power to the people (both radicals and those archconservatives, the community establishment), there is community consultation in which the psychiatrist becomes involved in many kinds of groups and organizations for various purposes, including that of involving his potential patients in efforts to improve their living conditions.[27]

There are three objections to this activity, two of them discussed above. First, it is essentially a reform activity for which a psychiatrist is not trained; second, it distracts him from his core activity, which is the care and treatment of the ill. Third, there is no evidence that any of these activities at any time prevented so much as one case of mental illness. Nobody, in fact, appears to be interested in trying to discover the effects of these efforts and it is very doubtful whether such a discovery could be made because a controlled experiment would be almost impossible to arrange.

It is hard to avoid noticing in reviewing the literature that both consultee-oriented and community consultation seem to be models for a pecking order with the psychiatrist at the top. Just as the psychiatrist does not ask the policeman for his advice, so he cannot give his advice to the one group of people who are convinced that their status is higher than his, that is, other practicing medical doctors. As Eisendorfer and Altrocchi [28] admit, medical doctors should not be included as consultees because they are "ambivalent to the process."

None of this should be taken as a criticism of programs of community development, restoration, and organization, unquestionably good things in their own right, but just as a reflection of the belief that psychiatrists have other things to do and perhaps also that their very presence unnecessarily suppresses the status of people such as social workers, labor organizers, and many others who are better trained for the job.

There Must Be a Way

I have taken a strong position against certain activities undertaken in the name of primary prevention because I think some psychiatrists have lost their way by allowing themselves to become mouthpieces of a popular morality.

In the past we have succeeded in preventing mental illnesses like pellagra, tertiary syphilis, and various toxic conditions, but we have done it in a thoughtful epidemiological way, discriminating between different forms of illness and combining knowledge about distribution with clinical explorations and then working to establish causal linkages between the environment, the individual, and the illness. An excellent summary of successes in primary prevention is given by Eisenberg.[29] Pointing out that psychiatric illnesses are no less psychiatric for having specific etiologies, Eisenberg lists the known successful strategies. These include genetic counseling, protection of the foetus and the neonate to avoid neurological damage, and the wider availability of acceptable birth control methods (on the grounds that there is some evidence that unwanted children are particularly liable to emotional disability). Since Eisenberg's review, this strategy has become more important because of evidence that in large families schizophrenics seem to be in the last half of the sibline,[30] because schizophrenia appears to be familial,[31] and because the fertility of schizophrenic women seems to have increased since the development of community care.[32] For all our efforts, however, that great foe is still untouched. As Ewalt and Maltsberger [33] say, "The present state of psychiatric knowledge does not permit the claim that we can prevent the development of schizophrenic illness in any given individual or population." It is in the area of this frustratingly resistant illness that we are most likely to go astray and to invent gratifying methods of prevention because we have no cures.

Summary

1. The effectiveness of popular strategies for the primary preventions of the major mental illnesses has not been tested.

2. These strategies remove needed manpower from the treatment of the mentally ill.

3. The moral and social problems that afflict our society should be attacked because they are insupportable, not because they cause mental illness, which has not been demonstrated.

NOTES

1. Eugene Bleuler, *Dementia Praecox or the Group of Schizophrenias* (New York: International Universities Press, 1950).

2. Elaine Cumming, "Unsolved Problems of Prevention," *Canada's Mental Health Supplement,* no. 56 (January–April 1968).

3. James A. Davis, *Education for Positive Mental Health* (Chicago: Aldine, 1965).

4. Just in passing, it might be noted that while such an upbringing was explicity contrasted with the strictness of the earlier behaviorists and the harshness of the Victorians, it was also implicitly contrasted with materialism: "They buy him a

roomful of toys but give him no love." Materialism has always been a bugaboo; the Victorians deplored it when they contrasted it with duty and honor, and even the materialistic 1920s paid lip service to "the best things in life are free." No matter what has been thought to be the good life, on the surface at least, materialism has been bad. It should also be noted that just as there is no compelling evidence that warmth prevents mental illness, there is none that materialism causes it.

5. Herbert Kaufman, "Administrative Decentralization and Political Power," *Public Administration Review* 29, no. 1 (January–February 1969): 3–14.

6. Kurt Lewin, *Field Theory in Social Sciences* (New York: Harper, 1951).

7. Erik Erickson, *Childhood and Society* (New York: Norton, 1950).

8. John Cumming and Elaine Cumming, *Ego and Milieu* (New York: Atherton, 1962), and Joint Information Service of the American Psychiatric Association and the National Association for Mental Health, *The Psychiatric Emergency* (Washington, D.C.: American Psychiatric Association, 1966).

9. Gerald Caplan, *Principles of Preventive Psychiatry* (New York: Basic Books, 1964).

10. Erich Lindemann, "Symptomatology and Management of Acute Grief," *American Journal of Psychiatry* 101 (1944): 141–148.

11. Phyllis Rolfe Silverman, "Services to the Widowed: First Steps in a Program of Preventive Intervention," *Community Mental Health Journal* 3, no. 1 (Spring 1967): 37–44.

12. Gerald Caplan, Edward A. Mason, and David M. Kaplan, "Four Studies of Crisis in Parents of Prematures," *Community Mental Health Journal* 1, no. 2 (Summer 1965): 149–161.

13. The psychiatrists' ability to predict simply shows that they are able to discriminate among people of different competencies on the basis of one sampling of behavior, itself no mean feat, but beside the point.

14. Harris B. Peck, "The Small Group: Core of the Community Mental Health Center," *Community Mental Health Journal* 4, no. 3 (June 1968): 191–200.

15. John W. Apple and Gilbert W. Beebe, "Preventive Psychiatry," *Journal of the American Medical Association* 131, no. 18 (1946): 1469–1475; Daniel H. Funkenstein, Stanley H. King, and Margaret E. Drolette, *Mastery of Stress* (Cambridge, Mass.: Harvard University Press, 1957); William W. Michaux et al., "The Psychopathology and Measurement of Environmental Stress," *Community Mental Health Journal* 3, no. 4 (Winter 1967): 358–372; and Jack L. Katz et al., "Stress, Distress, and Ego Defenses: Psychoendocrine Response to Impending Breast Tumor Biopsy," *Archives of General Psychiatry* 28, no. 2 (August 1970): 131–142.

16. Apple and Beebe, "Preventive Psychiatry."

17. For years the Mental Health Associations of the country distributed "Blondie" comics teaching us how to express our emotions instead of bottling them up.

18. John Arsenian, "Toward Prevention of Mental Illness in the United States," *Community Mental Health Journal* 1, no. 4 (Winter 1965): 320–325.

19. Bernard L. Bloom, "The 'Medical Model,' Miasma Theory, and Community Mental Health," *Community Mental Health Journal* 1, no. 4 (Winter 1965): 333–338.

20. Charles J. Rabiner et al., "Consultation or Direct Service," *American Journal of Psychiatry* 126, no. 9 (March 1970): 1321–1325.

21. Carroll M. Brodsky, "Decision-Making and Role Shifts as They Affect the Consultation Interface," *Archives of General Psychiatry* 23, no. 6 (December 1970): 559–565.

22. Ogura Kiyoshi and Virgil Bradley, "A Look at the Consultative Process: The Psychiatric Team and Community Agencies," *Psychiatric Quarterly Supplement* 41, pt. 1 (1967): 15–35.

23. L. S. Kubie, "The Retreat from Patients," *Archives of General Psychiatry* 24, no. 2 (February 1971): 98–106.

24. Davis, *Education for Positive Mental Health.*

25. J. C. Nunnally, Jr., *Popular Conceptions of Mental Health: Their Development and Change* (New York: Holt, Rinehart, 1961).

26. I. Janis, *Psychological Stress: Psychoanalytic and Behavioral Studies of Surgical Patients* (New York: Wiley, 1958).

27. Peck, "The Small Group."

28. Carl Eisendorfer, John Altrocchi, and Robert F. Young, "Principles of Community Mental Health in a Rural Setting: The Halifax County Program," *Community Mental Health Journal* 4, no. 3 (June 1968): 211–220.

29. Leon Eisenberg, "Preventive Psychiatry," *Annual Review of Medicine* 13 (1962): 343–360.

30. R. D. Hinshelwood, "The Evidence for a Birth Order Factor in Schizophrenia," *British Journal of Psychiatry* 117, no. 538 (1970): 293.

31. David Rosenthal and Seymour S. Kety, *The Transmission of Schizophrenia* (New York: Pergamon, 1968).
32. "Fertility of the Mentally Ill," *New Society* 15, no. 383 (1970): 183.
33. Jack R. Ewalt and John T. Maltsberger, "Prevention," in *The Schizophrenic Syndrome*, ed. L. Bellak and L. Loeb (New York: Grune-Stratton, 1969), pp. 757–775.

COMMENTARY

Elaine Cumming has provided a provocative and partisan critique of socially oriented preventive mental health efforts. From her perspective as a professor of sociology, she has noted the range of preventive efforts from the purely social to the purely biological, and argued strongly for limiting programmatic efforts to the latter and investing only in research in the area of social efforts.

The paper correctly points out that diverse and seemingly unrelated assaults upon mental disorders may all be grouped under the "primary prevention" label. Perhaps this is because the word "prevention" itself has been highly regarded in recent years, and has led advocates of various kinds of activities to select this affirmative label. Without narrowing and defining exactly what it is that we are criticizing, being for or against primary prevention is meaningless. Are we talking about political activity to bring about a more humane community? Plans to provide adequate employment, housing, and social resources to all members of the population? Do we wish to train teachers and parents in the principles of child development so that they can enhance the maturation of school-age children? Or do we feel that school age is too late and so advocate making nursery schools with diagnostic and therapeutic resources available to all children from age three on? Some say that even age three is too late for primary prevention, and prefer a major investment of resources in family planning and prenatal and postnatal care, with screening for the endocrine and anatomic disorders of infancy which can now be diagnosed and often treated. Again on the biological side, some advocate a major effort toward assuring adequate nutrition for pregnant women and for infants and young children.

With regard to preventive effort for adults, we may note that strong arguments for adequate housing, employment, and social resources are presented in Chapters 23 and 24. Epidemiologic studies have revealed a disproportionately high incidence of mental disorders among the unemployed, recently bereaved persons, and immigrants, to name but a few of the categories of adults who have thus come to be known as "target groups." Since first contact with such persons is usually made by community care givers such as the police, firemen, the clergy, and community leaders, many have recommended that they be trained to do basic problem identification, crisis counseling, and referral (when necessary) to professional agencies. In a related man-

ner, the use of mental health personnel to generate, train, and support self-help groups for the recently widowed, the elderly, the unemployed, the medically ill, the physically handicapped, homosexuals, drug abusers, alcoholics, and adolescents has been advocated.[1] Unfortunately, while there is considerable evidence, as reviewed in the prior two chapters, to support the notion that members of such groups are at relatively high risk of developing a mental disorder, little in the way of objective evidence is presently available to prove that current prevention efforts are successful. Much more study will be required to indicate which of these is both effective in reducing the incidence of breakdown in the target populations and also economically effective and therefore meriting community financial support.

In the paper which follows Alexander Leighton reviews some of these socially oriented preventive efforts from a very broad, community study perspective. His finding and recommendations are in provocative contrast to those offered by Dr. Cumming.

NOTE

1. Gerald Caplan, *Support Systems and Community Mental Health* (New York: Behavioral Publications, 1974).

CHAPTER 26

Primary Prevention—
A Positive View

INTRODUCTION

This brief paper was selected to serve as a counterweight to Cumming's position, in Chapter 25, opposing socially oriented prevention efforts. It was also chosen to introduce the reader to the long-term studies of Alexander Leighton and his multidisciplinary research group. For more than twenty years they have studied social, cultural, and psychiatric-psychological variables in several test communities. Their work, of magnificent theoretical and quantitative dimensions, has been reported extensively in books and journal articles. Perhaps their most widely known book is The Character of Danger.[1]

The following article describes how, using multiple investigatory techniques, the research group carried out serial studies of the Road, a community suffering from sociocultural disintegration, starting in 1950. The Road was long believed to be a community comprised primarily of mentally retarded persons; it was thought that the intellectual defect was being maintained by inbreeding. The results of multidisciplinary community studies were surprising. Following a field anthropologic study, the children's intelligence was tested. The tests disproved the notion, long held in neighboring towns, that they were "feebleminded." Following these early studies a program of community development was planned by some members of the research group and public officials, and initiated with residents of the community. These efforts at sociocultural improvements were designed to minimize the passivity and dependence of the residents by creating new opportunities for individual development and group activities. The effectiveness of these efforts is reported.

NOTE

1. D. C. Leighton, J. S. Harding, D. B. Macklin, A. M. Macmillan, and A. H. Leighton, *The Character of Danger* (New York: Basic Books, 1963).

SOME NOTES ON PREVENTIVE PSYCHIATRY

Alexander H. Leighton

This paper will be concerned with leads regarding causes of psychiatric disorder and with implications for prevention. The notion of cause employed is consonant with that of MacMahon, Pugh, and Ipsen when they say "A causal association may be defined as an association between two categories of events in which a change in the frequency or quality of one is observed to follow alteration in the other." [1]

For a variety of reasons which have been explained in other publications,[2] we [3] have been giving attention to a complex of societal phenomena to which we have attached the label "sociocultural disintegration." This is an approach which differs from most other epidemiological studies in that it does not give main emphasis to discrete experiential factors such as smoking, deficiency in diet, or loss of a parent, but rather to the functional state of a whole environmental system.

The system in question is the human community and for purposes of study and comparison we have examined a variety of more or less discrete small examples. These communities are visualized as semiorganic systems which perform various functions on which the survival and well-being of the group depend. Among the functions are the acquisition of food, shelter, and other material necessities; the organization and distribution of work; the indoctrination of children into the ways of the system; the use of leisure time; and processes of decision making on the part of the group when it is confronted with new situations.

The storage of resources against future need is also an important aspect of function. Such resources range from economic entities such as money, land, and possession to accumulated knowledge. Increases in the quantity and diversity of stored resources tend to increase the

"Some Notes on Preventive Psychiatry," *Canadian Psychiatric Association Journal* XII, 1967, pp. 543–550. Used by permission.

capacity of the group for taking advantage of opportunity and for coping with adversity.

With this model in view we selected ten criteria by which communities might be judged in terms of their sociocultural integration. These criteria, set forth in negative terms and therefore indicative of sociocultural disintegration, are: economic inadequacy, cultural confusion, widespread secularization, high frequency of broken homes, few and weak associations, few and weak leaders, few patterns of recreation, high frequency of interpersonal hostility, high frequency of crime and delinquency, and a weak and fragmented network of communications.

In the beginning these criteria were used as a guide in observing and describing several communities. Our method was chiefly that of the cultural anthropologist: field workers spent time in the communities talking with people and watching what was going on. They also systematically interviewed key informants, that is, persons who knew the communities well. On the basis of such information we classified the communities in a series ranging from high integration to low. In the course of doing this we discovered that independent observers easily agree on whether a particular community belongs at the bottom, in the middle, or at the top of the range.

From this start most of the criteria were resolved into several more precise and objective components that could be handled by quantitative methods. Participant observers, after spending some months in a community, were able to fill in a household survey that included such items as the number of "broken" families (defined as families with one parent absent, or families in which parents were constantly in conflict). Further, interviewing and observation throughout the communities made it possible to count leaders, if they existed, and to classify them by type. We used the same methods to estimate the extent and kinds of hostility among the people.

In addition we gave a questionnaire interview to a systematically selected sample of adults. On the basis of this questionnaire it was possible to assess such matters as participation in religious activities and sense of identity with an ethnic group. By using the questionnaire in conjunction with direct observation, we gathered data on the economic resources of each respondent in the sample. More recently we have been constructing an atlas of community activities and finding ways to estimate the amount of time a sample of individuals spends in each kind of activity.[4] These techniques are making it possible to state more precisely the differences in integration among communities and also in the same community at two different points in time. All these methodological steps present new questions and therefore new possibilities for advance in understanding the processes at work and the causal factors involved in the shifts of groups from integration to disintegration and vice versa.

The fact that our epidemiological investigations repeatedly found a high correlation or association between the prevalence of psychiatric disorders and extremes of disintegration has kept our interest alive.[5] Among the most salient questions that have arisen are those which have to do with whether a disintegrated community can be brought to a state of integration and, if so, whether this has any effect on the prevalence of psychiatric disorders. Such a transition from disintegration toward integration has occurred in one of the communities under our observation during the last sixteen years. A description of this will serve to illustrate more specifically what is meant by sociocultural disintegration and integration, and will provide a basis for some concluding remarks on the relationship between societal processes and the prevalence of psychiatric disorders.

In 1950 the group, which is called the "Road," consisted of 118 people living in twenty-nine houses.[6] Sixty-six of the residents were under the age of twenty-one. The dwellings, small and cramped, were scattered irregularly along a country road and were somewhat separated by fields and woods from the other communities of the region. The Road's economic base was obviously low; when the men worked they cut logs for pulp, dug clams, and hired out as day laborers. Many of the women were occasionally employed shucking clams at a plant in a nearby town. Family allowances played an important part in the life of the community.

The Road had an unenviable reputation in the surrounding countryside. If you asked about it you were almost invariably told that the people who lived there were mentally retarded. The informant would often add that they were the products of inbreeding, that insanity, alcoholism, and delinquency were rampant among them, that they were lazy and unreliable as employees, and that it was impossible to do anything to help them. Indeed, they were known throughout the county by an uncomplimentary nickname.

We began our study with an attempt to answer the question of whether or not the Road people did exhibit an unusually high prevalence of mental deficiency. After months of effort Macmillan won sufficient cooperation to be able to give intelligence tests to the children. For purposes of comparison he also tested children from five other rural sections who were generally regarded as normal in their sociological and psychological attributes.

When the intelligence scores of the Road children were projected against those from children in the "normal" communities, no difference could be found. In other words, the Road children as a group showed essentially the same range from stupidity to better-than-average intelligence which was shown by the other children. Since it is not likely that a group of inbreeding, constitutionally inferior adults would produce a child population with normal intelligence, we were led to conclude that whatever might be wrong with the people of the Road, it was not a biologically determined lack of intelligence. It seemed more plausible that there existed a set of patterns with which those who grew up in the neighborhood became inculcated—patterns that had properties considered indicative of mental handicap by those in the surrounding larger society.

With this start we began to study the Road in a broader frame of reference than that of mental deficiency. Historical investigation showed that the neighborhood had existed as a human group for more than 100 years. The original inhabitants had been workers in shipyards on the coast a few miles away or had hauled logs to the coast from the forested interior. At that time the shipyard community of "Port Harmony" was flourishing, and the Road shared in this economic and social well-being. The men of the Road were almost entirely Acadians who had moved in from some distance, attracted by the employment opportunities. As far as one can tell now, they came from normal farming families in which they were economically supernumerary children: offspring beyond the number the farms could support. In the beginning the men probably did not intend to stay permanently, and therefore they chose land that was both close to their work and cheap. It was cheap because it had a thin, rocky soil, mostly unsuitable for either farming or lumbering. With continuing employment and the passage of time, Acadian wives joined the men and families became established.

Cultural erosion and change began gradually. The Road people were employed by and surrounded by English-speaking Protestants and were separated from their own church and ancestral families by distance. Intermarriage took place bit by bit, and proselytizing by Protestants very likely loosened the hold of the Roman Catholic faith, even though it did not succeed in making any large number of converts. The measure of cultural confusion entering the lives of the people is indicated by the fact that although they stopped speaking French, the English they acquired was limited and had an accent that was a source of amusement to outsiders.

The real turning point for the Road, however, came at the beginning of the century. The coastal industry of building wooden ships collapsed and was not replaced by any comparable economic activity in the region. This change was part of the more general economic shift in North America from commerce to industry and from widely scattered small manufacturing enterprises in towns and villages to mass production in urban centers. People with education, fluency in English, and capital resources were able to move out of the region or otherwise adjust to these changes. Today the shipbuilding of Port Harmony is scarcely remembered; one has to look carefully to find a few waterlogged stumps of pilings where the wharves once stood.

The people of the Road thus suffered a precipitous loss of economic resource. Although some were able to move, enough of them remained to perpetuate the existence of the group, and deterioration set in. By 1950 their poverty was manifest in their low and undependable income, lack of capital, lack of property, and lack of credit. The educational level was nominally fourth or fifth grade, but among the adults were eight who could read and write little or not at all. The typical house was described as "one-and-a-half stories." It had three small rooms on the ground floor, while the "half" was a garret reached by a ladder. There the children usually slept, often on the floor. Cooking was done mostly on wood stoves, occasionally on oil stoves.

The houses had no electricity and no inside toilets. Furnishings were few and tawdry, although one house had a real living room with a woven-wicker settee and matching chairs. Only about half the families had vegetable gardens and most yards were unkept.

The families who lived in this physical setting showed a high prevalence of broken marriages, interparental strife, and child neglect. The last was often due to the fact that both parents were simultaneously away at work, leaving younger children to be cared for by siblings not much older. Between families there was a surprising degree of isolation. Individuals were not bound together in groups by any kind of formal social organization except the church, which they rarely attended.

Some informal organization was evident, primarily as house-to-house visiting by the women. The men of the neighborhood did not participate much in such visiting patterns but gathered to idle away spare hours at a filling station near the Road; they also hunted together and at times worked and camped near tidal flats some miles from the Road. The nearest thing to leadership outside the family was the role assumed by one man in assembling woodcutting teams and by one woman who did the same for clamshucking.

The Road was, in short, not really a community but a neighborhood based on exclusion. One often heard residents of nearby communities refer to Road people with such remarks as "They had better keep their place" and "We don't want them here." Attitudes of this kind put innumerable limitations on the people of the Road, making it difficult for them to obtain work, form friendships, and find mates. The mates were mostly from similarly depressed areas and so tended to perpetuate the character of the Road.

The sentiments prevailing among Road people reflected the disintegrated nature of the neighborhood. Although most of the values found in the larger society were also evident on the Road, expressions of them by Road residents were comparatively pale and lacking in commitment. An example was the merely nominal Catholicism of the Road people. In addition, the people voiced strong sentiments of self-disparagement, mistrust of each other, and distrust of outsiders, particularly those in positions of authority. Work was regarded as virtueless—a necessary evil to be avoided when possible. The people showed little in the way of foresight. They tended to regard the future as uncontrollable, an attitude reflected by the fact that most of them thought the best thing to do with a dollar was to spend it at once, because only in that way could they be assured of getting full use of it.

I should temper my description by noting that it leans toward caricature. There were a few residents of the Road who differed from the others in their attitudes. Among some of the women in particular there was a feeling that conditions could be improved and that education was a means to that end. (This view was not shared by the men and boys, who looked on escape from school as a sign of entry into manhood.) However, one must say that in spite of individual variations the people of the Road were in the grip of interlocking factors, internal and external, which tended to keep them mired. The people had few resources, to be sure, but it should also be noted that they made very poor use of the resources they did have—not only because they lacked knowledge, skills, manners, habits of cooperation, and leadership, but also because of their deeply rooted tendencies toward hostility, disparagement, and suspicion.

In 1950 Macmillan gave a report to county and provincial officials listing several needs that would have to be met if the disintegration of the Road were to be arrested and reversed. At the top of the list were three things: (1) the introduction of social organization and social values through the development of leadership; (2) education; and (3) improved economic opportunities. Officials gave attention to these recommendations and gradually, as the result of a series of steps, conditions along the Road began to improve.

The first step was an experiment undertaken by the official responsible for adult education in the area. He defined his objective as improving the manners and skills of the Road people so that they would be better able to get and hold jobs, not only locally but also in urban centers. He hoped to evolve a general formula whereby rural depressed areas of this sort might be helped. His intermediate goal was to establish adult-education classes in the local one-room school. As a step toward that end he decided to organize meetings at which motion pictures would be shown.

The second step was the appointment of a schoolteacher who was competent and aware of the Road's problems, a woman in marked contrast to the succession of substandard teachers who had come and gone at the school before. She and the adult-education official began by showing motion pictures to the school children during school hours. Then they sent the children home with the word that evening showings of motion pictures would be available at the school without charge.

Since there was no electricity in the school, the first film showings (at which attendance was fairly good) required a portable generator. Eventually the official pointed out that if the programs were to continue, the school ought to be electrified. He told the people that the regional department of education would meet half of the cost if the other half were raised locally. His reasoning in this move was that the people would have to develop internal leadership and gain experience in cooperation before any more ambitious program could succeed. He was aware that he ran the risk of having his undertaking collapse for want of interest in the wiring project. As it turned out, however, the people of the Road, canvassed by school children with a petition drafted by the teacher, raised their share of the money and enough more to pay for the electricity for the following year.

At this critical juncture the program did collapse because the adult educator was transferred to a different district. Such a turn of events was so thoroughly in keeping with the Road's chronic attitudes of mistrust and with the predictions of the venture's opponents on the Road that recovery seemed impossible. The schoolteacher, however, stepped into the breach by continuing to promote group activity, such as evening bingo games at the school to finance the purchase of new desks. It is possible that, being a woman, she was more effective than the adult educator would have been with the Road women, who had begun to take some interest in improving educational conditions in the neighborhood.

One of the teacher's most important moves was to bring up (at the suggestion of school authorities, who were influenced by Macmillan's report) the question of having the district admitted to the consolidated school of the region. Such admission meant the daily bus transportation of all children above the sixth grade to the consolidated school in a town some miles away, where the educational opportunities were considerably richer and the way was clear for going on to high school. It would also mean, of course, an increase in taxes for landowners in the school district.

That these were resisted is not surprising when one realizes that although most of the children in the school were from the Road, virtually all the taxes were paid by owners of the surrounding farms and woodlots, many of whom had no children in the school and most of whom saw no sense in spending money on the education of those they considered constitutionally incapable of benefiting from education. Ordinarily, few or no people from the Road appeared at public meetings, but at the meeting on this issue enough attended to swing the vote, and the Road became a part of the consolidated school system.

When the first group of Road children arrived at the consolidated school, the principal noted that they stood apart, said little, and were awkward. Moreover, their clothing was out of keeping with the fashions for young people and was often ill fitting. One day about five months later the principal noticed at an assembly that none of the Road children seemed to be present. He asked one of his assistants if they had stopped coming to school. The assistant replied that they were there but that they had now blended with the rest of the student body. The speed of this adjustment was doubtless facilitated by the fact that each year the new children entering the school included some from rural areas in which clothes, manners, and language were different from those of the student majority. Thus the situation was not one of a large gulf between the Road children and everyone else; rather there was a continuum with the Road children at one extreme.

We can suppose that the children began to bring new ideas about deportment, clothing, values, and motivation back to the Road neighborhood. No doubt this was resisted and treated with ridicule at first, but as the number of children going to and from the consolidated school increased they were able more and more to reinforce each other. There was a gradual but progressive impact that could never have been achieved if only a few people had been involved.

Coincident with these developments came an upswing in the availability of employment in the area. Of particular note in this connection was a nearby public works project which employed 300 to 400 men over a period of three years. One of the labor recruiters for the project came to the Road, and by this means many of the men found fairly steady work.

This employment had one unusual feature which introduced something new to life on the Road. The recruiter also acted as an agent for electrical appliances. He combined his recruiting on the Road with a sales campaign, offering appliances on the installment plan. Electricity had by this time come to the Road as part of the general power development of the county. As a result the purchases were by no means useless; in fact, it is reasonable to suppose they led to the development of some new trends in the economic life of the community. First, having acquired a washing machine, a refrigerator, a vacuum cleaner, or a television set, the Road dweller became accustomed to using them. In due course this had its effect on his values and habits. Television in particular appears to have been an influence in bringing the dress, speech, and manners of the Road more in line with those regarded with approval by the larger society. Second, since the appliances were removed if the payments were not kept up, the Road men became far more diligent on the job than had been their custom. Finally, and perhaps most important, the Road people discovered the principle of credit. From this start they went on to a greater use of the principle, thereby binding themselves more tightly to the wage economy and the values and motives that go with it.

Another important development took place when a few Road people found unskilled work in a city 800 miles away. Gradually residents of the Road adopted the custom of going to the city to work for a few months and then returning home. By 1957 there were twenty-one people from the Road in the city; by 1962 some individuals had made the circuit several times. This arrangement had the obvious advantage of bringing money to the Road. It also helped to reduce the fear of the unknown in a city which had characterized many of the Road people.

As a result of all these influences the Road differed considerably at the end of ten years. This has been maintained so that now, fifteen years later, the houses, although still small, are larger than they used to be. Nearly all are neatly painted and have lawns, gardens, and occasionally ornamental shrubbery. Almost every family has a comfortably furnished living room, and the furnishings of the other rooms have improved comparably.

Paralleling these physical changes are changes in the situation and attitudes of the people. The level of education has risen markedly: Many of the children go beyond sixth grade and some continue through high school. It is the exceptional person today who has manners and clothing that set him off from the average of the county. Many of the adults hold semiskilled jobs, and several of the men have joined in business ventures requiring capital and cooperation. There has been a notable reduction in idleness, drunkenness, and brawling. One also finds the emergence of values oriented to the future and concerned with responsibility. People from the Road now participate in formal organizations, such as the church and the Home and School association. Various informal organizations have sprung up.

The changes on the Road are recognized in the surrounding areas, often with expressions of amazement. The benefits of this recognition include the lowering of barriers to friendship and employment. Thus the advances taking place on the Road are being reinforced by the surrounding society.

The prevalence of psychiatric disorders on the Road turned out to be much lower when resurveyed in 1962 than it had been in 1952. Thus improvement in mental health closely paralleled the growing integration of the community.

Two other communities were kept under paralleled study during the same period of time. Although exposed to all the same opportunities in education and employment they did not shift significantly toward either integration or reduced frequency of psychiatric disorder. This leads us to think that the initial push by the two teachers toward the development of social organization and social competence was of critical importance.

In summary, the people of the disintegrated communities find themselves in the grip of two interlocking and self-defeating forces, one sociocultural, the other psychological. As a result, these people do not make adequate use of the admittedly meager resources available to them. Even more significant for the success of any "war on poverty," they are not in a position to make adequate use of the resources that might be offered them in a development program. Thus, increased economic and educational opportunities are not enough to bring about a turn for the better in a disintegrated community, although such opportunities are essential to the process. What is needed in addition is the development of patterns of social functioning: leadership, fellowship, and practice in acting together cooperatively. In other words, it is necessary that the offers of better education and of training in marketable skills go hand in hand with help in learning the elements of human relations. Rooted in this necessity is the requirement that the people be enabled to gain confidence that some things can be done to better their lot; that they be assisted in modifying unrealistic or nihilistic views of the world and that they be encouraged to develop motivation. Without social and psychological changes of this kind the people will retain their inability to make adequate use of educational and employment opportunities.

And what of preventive psychiatry? Is this to be left to economists, educators, sociologists, and psychologists? Not "left to them," but rather "entered into with them." At the present time we have no firmer bases for conclusions than leads from exploratory studies, and much more work is obviously necessary. But if the leads turn out to have validity and if sociocultural disintegration becomes clearly identified as a form of societal pathology that has grave consequences for psychological health, then it will also be clear that preventive psychiatry, in order to be effective, must be a component in a coherent and congruent program which includes numbers of professions and disciplines.

There is, however, one further point to be made, and that concerns the role of therapeutic psychiatry in preventive effort. All the indications we have at present suggest that once sociocultural disintegration starts bringing about an increase of impairing and disabling psychiatric disorders, then this prevalence itself becomes a factor in the perpetuation of disintegration. Thus, a set of mutually enhancing noxious relationships becomes established. The story of the Road indicates that measures aimed at social organization, education, and economic opportunity can result in improved integration and improved mental health. But there is also the possibility that if therapeutic measures had been available and utilized by those in the group who needed them most, reduced anxieties, apathies, and depressive states would have made the shift toward integration occur much faster.

Summary

An epidemiological approach is described in detail, giving main emphasis to the functional state of a whole environmental system. Criteria were established by which communities were judged in terms of their sociocultural integration. A high correlation between the prevalence of psychiatric disorders and extremes of disintegration was found. By inducing in one community—the Road—patterns of social functioning including group action and local leadership, changes in the situation and attitudes of the people were promoted. On a resurvey after one decade the prevalence of psychiatric disorders turned out to be much lower than the initial survey.

NOTES

1. B. MacMahon, T. F. Pugh, and J. Ipsen, *Epidemiologic Methods* (Boston: Little, Brown, 1960).

2. A. H. Leighton, *My Name is Legion: Foundations for a Theory of Man in Relation to Culture*, The Stirling County Study of Psychiatric Disorder and Sociocultural Environment, vol. 1 (New York: Basic Books, 1959).

3. M. Beiser, "Poverty, Social Disintegration, and Personality," *Journal of Social Issues* 21, no. 1 (January 1965): 56–78, and C. C. Hughes et al., *People of Cove and Woodlot: Communities from the Viewpoint of Social Psychiatry*, The Stirling County Study of Psychiatric Disorder and Sociocultural Environment, vol. 2 (New York: Basic Books, 1960).

4. R. G. Baker and H. F. Wright, *Midwest and Its Children* (Evanston, Ill.: Row, Peterson, 1954).

5. A. H. Leighton, D. C. Leighton, and R. A. Danley, "Validity in Mental Health Surveys," *Canadian Psychiatric Association Journal* 11, no. 3 (May–June 1966): 167–178.

6. The foundations of this study and basic observations were conducted by the late Allister Miles Macmillan. Other participants, especially in later observations and analysis, were I. Thomas Stone, A. L. Nangeroni, D. C. Leighton, and R. A. Danley.

COMMENTARY

Leighton's provocative paper has examined efforts aimed at minimizing sociocultural disorganization in the test community—the Road—over time. As programs of community improvement and sociocultural development continued over a period of several years, the apparent differences between residents of the Road and their neighbors diminished or disappeared.

Leighton concludes that, as sociocultural disorganization decreased over time, the measured prevalence of psychiatric disorder also decreased. Although Leighton does not note the correction, the description of the "psychopathologic" state commonly found among residents of the Road suggests a striking parallel to the condition portrayed by Ernest Gruenberg in his description of the social breakdown syndrome.[1] This syndrome was described by Gruenberg as a frequent end product of years of residence in large mental hospitals.[2] He feels it is often incorrectly viewed as the end stage of schizophrenia. The three adjectives most descriptive of the syndrome are apathy, hostility, *and* negativism. *Note how well this fits Leighton's description of how the "psychological climate in the disintegrated neighborhoods can be represented by such words as apathy, interpersonal hostility, anxiety, depression, suspicion, and an unrealistic view of human affairs. This condition often runs to extremes in certain individuals, as shown by our findings of a high prevalence of psychiatric disorder in the Road and other disintegrated communities." Leighton's description invites a fascinating speculation: Were these individuals, labeled by Leighton as having "psychiatric disorder," really suffering from a socially induced social-psychological condition which Gruenberg calls social breakdown syndrome? Are both talking about the same thing?*

Since this paper, in the interest of brevity, omits a description of the method of determining "psychiatric disorder," a note may be helpful. The Leighton group measures "psychiatric disorder" by means of a symptom checklist completed by a trained interviewer who is usually not a psychiatrist. These forms are then reviewed by a psychiatrist. There is little concern about making a formal, specific psychiatric diagnosis; instead, symptoms are seen as additive, with a large number of them defined as "psychiatric disorder." [3] This procedure has been criticized by investigators who do not find direct linear correlations between signs and symptoms of mental disease, problems in living, and major psychiatric disorders (psychoses). How does this criticism fit in with your own clinical experience?

Further light may be shed on this relationship by referring back to Chapter 24; in his complementary formulation Fried suggests that "the greater the difficulty in establishing social solidarity, the more the individual must rely upon himself and his own resources and regulatory mechanisms." Later in the same paper Fried states, "Under conditions of intensified social deprivation, whether due to loss of employment, marital disruption [or other causes] . . . , there is simultaneously an intensified need for group resources and a more perceptible inability of the group to meet these needs."

Leighton's and Fried's papers are well considered together; each seems to illustrate and enhance the utility of the other's constructs. If after reading Leighton the reader begins to get the heady feeling that the key to effective prevention—social reorganization—is in his or her hand, we suggest that he or she reserve judgment while reviewing Dr. Cumming's penetrating questions, and plunge on ahead to incorporate the ideas and evidence offered by the other authors in this part.

NOTES

1. Ernest M. Gruenberg, Richard Kasius, and Matthew Huxley, "Objective Appraisal of Deterioration in a Group of Long-stay Hospital Patients," *Milbank Memorial Fund Quarterly* 40 (1962): 90; Ernest M. Gruenberg, "Can the Reorganization of Psychiatric Services Prevent Some Cases of Social Breakdown?" in *Psychiatry in Transition,* ed. A. B. Stokes (Toronto: University of Toronto Press, 1966–1967).

2. Gruenberg has since reported new cases of this syndrome developing in *community settings* in a paper presented to the American Psychiatric Association in May 1973, "Social Breakdown Syndrome in the Community in Honolulu, Hawaii."

3. For discussion purposes, Leighton's sophisticated and complex technique of correlating symptoms and psychiatric impairment has been greatly oversimplified. A full exposition can be found in A. H. Leighton, *My Name is Legion,* vol. 1 *The Stirling County Study of Psychiatric Disorder and Sociocultural Environment* (New York: Basic Books, 1959).

CHAPTER 27

Emergency Treatment

INTRODUCTION

The following paper reviews the theoretical underpinnings of the various types of crisis intervention and psychiatric emergency services that have developed in recent years, and considers briefly some of the evaluative literature in the field.

From the psychoanalytic perspective, a crisis may be seen as arising from an earlier core conflict (childhood neurosis) which has been reactivated by present intrapsychic or external circumstances. Alternatively, crisis may be interpreted as an acute loss of equilibrium in the individual's social system, resulting in interpersonal needs being unmet; for example, breakdown of needed communications with significant others may result from dysfunctional social relations. These two approaches are not mutually exclusive, but they do suggest different directions that may be taken in seeking resolution. If the crisis is seen as the renaissance of a core conflict it may be desirable to engage in psychotherapy directed toward dealing with the original conflict. If, on the other hand, the crisis is interpreted as a signal that interpersonal needs are not now being met, then psychotherapy and social interventions which encourage those behaviors which will most quickly lead to the regaining of adequate social relationships and communication would seem to be in order.

Many contemporary crisis intervention approaches accept as valid the goal often sought by clients by offering brief, intensive intervention aimed at restoring the social support system. When this approach is taken, longer-term psychotherapy may be offered postcrisis if a higher level of functioning or a greater degree of conflict resolution is desired by the client.

A REVIEW OF
CRISIS INTERVENTION PROGRAMS

Stephen L. Schwartz

Definition

In the 1960, third edition of the *Psychiatric Dictionary* edited by Hinsie and Campbell, the term "crisis intervention" is not included. It would appear that this was a concept which, though discussed and practiced, was not sufficiently reified prior to 1960 to be included in this fairly comprehensive text. However, by 1970, the fourth edition of the *Psychiatric Dictionary* does list *crisis intervention*. It is included as one of several models of community psychiatry:

> In the crisis intervention model the focus is on transitional—developmental and accidental—demands for novel adaptational responses. Because minimal intervention at such times tends to achieve maximal and optimal effects, such a model is more readily applicable to population groups than the medical model.[1]

A review of the literature indicates that crisis and crisis intervention are used in three ways:

1. Psychiatric emergencies. The full-blown manifestation of psychiatric illness in previously well individuals or acute exacerbations in the course of chronic psychiatric illness.[2]
2. Accidental crises. Periods of acute disorganization of affective, cognitive, and behavioral functioning, precipitated by a stressful life experience. The event may represent a loss, threat, challenge, and even an apparent gain but containing latent risks. Examples include death of loved ones, illness, accidents, surgery, and loss or change of jobs.
3. Developmental crises. Periods of acute disorganization of functioning transitional between one developmental phase and another. Examples include entering school, matriculation at college, getting married, and becoming a parent.

According to Caplan, developmental and accidental crises both refer to periods of acute psychological upset, lasting one to five weeks, not signs of mental disorder in themselves, but the manifestations of adjustment and adaptation struggles in the face of a temporarily insoluble problem. They have been novel situations that the individual has not been able to handle quickly with his existing coping and defense mechanisms. The problems are serious and unavoidable. As adjustment and adaptation struggles, they present both an opportunity for

Stephen L. Schwartz, "A Review of Crisis Intervention Programs," *Psychiatric Quarterly* XLV, 1971, pp. 498–507. Used by permission.

personality growth and the danger of increased vulnerability to mental disorder, the outcome depending to a degree on how the situation is handled.[3]

Characteristics of Crises

Thus crisis is viewed as a marked and moderately prolonged disruption in homeostasis. Relative to the seriousness of the problem, the individual's usual coping mechanisms are not immediately adequate. The disequilibrium of emotional upset ensues. Classically, four phases have been described in the life cycle of a crisis: [4]

1. An initial phase in which an individual, responding to the problem and the tension generated thereby, attempts to solve the problem by his usual problem-solving techniques.
2. If unsuccessful, a second phase is entered. Tension increases, producing emotional upset. Feelings of anxiety, guilt, shame, fear, and helplessness may be experienced. Ineffective and disorganized functioning occur. There may be successive abortive trial and error attempts to solve the problem. An individual may seek to discharge tension through activity unrelated to solving the problem, e.g., getting drunk.
3. With the continued failure to solve the problem, rising tension acts to stimulate renewed problem-solving efforts and resources. The problem may be reexamined and redefined to be amenable to solution. Novel solutions may be tried. During this phase, the problem may be solved. The solution may involve acceptance of previously unacceptable aspects of the problem. However solved, homeostasis is restored, possibly at a higher level than before.
4. Lack of solution and continued tension characterize a fourth phase with clinical evidence of major disorganization.

In addition to these phases, there are certain characteristics of crisis which are particularly relevant for therapeutic intervention: [5]

a. The outcome is not solely determined by antecedent factors. That is, our fates are not sealed, but subject to our own action as well as external intervention.
b. During crisis, an individual experiences increased dependency feelings, a wish to be helped, and signals this to his environment.
c. The individual in crisis is more open to the influence of others. As indicated in the initial definition, minimal intervention at such times tends to achieve maximal effects.

Primary Prevention Programs

Intervention in the developmental and accidental crises of individuals not previously regarded as psychiatrically ill constitutes efforts at primary prevention. The mental health professional may intervene directly with the individuals in crisis, or may act through direct personal contact with other care-giving persons. Such intervention involves gaining access to a high-risk population, e.g., college freshmen, surgical patients, new mothers, recently bereaved persons, and identifying those individuals who are coping poorly. Through individual and small group intervention, efforts are made to enlarge understanding, assist the expression of feelings, point out areas for exploration, reexamine the problem in reality terms, open channels to sources of help, and reconvene the individual's social supportive matrix—the family—to assist healthy coping.

Such a program of intervention was first used systematically by Lindemann [6] in 1944. Survivors of the Coconut Grove fire had to confront accidental crises as a result of their own injuries, the deaths of loved ones in the fire, and their feelings of guilt and shame.

Another program designed to intervene in the crisis period of recently bereaved persons was initiated by Caplan. In this program the mental health professional trained a group of widows in the recognition of good and bad coping techniques of mourning, and in the techniques of assisting good coping. These widows, following their training, were then placed in contact with recently bereaved women. An important aspect of intervention by someone other than the mental health professional involves adequate support of the care givers. This relates to dealing with poor results as well as their own involvement in the crises. In the case of the widow care givers, a recrudescence of their own grief was noted after a period of working with recent widows.

An elaborate and sophisticated program of intervention in a developmental crisis is a component of the Peace Corps program. A particular technique of "anticipatory guidance" has proven to be of value. Present experiences, e.g., leaving home and family to attend the training center, are used to anticipate and guide the candidate through the crises of separation and a strange environment with novel tasks to be encountered in foreign lands.

A vast opportunity for intervention in developmental and accidental crises is available to every physician.[7] No other single professional is exposed to as many people facing crisis. Examples include the effect of illness and surgery on patients and their families, the separation of parents and children during hospitalization, wanted and unwanted pregnancy, abortion, and bereavement.

Research in intervention programs has uncovered a series of general principles of therapeutic value in dealing with individuals in crisis: [8]

1. Help the individual to face the crisis. Defenses of denial or avoidance only delay and ultimately worsen the process, e.g., delayed grief reactions.
2. Assist in the individual to face the crisis in manageable doses. Individuals facing crisis must not persist to exhaustion. Short retreats from confrontation are restorative of function, but must be limited to avoid denial and regression. The brief, symptomatic use of medication should be considered.
3. Assist fact finding. Help the individual examine the problem in a reality-based frame of reference. Studies of the psychiatric problems

of hospitalized individuals reveal cognitive defects to their illnesses to be a significant factor in emotional decompensation.[9]

4. Avoid false reassurance. Everything may well not turn out all right. However, the reassurance of faith in an individual's ability to handle the crisis is of value.

5. Discourage projection. The blaming of others is of little value in crisis resolution.

6. Help the individual to accept help. The acceptance of appropriate support from an individual's social supporting matrix, especially his family, assists his efforts at restoring homeostasis.

7. Assist with everyday tasks. Examples include arrangements for a homemaker in a family during the hospitalization of a mother, as well as the help of a husband or mother during the immediate postnatal period of a new mother.

Secondary Prevention Programs

In the past few years, crisis intervention has become spoken of, increasingly, in the sense of intervening in the disequilibrium of overtly psychiatrically ill individuals. Efforts are aimed at case finding and treating the patient early in the course of his illness, whether this is a first occurrence or an exacerbation in a chronic process. The previously noted principles about crisis and intervention remain applicable; however, the major focus is one of care delivery and shortening of the acute process. The goal is usually restoration of the premorbid level of functioning or limiting and minimizing disability. There is little attention to the concept of crisis as a stimulus producing a higher level of functioning homeostasis.

Definitions of crises or emergencies vary widely. They include objective behavioral manifestations, subjective feeling states, and traditional psychiatric concepts of emergencies. In practice, pragmatically, these definitions are of little value. The clinician faced with an individual seeking help, a family disturbed by one of its members, or representatives of social or legal agencies troubled by a client has an emergency requiring response regardless of prior definitions.

Existing programs can be divided into two main areas: [10] (1) the avoidance of hospitalization; and (2) shortening of hospitalization.

Programs to Avoid Hospitalization

Four approaches used singly and together are practiced to avoid hospitalizing patients. These include walk-in clinics, home visits, telephone hot lines, and programs of family intervention.

1. *Walk-in clinics* are organized operationally in one of three modes: [11] twenty-four-hour psychiatric consultation to the emergency room of a general hospital; a twenty-four-hour clinic specially staffed

with various mental health personnel; a combined approach using a special clinic during the day with psychiatric consultation available to medical personnel during the night.

Examination of walk-in psychiatric emergency clinics reveals multiple qualities held in common. They each strive to be readily available and accessible. This relates to hours of operation, absence of waiting lists, proximity to target population, geographic considerations including ground level location and availability of public transportation, and child care programs for mothers seeking help. A multidisciplinary team approach is characteristic, with an attempt to avoid defining clinical roles solely on the basis of a worker's professional discipline. Expectations regarding the duration of intervention are altered in the direction of sharply limiting the total treatment program. Allied to this is a shift in the therapeutic orientation from an extended in-depth understanding of the past to an action-oriented, problem-solving approach to the here and now. Engagement with the patient's family and other significant persons in his supporting social matrix is considered an important aspect of intervention.

Problems encountered have related to lack of concordance between the therapist's view of the treatment process and the patient's expectation of how the therapist would act. A similar lack of concordance relative to treatment goal has also been noted. Questions have arisen about the very value of such intervention. Is a patient population of recidivists being created? Other problems have related to the anxieties stimulated in professionals called upon to intervene in problems not traditionally considered within their area of professional expertness.

2. *Home visits* [12] can be useful in several areas of emergency care, such as relief of acute symptoms, crisis intervention, prevention of hospitalization, facilitation of hospitalization if necessary, emergency evaluation, and reaching out to an otherwise unavailable patient. Specific examples of situations warranting a home visit include instances in which it is impossible to induce a patient or family to come in to the clinic, the follow-up of ambulatory patients who fail to keep visits, initial requests for hospitalization, as a component part of the routine care of ambulatory patients, and in geriatric cases.

Problems encountered have included questions of who is to make the visit, flexibility of administrative policies, availability of staff, transportation, and economic considerations. The advantages that accrue to such a program consist of the more complete clinical picture gained from engaging the patient in his natural environment, the ready availability of the family to supply information as well as assist in the treatment program, and the economic savings if hospitalization can be avoided.

3. *Telephone hot lines* are an integral part of crisis intervention programs. The pioneering work in the use of the telephone as a therapeutic tool, with techniques able to be taught to persons of varied levels of training, has been reported by the Los Angeles Suicide Prevention Center.[13] Hot lines have been established to deal with both special problems, e.g., drug abuse, and the whole area of people in distress. It

is a convenient vehicle of entrance for individuals unwilling or unable to present themselves in person.

4. *Family intervention programs* are again an aspect of most efforts at crisis intervention. The need to involve family if rapid resolution is to be achieved has become a part of standard operation. In most instances this is done as a matter of course with little effort at research evaluation. However, in an effort to evaluate such intervention, an elaborate research and treatment program was undertaken by Langsley [14] at Colorado Psychiatric Hospital. One hundred and fifty patients, deemed in need of immediate hospitalization, were assigned to outpatient family crisis therapy, while 150 similar patients were hospitalized. After six months twice as many of the originally hospitalized patients had to be rehospitalized as compared to the group in family crisis therapy. This difference persisted after eighteen months of study. In addition, those patients originally hospitalized, when rehospitalized, stayed an average of twice as long as those in the family program. On various tests measuring functioning capacity, the group in family crisis therapy did as well as or better than the hospitalized group. On a cost basis, the family crisis program was one-sixth as expensive as the comparison hospitalization program.

Programs to Shorten Hospitalization

Several programs of treatment and research have been undertaken to shorten psychiatric hospitalization without sacrificing the restorative value of such care. Review of reports coming from such programs reveal· not only a high degree of effectiveness but a set of operational practices held in common.

The units are relatively small, ranging from three to eleven beds, and operated by a small, multidisciplinary staff. The low patient population permits intensive, united staff intervention. The use of a small staff encourages an intimate working relationship with a minimum of communication problems. It also fosters a special esprit of mutual responsibility and status, relieving the psychiatrist of inappropriate totem responsibility. The multidisciplinary approach offers the patient help in the many social and psychologic areas that are not amenable to purely psychiatric intervention.

A definite time limit to hospitalization is set. Sharply defined goals are established. The setting of a time limit works an attitudinal change in both the patient and staff. Each minute is important. Discharge planning is a part of admission procedure. Nights and weekends are utilized. The message conveyed to the patient is that he is a person able to and expected to handle his life. Responsibility is restored to the patient; dependency and regressive prolongation of the sick role is discouraged. The expectation of rapid restoration is ever present.

The active involvement of the patient's important others is pursued. Family is brought into the therapy. Family dynamics are explored and staff intervenes in pathologic and pathogenic family functioning. Healthy family functioning is supported to assist the patient's restoration of homeostasis.

A program of intensive intervention has been studied at the Yale-Connecticut Mental Health Center.[15] Patients deemed in need of hospitalization were offered conventional psychiatric hospitalization or a special contract. The contract consisted of three days of inpatient care on the emergency treatment unit plus thirty days of follow-up outpatient care by the same personnel. The unit contains seven beds and admits about 350 patients annually for seventy-two-hour intervention. Day shift staffing consists of two nurses, two aides, a social worker, a psychiatric service chief, and two half-time, second-year, psychiatric residents. Admission diagnoses of psychosis or borderline psychosis were present in 48 percent of cases. Suicidal behaviors were present in 50 percent. The unit was open and located on ground level with patients permitted freedom of movement.

The general operational practices noted above included the reinforcement of self-reliance "by focusing on the patient's responsibility for his life, in particular for discharge plans, and for what is to happen to him once he leaves,[16] thereby maximizing autonomy. There are minimal institutional restrictions, combined with a highly structured program to minimize regression and dependency. The focus is on recent problems, assisting the patient to evolve adequate coping and problem-solving capacities. The family is involved early and intensively. Several staff members have scheduled meetings with the patient daily, complemented by multiple group techniques. Psychotropic agents are used to diminish target symptoms.

Follow-up of the first 100 cases indicates that 18 percent were transferred to longer inpatient care immediately after three days, with another 19 percent being hospitalized within one year of discharge. Thus after one year 63 percent did not require further hospitalization. A two-year follow-up revealed 6 percent more hospitalized. This compared favorably with other recent follow-up studies of hospitalization periods ranging from three weeks to eight months.

Another program of short-term hospitalization has been evolved in the Emergency Psychiatric Service at Colorado General Hospital,[17] in which hospitalization of three to seven days was considered as the "beginning of crisis therapy for patients who the evaluating team feels cannot be treated initially on an outpatient basis." The unit consisted of eleven beds. Basic operational principles were: (1) limited goals, with emphasis on the here and now; (2) immediate formulation and planning; (3) focus on termination from the beginning; (4) involvement of significant others; (5) flexibility; and (6) team approach." [18]

A one-year follow-up of 100 patients indicated that 16 percent were transferred for longer care following the crisis admission. During the first six months following discharge, 11 percent more were hospitalized and another 3 percent during the second six months. Thus at one year following crisis admission, 70 percent did not require further hospitalization.

Summary

Review of the denotative usage of the term "crisis" in the psychiatric literature of the past twenty-five years indicates three distinct concepts: (1) developmental crises; (2) accidental crises; and (3) the acute onset of psychiatric disability or acute exacerbations in the course of chronic disability. However, common to all is a body of crisis theory embracing the characteristics of crisis itself, the progressive stages of individual responses to crisis, and general principles of crisis intervention.

Programs of crisis intervention were reviewed from the vantage of primary and secondary prevention. Intervention in the developmental and/or accidental crises of heretofore healthy individuals, i.e., primary prevention, was described. Descriptions of programs of secondary prevention dealing with the acute onset or recurrence of psychiatric disability were divided into programs to avoid hospitalization and programs to shorten hospitalization.

In conclusion, the goal of crisis intervention is never merely the resolution of the crisis. Crisis, by definition, is always terminable. Intervention seeks as its goal a higher order of resolution than would be provided by nature or chance alone.

· *NOTES*

1. L. E. Hinsie and R. J. Campbell, *Psychiatric Dictionary*, 4th ed. (New York: Oxford University Press, 1970), p. 606.
2. L. Bellack et al., "Psychiatry in the Medical-Surgical Emergency Clinic," *Archives of General Psychiatry* 10 (1964): 267–269; J. V. Coleman, "Research in Walk-in Psychiatric Services in General Hospitals," *American Journal of Psychiatry* 124 (1968): 1668–1673; L. Bellack, "A General Hospital as a Focus of Community Psychiatry," *Journal of the American Medical Association* 174 (1960): 2214–2217; J. V. Coleman and P. Errera, "The General Hospital Emergency Room and Its Psychiatric Problems," *American Journal of Public Health* 53 (1963): 1294–1301; and W. B. Miller, "A Psychiatric Emergency Service and Some Treatment Concepts," *American Journal of Psychiatry* 124 (1968): 924–933.
3. G. Caplan, *Principles of Preventive Psychiatry* (New York: Basic Books, 1964), pp. 35–36.
4. Ibid., pp. 40–41.
5. Ibid., pp. 53–54.
6. E. Lindemann, "Symptomatology and Management of Acute Grief," *American Journal of Psychiatry* 101 (1944): 141–148.
7. G. Caplan, "Practical Steps for the Family Physician in the Prevention of Emotional Disorders," *Journal of the American Medical Association* 170 (1959): 1497–1506.
8. Caplan, *Principles of Preventive Psychiatry*, pp. 293–296.
9. E. H. Stein, J. Murdaugh, and J. A. Macleod, "Brief Psychotherapy of Psy-

chiatric Reactions to Physical Illness," *American Journal of Psychiatry* 125 (1969): 1040–1047.

    10. J. F. Wilder, "Crisis Intervention Programs" (Paper presented to Twenty-third Institute on Hospital and Community Psychiatry, Seattle, Washington, September 1971).

    11. *Emergency Services,* U.S. Public Health Service Pub. No. 1477 (Washington, D.C.: Government Printing Office, 1968).

    12. L. D. Hankoff, *Emergency Psychiatric Treatment* (Springfield, Ill.: Charles C Thomas, 1969), pp. 29–34.

    13. R. E. Litman, E. S. Shneidman, and N. L. Farberow, "Los Angeles Suicide Prevention Center," *American Journal of Psychiatry* 117 (1969): 1084–1087; M. N. Kaphan and R. E. Litman, "Telephone Appraisal of 100 Suicidal Emergencies," *American Journal of Psychotherapy* 16 (1962): 591–599; and R. E. Litman et al., "Suicide Prevention Telephone Service," *Journal of the American Medical Association* 192 (1965): 107–111.

    14. D. G. Langsley, P. Machotka, and K. Flomenhaft, "Avoiding Mental Hospital Admissions: A Follow-up Study," *American Journal of Psychiatry* 127 (1971): 1391–1394.

    15. G. Weisman, A. Feirstein, and C. Thomas, "Three-day Hospitalization— A Model for Intensive Intervention," *Archives of General Psychiatry* 21 (1969): 620–629.

    16. Ibid., p. 621.

    17. M. W. Rhine and P. Mayerson, "Crisis Hospitalization Within a Psychiatric Emergency Service," *American Journal of Psychiatry* 127 (1971): 1386–1391.

    18. Ibid., p. 1387.

COMMENTARY

Schwartz has defined three types of crisis: the psychiatric emergency, the accidental crisis precipitated by a major acute life stress, and the developmental crisis. He has suggested the possibility that therapeutic intervention, particularly in a developmental crisis, may result in a higher level of functioning than existed prior to the crisis.

Events which might precipitate either an accidental or a developmental crisis can be expected to occur in everyone's life, including those who have no psychiatric disorder. Presumably the degree of distress, disorganization, and success of coping efforts in each situation will depend significantly on resources made available to the individual by his or her primary group relationships, as well as by his or her personal psychological resources. Thus we might anticipate that immigrants, the recently bereaved, persons who have recently lost their jobs and thereby lost both primary group relationships and income, and persons from disorganized communities might be at high risk. Such persons might suffer severe distress and require special assistance when confronted with an accidental or developmental crisis. Much sociological and epidemiological literature emphasizes and illustrates this point. Some of these data are reviewed and discussed in Chapters 4, 7, 21, 23, 24 and 26.

Much work in this area has been organized and summarized by Holmes and Rahe, who have developed a life stress table.[1] They give point values to specific life stresses—marriage, divorce, moving, loss of employment, death of parent—and suggest that, if at all possible, decisions should be avoided which would lead to exceedingly large point accumulations. They thus provide a framework for professionals to use in quantifying stress in their patients. Can this approach also lead to a community education approach to crisis prevention?

By implication, Schwartz offers supportive arguments for providing primary psychiatric hospitalization in a short-stay community hospital and for the location of crisis-evaluation-triage-acute intervention services in easily accessible community locations, rather than at a hospital which can conveniently offer only inpatient admission. How does this recommendation fit in with your own experience? Do you see any problems in its implementation?

The idea of providing brief intervention to a large number of patients may run counter to the view that the essential training to become a good clinician consists of spending a great deal of time with a very few patients. In programs guided by this kind of thinking there indeed may be a conflict between the crisis intervention service and training goals. The editors hold a contrary view. From our own clinical and teaching experience we have found that gaining skill and experience in crisis intervention can provide several training benefits, if certain conditions are met. The teaching staff must themselves hold the work as interesting, important, and valuable for training: their attitudes are readily transmitted to trainees. For example, assigning first-year psychiatric residents to the emergency room without experienced consultation and supervision severely limits the educational value of the work. It also angers the residents because they know that they cannot provide adequately for the patients' needs, and it denigrates the whole experience as a "scut" assignment. The simple addition of morning rounds in the emergency room, conducted by an experienced clinical teacher who reviews the prior night's emergencies, can reveal the drama as well as the didactic and service potentials of this kind of work. Beyond the emergency setting, we have found that crisis-handling skills and knowledge, once acquired, are fundamentally useful in all diagnostic and therapeutic aspects of mental health work.

NOTE

1. Thomas H. Holmes and Richard H. Rahe, "The Social Readjustment Rating Scale," *Journal of Psychosomatic Research* 11 (1967): 213–218.

CHAPTER 28

The Consequences of
Evaluative Research

INTRODUCTION

This book has tried to make the point that the mental health system is constantly being pressured and realigned by changing social values and expectations. A reciprocal observation can be made: Mental health is not as much or as quickly changed by objective new scientific knowledge as we might expect or like to think.

The following paper is a synopsis of a great deal of research on the treatment of schizophrenia carried out by Dr. May and his colleagues in California. It summarizes their research findings very briefly; a fuller report is available in a book.[1] The research has compared the outcome of five commonly used methods of treating hospitalized schizophrenic patients. These were psychotherapy alone, trifluoperazine (Stelazine), a combination of psychotherapy and trifloperazine, electroshock therapy, and hospital milieu therapy. Length of hospital treatment and cost of treating each patient were studied as the primary outcome variables. The distinctly different results with the various treatment regimens suggest that electroshock therapy, psychotherapy without drug, and milieu therapy alone should be discarded in ordinary cases. Drug treatment, with or without psychotherapy, led to a significantly more rapid restoration of function, as evidenced by release from the hospital.

In his discussion Dr. May makes the point that as of the time he was writing (1969), treatment practices reflected little use of these findings. This was true despite the fact that the data were by then widely available in the psychiatric literature, having been corroborated by other investigators who also had reported their work at professional conferences and in journals. Dr. May concludes by offering his personal suggestions as to how the treatment of schizophrenics might be improved.

NOTE

1. Philip R. A. May, *Treatment of Schizophrenia* (New York: Science House, 1968).

MODIFYING HEALTH CARE SERVICES FOR SCHIZOPHRENIC PATIENTS

Philip R. A. May

For some years I have been engaged in long-term research comparing the outcome of five commonly used methods of treating hospitalized schizophrenic patients—individual psychotherapy; an antipsychotic drug, trifluoperazine; [1] a combination of psychotherapy and trifluoperazine; electroconvulsive therapy; and milieu alone without any of the other treatments. Details of the study, a description of the patient sample, and the statistical techniques used have been published elsewhere.[2] My purpose here is to discuss the implications of our findings and follow-up experience for modifying health-care services to meet the long-range needs of similar patients. That is possible because we recorded the information needed to estimate the cost of treating each patient.

At Camarillo State Hospital, we assigned 228 first-admission schizophrenics with an "average" prognosis to one of the five methods. They were assigned randomly to try to equalize the makeup of the treatment groups as much as possible. Both before and after treatment, each patient had a comprehensive multidisciplinary work-up. The treatments were given either by psychiatric residents or by psychiatrists who had completed their training and had up to three years of subsequent experience. They were supervised by senior psychiatrists who were experienced in the particular treatment that was being given. Each form of treatment was given a fair trial, under good realistic conditions, either until the patient was improved enough to be released or until

Hospital & Community Psychiatry XX, December 1969, pp. 17–22. Condensed version reprinted with permission of *Hospital & Community Psychiatry*, a journal of the American Psychiatric Association.

treatment had been given from six to twelve months and therapists and supervisors agreed it had been a failure.

Our findings apply only to hospital patients who are diagnosed as schizophrenic; they do not apply to the treatment of any other mental disorders. In general, I would say that they reflect the immediate outcome for most first-admission schizophrenic patients in most hospitals when they receive suitable, realistic amounts of the treatments. The outcomes are those to be expected when the patients are treated by an ordinary therapist—not by one of the relatively few who are unusually gifted and experienced in treating psychotic patients, nor by one of those, also relatively rare, who are both incompetent and unsupervised. Indeed, our findings may even apply to patients treated by gifted therapists.

Of the forty-eight patients treated with drugs, forty-six, or 95.8 percent, were released within a year, and were treated at an average cost of $2,680 each. Of the forty-four patients who received drugs and psychotherapy, forty-two, or 95.5 percent, were released within a year, and the average cost was $3,290. Of the forty-seven who received electroconvulsive therapy, thirty-seven, or 78.7 percent, were released within a year; the average cost was $2,810. Of the forty-six treated with psychotherapy alone, thirty, or 65.2 percent, were released within a year, and the average cost was $4,470. Of the forty-three who received milieu therapy alone, twenty-five, or 58.1 percent, were released within a year, and the average cost was $3,390. The costs given here do not include the cost of treating the failures.

Those figures show that the two most effective of the five treatments were the drug alone and psychotherapy plus the drug. The differences in outcome between those two methods were small and insignificant. Psychotherapy alone and milieu alone were clearly the least effective and the most expensive methods, with little to choose between them. Electroconvulsive therapy fell in the middle.

By almost all criteria, including the opinions of the patients, nurses, physicians, and psychoanalysts, the drug had a powerful, beneficial effect, while the effect of psychotherapy was insignificant. There was no evidence of antagonism between drug and psychotherapy; on the contrary, if anything, the two seemed to potentiate one another's benefits. Thus our results, which are consistent with the results of others, indicate that we can dismiss the fairy tale that drugs should be avoided for hospitalized schizophrenic patients because they interfere with psychotherapy.

Our study demonstrates to my satisfaction that the ataraxic drugs are the most effective single form of treatment for the general run of hospitalized schizophrenic patients, and also are the cheapest. It is particularly impressive that all clinical judgments, as well as the psychometric, movement, and cost measures, support those findings. Such sweeping agreement indicates that antipsychotic drugs offer more than relief from symptoms. Indeed, the drug produced such a marked improvement in reality testing that patients treated with the drug alone actually developed more insight than did those treated with psychotherapy alone. Apparently the nature of the effect of ataraxic drugs has been subject to some misconceptions. The balance of evidence favors the view that drug-induced restitution is primarily a matter of improved ego functioning, and that any affective change is secondary and of secondary importance. In my opinion, the specific effect of ataraxic drugs on anxiety or aggression is a myth.[3]

Our results do not imply that all hospitalized schizophrenics should be given ataraxic drugs indiscriminately. Patients who are already on the way to restitution during their initial evaluation period should not receive any specific treatment, unless there is good probability that additional treatment will either improve their final condition or lessen the financial burden of their illness. But for the general run of schizophrenic patients drug therapy is undoubtedly the single treatment of choice at present.

Judging from our results, which are consistent with the few other reports available,[4] the value of psychotherapy for hospitalized schizophrenics has been greatly exaggerated. At this stage of the illness, individual psychotherapy without ataraxic drugs is expensive and ineffective, and apparently adds little or nothing to conservative milieu therapy. Is there anything to be gained by adding it to drug therapy? All in all, we found that the addition does not seem to offer much advantage. By comparison with patients receiving the drug alone, patients receiving individual psychotherapy as well are likely to have their hospital stay prolonged, and as a result the cost of treatment will be increased. Some may perhaps show some very slight additional clinical benefit in a few areas, but the difference is unlikely to be impressive.

Milieu therapy alone is expensive and relativly ineffective. It obviously is fiscally unsound to rely on milieu therapy without also providing specific methods of treatment. For the benefit of those who make decisions about treatment programs and budgeting, a concrete illustration may drive home the point. In 1966, a total of 3,253 schizophrenics between the ages of sixteen and forty-four were admitted for the first time to psychiatric hospitals operated by the California Department of Mental Hygiene. Assuming that by and large we may reasonably apply the findings for our group directly to that group, it would have cost $10,640,000 less—and led to better results—to treat them with the drug plus a decent milieu than it would have to treat them with milieu alone.

In this connection, the paucity of controlled research on psychosocial methods of treating schizophrenia should be a matter of concern. I have the impression that "therapeutic milieu" has become a sacred cow, supported more by uncontrolled staff proclamation than by objectively determined therapeutic benefits. We must be alert to the possibility that professional energies and skills may be diverted into appealing but costly high-prestige activities that, although no doubt satisfying, rewarding, and of considerable value for staff morale, may be of little value to patients—in some cases perhaps even detrimental.

Obviously each hospital provides some level of care. The question is what can be gained from each additional expenditure of time and effort over and above reasonable routine care. It has been widely assumed that differences in outcome between hospitals can be attributed to the hospital milieu. Yet the only objective study of that matter showed that the differences were primarily due to the admission of patients with better prognoses, and that ward atmosphere, hospital policy, and philosophy toward treatment contributed nothing further.[5] A therapeutic milieu can be extremely expensive in personnel time and therefore cost. It would seem more prudent to spend the money and the time to benefit patients in some other way, especially when ataraxic drugs are used. Our findings and those of other investigators indicate that the results of drug therapy are equally good at all levels of care except, of course, under virtual neglect or minimal custodial care.

Psychiatry suffers from a gulf between research and application. Pertinent to that problem is a recent report made for the U.S. Navy, which emphasizes the alarming schism between the ivory tower of psychological research and the realities of training. Research in modern learning, the authors found, has little impact on educational technology or training practices, because few psychologists attempt to apply research findings to educating or training people. "The scarcest quantity in the United States is at the interface between research and application," they write. "Research is generally simple. We must not perpetuate the notion that we must put our best people into research. A good researcher is not necessarily a good interfacer."

The report recommends that a new class of professionals should act, at the interface, as constructive critics to define the problems of the classroom for research investigators and interpret research findings to the educators—thus functioning like industrial engineers.[6] I would recommend that administrators of health care and health care research read the report very carefully, because a similar problem exists in psychiatry. We need health care engineers, people who can speak three "languages"—research, clinical practice, and simple English—not only to galvanize investigators into research that is relevant but, far more important, to translate research findings into tactics and strategy for action.

I see the translation of research findings into effective action as one of the major problems for health care delivery systems. Publication in learned journals will not accomplish very much; there is already a vast information overload. Computerized information storage and retrieval systems do not offer the answer. The fundamental tasks are to sift out reliable information that is relevant for treatment, think through how to apply it, and then communicate the practical applications in simple English to clinicians. All those are tasks for a health care engineer—not for a machine or, for that matter, a researcher.

We do not have a health care engineer in our line-item budget in California, nor, I believe, does he exist anywhere else. My first recommendation therefore is to establish this new career category and department, called psychiatric research liaison or health care engineering, with a purely staff function.

In the meantime, I will feel free to stick my neck out and review somewhat sketchily what I believe are the program implications of our findings, taken in conjunction with other relevant research. My discussion will focus on patients who must be admitted to a hospital, although obviously a considerable number can be successfully managed as outpatients without ever being admitted to a hospital.

Our results indicate that drug therapy, properly supervised by experienced consultants, can move the average schizophrenic patient rapidly from inpatient care to aftercare. Formal psychotherapy or an elaborate, expensive therapeutic milieu is not important for such patients during their hospital stay. The essential thing is for the staff to prepare the patient and his family for psychotherapy, psychotherapeutic management, rehabilitation, and continuing drug therapy after he is released. The goal of hospital treatment should be discharge at the earliest reasonable moment to an aftercare unit.

In the hospital phase, therefore, treatment of the schizophrenic patient should be concentrated on psychiatric first aid and restitution. By contrast, the ultimate goal of outpatient treatment is stabilization of the personality. It is during that stabilization phase—not during hospital treatment—that psychotherapy, social therapy, and rehabilitation are likely to be most helpful. The treatment strategy should center around careful integration of hospital care and aftercare. If the delivery system provides continuity of inpatient and outpatient care by the same treatment team, the transition will be easier and more effective than if care is fragmented so that a different therapist treats patients after their release. If that is not possible, matters will be improved somewhat if a patient can be returned to a therapist who treated him before admission. Failing that, another possible approach might be to arrange for the new outpatient therapist to see the patient in the hospital a few times to initiate their relationship.

Great efforts have been made in the past to raise the levels of ward staffing and hospital medical care, while outpatient and community care have received much less attention. However, with the proper use of ataraxic drugs and psychotherapeutic management, expensive and time-consuming techniques of psychotherapy and milieu therapy are not required for the average schizophrenic patient. Indeed, they are likely to prolong hospital stay and increase cost. Because research has demonstrated conclusively that adequate aftercare is essential to successful treatment outcome,[7] the time has come to reexamine our distribution of personnel on the basis of cost efficiency.

To maximize long-term results, efforts should be diverted into the most profitable channels—on the one hand, providing a larger number of home visits, immediate outpatient aftercare, and community rehabilitation for those who are released and, at the other extreme, intensifying research into the cause of treatment failures and how best to manage them. Traditionally hospital programs have focused staff attention and treatment resources on acutely ill patients. By contrast, avoiding unnecessary treatment for those who will do well without it and vigorously applying drug therapy plus psychotherapeutic management for those who do need treatment should make it possible to redistribute staff to provide a higher level of hospital care for the nonresponders, as well as better aftercare for those who have been released.

The time has come for us to reappraise our current practice of transferring to less well staffed continued-care units those who have failed to respond to intensive treatment. For patients who do not respond to drugs—say, after six months at a normally effective dosage —or who are not well on the way to discharge within a year, it may be better strategy to transfer them to a special research unit, with better facilities and staffing than the rest of the hospital. That unit should be able to give any form of treatment including behavior therapy, individual psychotherapy, electroconvulsive therapy, and specialized techniques of milieu therapy and sociotherapy, as well as to test the most recent research developments.

Using individual psychotherapy as a research technique might lead to better understanding and therefore more effective treatment of chronic patients and of those who have failed to respond to adequate drug therapy and psychotherapeutic management. Radical as this proposal may seem, it makes more financial and clinical sense, in the light of our findings, than the prevalent custom of using individual psychotherapy indiscriminately or reserving it for patients with a good prognosis. The failures need all the help they can get, and the extra cost of psychotherapy may be offset by a saving if the patient responds sufficiently to be discharged.

Admission and release of patients are critical transition points, where a great deal of time and effort can be wasted and previous efforts put to naught. If there is no continuity of inpatient and outpatient responsibility by the same clinical team, the impact of the transitions on the patient can be lessened by placing full responsibility for all transactions in the hands of those who will be responsible for his outpatient care. I make that recommendation because I hope that an increasing proportion of our hospital treatment efforts will be devoted to outpatient service.

At intake a special effort should be made to identify patients who are likely to restitute fairly quickly without any special treatment or who should not be admitted at all. In my experience, most hospital staff are oriented to admission and leisurely evaluation rather than to crisis care. Hence I make three recommendations. First, when the same therapist is to look after the patient in and out of the hospital, he should whenever possible conduct screening interviews at the patient's home or at an office some distance from the hospital. Second, when treatment must be fragmented between inpatient and outpatient services, admission to the hospital should be the responsibility not of the hospital inpatient service, but of a well-staffed unit oriented to the community. And third, that community-oriented screening unit should be assigned a few overnight beds and appropriate personnel in a separate area to be used flexibly for short-term crisis intervention without formally admitting the patient to the inpatient service.

If I had to select the phase of treatment most in need of improvement, it would be the release phase, the transition of the patient from hospital to community. Weeks or months of hard work can be quickly undone by failure in such simple matters as providing drugs and instructions about how they should be taken, eliciting family cooperation, and arranging for the patient to return for follow-up interviews. From our own experience in trying to follow up the patients in our research project, I would say that aftercare should start by establishing a follow-up relationship when the patient is first admitted.

Every possible administrative device is needed to strengthen continuity of care and to support the patient and his family during the discharge period. In the pressure of events surroundings release, there are many opportunities for errors and omissions that can be costly to the patient's eventual adjustment.

When the patient is discharged from the hospital, he faces a profound readjustment. At this time, changes in drug dosage are likely to be made, which may create additional problems. Studies have shown that unless special precautions are taken, any behavioral improvement the patient may have made while he was on drugs may be lost when he comes off them. To avoid that crisis, extra caution and concerted therapeutic efforts are needed. Sensitive adjustment of drug dosage to the optimal level must be combined with the establishment of a stable therapeutic contact to help the patient work toward the eventual goal of stabilizing his personality and mastering his illness.

Discharge should be treated as a family crisis too, and a home visit should be made to the family before the patient is released. The patient himself should be seen the day after his release, preferably in his own home. Any problems should be dealt with at once—for instance, ensuring the drug prescriptions can be filled at once and outside regular working hours. Contacts should be frequent during the first week or so, and taper off gradually as the crisis period passes.

Most outpatient clinics are reluctant to accept schizophrenic patients, and their staff members are relatively inexperienced in prescribing drugs for them. Because there is little immediate prospect of change in this respect, a reasonable level of care can be provided for such patients only if the responsibility, as well as the necessary personnel and financial support, is given to a special aftercare unit, even if such a unit might have to be located in a traditional outpatient clinic. Wherever the aftercare unit is located, its administrator will face a major interdisciplinary problem. He must structure the relationship among the various disciplines so that each patient will receive the optimum blend of psychotherapy, sociotherapy, rehabilitation, and drug therapy. Unless such amicable staff relationships can be developed, the result will be a program rigidly structured along doctrinaire lines.

If my proposed functional reorganizations were adopted, the table of organization for delivering health-care services to schizophrenics, exaggerated for dramatic purposes, would look something like Figure 1. Its central message is that the hospital is primarily responsible for delivering aftercare, and that inpatient functions are secondary. That is a radical departure from tradition, for the inpatient service is traditionally supreme. But perhaps the time has come to break with that tradition.

FIGURE 1

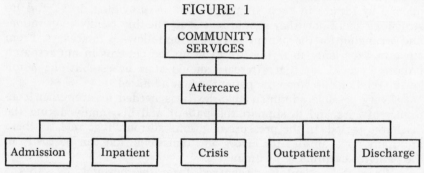

I would like to comment about the directions of future research. A review of the literature on psychiatric care shows that, with the exception of our own project, there has not been a single controlled study in which the cost of treatment was determined. Statistics abound, but statistical thinking has been virtually negligible; cost assessment by administrators is still fixated at the primitive, indeed archaic, level of cost per diem for the average patient, instead of directed at the cost per patient for various types of patients.

As our work has shown, modern computer capacities make it possible to include detailed cost comparisons in a clinical research project. Such comparisons add an important dimension to treatment evaluations. They enable the researcher to provide accountants, politicians, and health care administrators with realistic data to replace the misleading ratios and indexes that have been employed in the past.

Our study was a tentative exploration. I hope it will stimulate discussion and that other investigators will be encouraged to include cost comparisons in their investigations. Indeed, administrators should insist that cost comparison be part of any study of the outcomes of major treatments. And researchers should insist that they be provided with the management analysis and accounting services that are needed for such a venture.

NOTES

1. Stelazine, manufactured by Smith Kline & French, Inc., Philadelphia.

2. Philip R. A. May, *Treatment of Schizophrenia* (New York: Science House, 1968).

3. Philip R. A. May, "Anti-Psychotic Drugs and Other Forms of Therapy," in *Psychopharmacology: Review of Progress, 1957–1967,* ed. Daniel H. Efron et al., PHS Pub. No. 1836 (Washington, D.C.: Government Printing Office, 1968), pp. 1155–1176.

4. E. H. Uhlenhuth, Ronald S. Lipman, and Lino Covi, "Combined Pharmacotherapy and Psychotherapy: Controlled Studies," *Journal of Nervous and Mental Disease* 148 (January 1969): 52–64.

5. S. C. Goldberg, "Hospital Differences in Outcome as a Function of Patient, Ward, and Hospital Characteristics" (Paper read at the annual meeting of the American College of Neuropsychopharmacology, San Juan, Puerto Rico, December 1968).

6. R. R. Mackie and P. R. Christensen, *Translation and Application of Psychological Research,* Technical Report 716-1, prepared for personnel and training branch, psychological sciences division, Office of Naval Research, Department of the Navy, by Human Factors Research, Inc., Goleta, California, 1967.

7. Jacqueline Grad and Peter Sainsbury, "An Evaluation of Community Care: A Preliminary Report," *Proceedings of the Third World Congress of Psychiatry, Montreal* 1 (1961): 288–295; idem, "Problems of Caring for the Mentally Ill at Home," *Proceedings of the Royal Society of Medicine* 59 (January 1966): 20–23; idem, "The Effects That Patients Have on Their Families in a Community Care and a Control Psychiatric Service: A Two-Year Follow-up," *British Journal of Psychiatry* 114 (March 1968): 265–278; Else B. Kris, "Five Years' Experience With the Use of Drugs and Psychotherapy in a Community Aftercare Clinic," *American Journal of Public Health,* suppl. vol. 52 (September 1962): 9–12; idem, "Aftercare and Rehabilitation of the Mentally Ill," *Current Therapeutic Research* 5 (January 1963): 451–462; and Benjamin Pasamanick, Frank R. Scarpitti, and Simon Dinitz, *Schizophrenics in the Community* (New York: Appleton-Century-Crofts, 1967).

COMMENTARY

May has noted that treatment of our most common major psychiatric disorder—schizophrenia—continues to be misdirected from a scientific perspective, despite the fact that knowledge of how to treat it more effectively has been available to mental health workers and planners for years. Interestingly, he avoided analysis of the possible reasons why this might be the case, and proceeded immediately to suggest a possible solution—the "health care engineer." Problem solving without prior problem identification and analysis is not always the best path to success. Can you offer reasons that might explain why clinicians ignore this kind of research as they select treatment modalities?

It is now several years since May suggested that we should have health care engineers who would carry out liaison between research and treatment services. It has been as long since he argued so tellingly for an emphasis on brief hospitalization aimed solely at restoration of function, followed by careful planning to minimize the crisis of discharge, and an intense concentration on the provision of a full range of services in the posthospital period of community readjustment. Many of these same suggestions have been made anew in Chapter 15 and are just as relevant now as they were in 1969, since, unfortunately, they are so little followed in practice.

One recommendation has been followed: The length of inpatient stay has been shortened considerably in recent years. A review of the factors leading to this change suggests that social and economic pressures have been at least as influential as research findings. (Can you suggest other factors which have contributed to shortened hospitalization?) This seems to be supported by the observation that May's other major recommendations—for treating discharge as a crisis, for continuity of care, and for providing much more support during community readjustment—have generally not been followed. Indeed, the coupling of these two factors—shortened hospitalization and lack of adequate community aftercare services—presents us with a new social dilemma today. The solution to this may come from the societal pressures it has generated. As pointed out in Chapter 29, society may force the mental health system to follow May's recommendations in order to restore the "peace of mind" of the community. Such an outcome will still leave us with a haunting question: Why are the mental health sciences so slow to change when confronted with objective reasons to change?

CHAPTER 29

The Individual and Society: Maintaining Equity

Biologists, theologians, lawyers, politicians and artists can all agree that much of what makes life interesting is concerned with the maintenance of equity between the individual and society.

—ROBERT MORISON [1]

INTRODUCTION

Morison notes a current trend away from concern with the individual's duties to society, and toward the individual's claims upon it. To illustrate this shift he lists some newly developing "rights"—claims on society—which are becoming part of our social order. Among others he mentions the right to a job, to health, and to be supported at public expense for the first and last thirds of one's life.

In the paper which follows Bert Pepper examines the interplay between two elements of the mental health treatment system: the laws and social institutions which bring about involuntary hospitalization, and the fifteen-year-old movement to seek a "right to treatment" for patients so confined. He sees these as intertwined elements, and begins by providing a brief historical review of social and legal developments since the mid-nineteenth century which led to development of the large state hospital system. In the process he examines both the real and the purported uses of involuntary hospitalization. After noting how few of the involuntarily hospitalized mentally ill are indeed dangerous, the author concludes that many have been hospitalized to provide social control, rather than to protect the public or the patient from harm. He notes further that when commitment has been justi-

fied on the claim that treatment is needed but none is being provided, social control and removal of deviants from the community can again be identified as a real function of hospitalization.

The paper reviews a few recent landmark cases seeking judicial standing for the right to treatment, including the first Supreme Court decision on the right of the mentally ill to their liberty—O'Connor v. Donaldson. Dr. Pepper speculates about possible future developments in the courts, including the right to treatment in the community for patients who do not require hospitalization. The right to refuse treatment is also considered.

Except for a few psychiatrists who have specialized in forensic work, there has long been a chasm between the majority of mental health professionals and the legal system. In the past, most mental health professionals have preferred to keep far away from the courtroom. However, as some therapeutic personnel and some lawyers have recently identified a community of interests—either in attacking involuntary hospitalization or in seeking affirmation of a constitutional right to treatment—new and powerful coalitions have been formed. Interdisciplinary teams have collaborated in producing the effective amici curiae (friends of the court) advisory briefs which have succeeded, in less than a decade, in bringing these cases through the lower federal courts and, in 1975, to a unanimous Supreme Court decision affirming the basic right to liberty of mentally ill persons.

NOTE

1. Robert S. Morison, "Rights and Responsibilities: Redressing the Uneasy Balance," *Hastings Center Report* 4, no. 2 (April 1974): 1–4.

THE TREATMENT SYSTEM AS SOCIAL POLICY—CIVIL COMMITMENT AND RIGHT TO TREATMENT

Bert Pepper

Introduction

Psychiatric Diagnosis and Social Function. A common and important characteristic of seriously mentally disordered persons is that they do not make good use of social mechanisms and institutions.

They are less able to organize themselves into goal-oriented self-help groups than other minorities, such as women, alcoholics, blacks, or prisoners. In fact, as of 1976, patient "liberation" groups, while they do exist in a few cosmopolitan centers like New York and San Francisco, are not yet a significant force in the struggle for patient rights and liberties. Individual patients are, of course, deeply involved in these issues, but this is usually in a collaborative involvement with sympathetic lawyers and psychiatrists, rather than a self-initiated, collaborative effort with other patients.

A distinctive perspective on the poor social functioning of many mentally disordered persons is offered by theorists of labeling, who consider a psychiatric diagnosis of "psychosis" to be a label for markedly socially deviant behavior. Put differently, they view the lack of social abilities as more than simply one characteristic of the mentally ill, but as the primary and most consequential characteristic. For example, Scheff (Chapter 18) has described schizophrenics as the ultimate residual group, drawn from all of society's residual members.

Edwin Lemert [1] has suggested that *mental illness* may be more a social status than a disease. The role of *mental patient,* as analyzed by Erving Goffman,[2] Thomas Scheff,[3] and by David Rosenhan in Chapter 20 of this book, has some characteristics of being *ascribed* rather than *achieved.* Ascribed roles are arbitrarily assigned on the basis of one or more external characteristics: age, sex, a single episode of bizarre behavior. (For a fuller explanation of these terms, see Chapter 4.)

The Judiciary: Social Engine or Brake? One of the major social functions of the judiciary system seems to be to conserve the status quo. When necessary, the courts permit the development of a new balance point and a new status quo by permitting that *least* amount of social change necessary to deal with conflict, unrest, and pressure for rearrangement of the social order. The Supreme Court's decision in *O'Connor* v. *Donaldson,* which will be discussed later, is a good example of this. The executive and legislative branches of government may each, at different times, act as *either* conservative *or* reforming social forces. However, the judiciary is expected to function as a steering guide and gyroscope which smooths out the rate of social change and prevents sharp alterations of direction. If social change were likened to a locomotive, the legislative branch would be the engine, the executive branch the engineer, and the judiciary branch would be both the minimum and maximum speed limit and the tracks. This analysis of functional relationships is supported by the observation that members of the executive and legislative branches are elected for relatively brief and finite terms of office, to allow for changes in social direction. Judges, on the other hand, are elected or appointed for longer terms or for life, to enhance their stabilizing function and their independence from current tides of change.

Apparently paradoxically, the judiciary seems at present to be playing the active role in promoting social change, as in right-to-treatment cases and in the whole field of the civil rights and liberties of minority members of society. In fact, it may simply be that the courts are preventing a sharp deceleration of motion in this direction which our society has been taking, with gradually increasing force, for more than a century. In this case, the "conservative" role of the judiciary may be to *conserve* the developed energy and direction of social change.

Historic Overview

Reports of treatment effectiveness of American mental institutions in the early and middle 1800s often claimed nearly perfect cure rates; [4] some claimed to cure 100 percent of their patients. This false optimism ended about a century ago, when it was shown by Pliny Earle [5] and others that such outcome reports were largely the result of inaccurate recording and incorrect statistical methods. For example, it was common to count each discharge as a cure; sometimes a single patient was cured a dozen times.

The last quarter of the nineteenth century saw the pendulum swing too far in the opposite direction, and a pessimistic attitude developed toward the likelihood of cure of the mentally ill. Immutable constitutional, hereditary, and organic factors were felt to be the paramount causes of mental disorders. This was also the time of the development of large state mental institutions, and the demise of execrable local care in county and municipal poorhouses, workhouses, and jails. The main thrust toward large state hospitals came from the pioneering work of Dorothea Lynde Dix, whose crusade for the state governments to take over responsibility for the mentally ill from local governments began in 1845. She is credited with the establishment of many state hospitals, including Bryce Hospital in Alabama in 1861. More will be said of Bryce below.

Laws Governing the Mentally Ill. Laws concerning involuntary admissions to mental hospitals were practically nonexistent in the United States in the middle of the nineteenth century. [6] As the state hospitals grew in size and number, a reform movement in the 1860–1870 period helped fill the void by successfully lobbying for the passage of commitment laws in many states. [7] Following the criminal law model, these were focused on assuring that no one would be involuntarily confined who was actually sane. However, there was little concern for what might happen afterward to those persons found to be mentally ill and therefore "properly" hospitalized initially. These laws concentrated on such factors as assuring a proper judicial procedure on demand of the patient, requiring a sworn complaint for the initiation of commitment procedures, and providing criminal penalties for attempting wrongfully to cause a person to be committed. We thus note that current right-to-treatment suits are roughly a centennial memorial to these earlier legal efforts to protect the rights of the involuntarily committed mentally ill.

Ross [8] notes two major legal grounds for involuntary hospitalization:

1. *Police power:* the right and responsibility of the state to protect society from dangerous persons.
2. *Parens patriae:* the state's duty to help and protect those persons who, because of incapacity, are unable to care for themselves. Current legal philosophy often challenges the constitutional validity of this old English concept when it extends beyond protecting the *life* of the individual.

Social Practice versus the Law. Under the various involuntary commitment laws of the states it became usual for a functional social-medical-legal system to develop by the inclusion of: (1) prospective patients' relatives, who initiated complaints; (2) community physicians who performed certifying examinations; (3) the police; (4) lower court judges and clerks; (5) psychiatrists and other physicians employed by these courts on a part-time basis to perform commitment examinations; and (6) state mental hospitals. The informal operating system created by these elements made it likely that anyone engaging it would likely be hospitalized; like a Venus' fly-trap, contact initiated a uniform response. It seemed to utilize an operational assumption that it was relatively harmless to hospitalize when not really necessary, but relatively dangerous *not* to hospitalize when probably necessary. In other words, the system was biased toward the production of false positives (admissions) in order to avoid false negatives (dangerous persons at large in the community).

As this systematic bias has reached public awareness, involuntary hospitalization procedures have come to be seen and described as mechanisms for the social exclusion and social control of behaviorally deviant *as well as* dangerous individuals. Thus publicly employed psychiatrists—working either in the courts or in mental hospitals—have been described as agents of social control by Szasz (Chapter 17) and some others. Scheff [9] found strong support for these views in a detailed study of commitment procedures in a midwestern state. The four courts he studied seldom released prospective patients. The legal procedures and psychiatric examinations were carried out in such a perfunctory manner as to suggest that the medical recommendation and judicial decision to retain patients in the hospital were routine, largely based on a presumption that *illness must be present since a complaint had been made.* Scheff dramatized and exemplifies his conclusion by reporting a case in which the medical examiner recommended retention in the hospital for thirty days of observation, even though he had *not* thought the individual to be mentally ill; he believed that the young man could not get along with his parents and might get into trouble. "We always make the conservative decision. I had rather play if safe. There's no harm in doing it that way."

Lest the reader assume that Scheff's findings were not typical, I must add that I have observed identical situations in several states over the last two decades.

The Social Function of State Hospitals. The 1860–1960 period may well be described historically as the century of the state mental hospital in America. As these institutions grew in size and number they became, along with prisons, a major social resource for the control and disposition of deviant and unwanted persons. The nature of their clientele was such that society did not find it necessary or important to provide them with the funds and other resources that would have been necessary if they were really intended to serve as active treatment hospitals. Indeed, many of their buildings were actually built by patient labor, and until the mid-twentieth century their operating budgets consisted largely of salaries for the small number of staff provided to oversee the toiling of the patients. Such institutional peonage has continued to the present: The United States Department of Labor was *required* to take action against state hospitals on this matter by a 1973 federal court decision.[10] Stonewall Stickney [11] has pointed out that as early as 1875 Dr. Bryce was complaining that the Alabama state mental hospital which he directed was failing to meet the goals set by the Dorothea Dix reform movement, which had led to its creation. Specifically, he complained that the hospital was being subverted from its treatment purposes by the commitment of paupers, the elderly, mentally defective persons, harmless eccentrics, alcoholics, and vagrants. Bryce was unable to stem the tide of these admissions because of a gentlemen's agreement among community physicians, judges, and families, all of whom found it convenient to send unwanted persons off to the state hospital. It had become necessary to do this because the county almshouses, old folks homes, and poor farms were no longer available. The function of social exclusion, it would seem, has been part of our social system for a long time.

Recent Legal Challenges to Involuntary Commitment

The Courts Interfere with Traditions.   In the last few years there have been landmark cases in many state and federal courts which challenge the manner in which society exercises its *parens patriae* and *police powers* in cases of alleged mental illness. For example, in *Lessard* v. *Schmidt* a federal court held that individuals threatened with involuntary commitment are entitled to all constitutional procedural safeguards *as if the matter were criminal rather than civil.* [12]

In another key 1972 decision the Supreme Court ordered a halt to the use of *incompetency to stand trial* as a basis for indefinite commitment.[13] It is noteworthy that the chief justice of the Supreme Court, in rendering the Jackson decision, expressed surprise that the constitutional limitations on a state's power to commit the mentally ill had not been tested more frequently in court. His comment can be taken as suggesting that the judiciary branch is ready to entertain a change in the legal status quo because of a changed societal attitude toward restrictions of individual liberty.

In June 1975 the Supreme Court ruled on the appeal in *O'Connor*

v. *Donaldson*.[14] It held that even when a person was properly and legally committed initially, involuntary hospitalization cannot be continued indefinitely if the individual is not dangerous, has family or friends who are willing to provide care in the community, and is receiving only custodial care. The Supreme Court specifically refused to rule on the right-to-treatment issue in this case; more will be said of *Donaldson* later in this paper.

The States React to the Courts. In response to the kind of court decisions noted above, many states are now revising their involuntary commitment procedures by amending their laws or adopting new regulations. For example, Maryland, challenged by a federal suit, implemented a new regulation in 1973.[15] It provides for an impartial hearing within five days of the time that an individual is involuntarily brought *for observation* to a mental hospital, on complaint of a relative and *with certification by two physicians*. The hearing officer must find that three conditions all exist: (1) mental disorder is present; (2) the individual requires inpatient care or treatment; and (3) the individual presents a danger to the life or safety of self or others. If all three conditions are not met the person is released immediately, the record of what has transpired prior to the hearing is sealed, and the individual can legally deny ever having been a patient in a mental hospital.[16] Virginia [17] has taken the legislative approach; a new commitment and patient's rights law went into effect in September 1974. It provides the individual with the right to counsel, to obtain independent medical evaluation, and to appeal. It also provides that all patients admitted under earlier procedures and not charged with a crime must be reclassified to voluntary status within sixty days, unless a commitment hearing is held under the standards of the new law. Note the intent to apply the new social rules to those admitted under the old ones.[18]

Virginia and Maryland have been used as examples of the current nation-wide ferment over laws and procedures governing involuntary commitment. Activity on this matter is so intense that in 1974 the National Association of Attorneys General circulated a memorandum to its membership entitled "Memo on Current Mental Hospital Decisions." The document covers key right-to-treatment cases, as well as cases on involuntary commitment, the right to privacy in a hospital, the right to refuse medication on religious grounds, and the right of a hospitalized patient to be compensated for labor. It appears that each state's legal apparatus is currently experiencing strong pressures to assure patients' rights and liberties.

A New Social Problem Emerges. As action causes reaction, so social change stimulates its own ripple effect. Current concern for civil liberty has produced new rules which result in the discharge or non-commitment of many persons. As a result, numerous individuals who can be diagnosed as seriously mentally ill, and who display significantly deviant and/or dependent behaviors, are now living and visible in our communities. This has caused new trends and counterforces, one of which is a renewed effort to get them committed to mental hospitals. This is being strongly resisted by the judiciary which, now maintaining the *new* status quo, says that they can't be "put away" just because they upset, inconvenience, and make demands upon the community. Another reaction is an urgent call for local mental health services for such persons, including supportive residential programs in the community. The mental health system's present inability to satisfy these new societal expectations and demands has caused an acute loss of equilibrium in several state mental health departments, and may be a cause of the rapid turnover of state mental health commissioners. The average commissioner's tenure dropped from about eight years in the 1950s to three years in the 1970s. The subject of community treatment will be discussed further in the next section.

The Right to Treatment

The New History.   Stone [19] suggests that during the decade of the 1960s civil libertarians concentrated on fighting the legal basis of involuntary hospitalization laws and procedures. However, a new strategy to improve the lot of the mentally ill was signaled in 1960 when Morton Birnbaum, a lawyer and physician, published an editorial in the *American Bar Association Journal* [20] condemning overcrowding and understaffing in our public mental hospitals. He called this "a wrong which demands correction." This landmark article advocated the recognition and implementation of the constitutional right of an involuntarily committed patient to adequate care and treatment. For simplicity Birnbaum referred to this as the *right to treatment*.

For several years no court decisions upheld Birnbaum's suggested right, even though he persisted by bringing a number of test cases. His goal was not to do away with mental hospitals or with involuntary admission; he simply wanted to bring public attention to bear on the inadequate care being provided in public mental hospitals, as a means of increasing funding. His efforts have been joined by others with a different goal—to make it impossible for the states to continue operating mental hospitals for involuntary patients, by making the costs of staffing prohibitive.[20a]

The first breakthrough for the right to treatment came in 1966, when the United States Court of Appeals for the District of Columbia decided *Rouse* v. *Cameron*.[21] Rouse had been charged with carrying a dangerous weapon—a misdemeanor carrying a maximum jail sentence of one year. He was found not guilty by reason of insanity, and by the time of his court appearance on a writ of habeas corpus [22] had been in St. Elizabeth's Hospital for four years.[23] Although the district court had refused to consider the lack-of-treatment issue, and had denied the petition, on appeal Judge Bazelon reasoned that since he had been deprived of liberty for three additional years, with no end in sight, the only justification for such lengthy confinement was the need for treatment.[24]

Partners for Social Change.   Another breakthrough for the right to treatment came in *Wyatt* v. *Stickney* [25] in 1970. In that case, brought in federal district court in Alabama as a class action ("on behalf of all other persons similarly afflicted"), Judge Johnson held that persons involuntarily confined in hospitals for the mentally ill or mentally retarded have a *constitutional right to adequate treatment and habilitation.* This case was also important because it saw a new coalition develop. Several powerful national groups lent their resources to Dr. Birnbaum and the original plaintiffs by offering to serve as amici curiae (friends of the court). In fact, although the initial complaint against the Alabama mental hospital system was brought by a group of professional employees who were protesting the loss of their jobs because of budget cuts, the main effort of the suit was eventually carried by the amici— the American Civil Liberties Union, the American Orthopsychiatric Association, the American Psychological Association, and others. [26]

Legal Basis of the Right to Treatment. There are three basic *constitutional* provisions which may be called upon in the establishment of a right to treatment: [27]

1. *Due process*—No person may be deprived of liberty without due process of law, according to the Fourteenth Amendment to the Constitution.
2. *Equal protections of the laws*—Under this aspect of the Fourteenth Amendment the courts must review classifications of persons for reasonableness. If mentally handicapped persons are classified as such and then required to be hospitalized involuntarily *for treatment,* then the actual provision of treatment is required if this classification is to stand up to a reasonableness test.
3. *Cruel and unusual punishment*—This is prohibited by the Eighth Amendment: involuntary civil commitment without treatment may amount to punishment.

Johnson, ruling in the Wyatt case, was the first federal judge to find a constitutional basis for the right to treatment:

> To deprive any citizen of his or her liberty upon the altruistic theory that the confinement is for humane and therapeutic reasons, and then fail to provide adequate treatment vitiates the very fundamentals of due process. [28]

Johnson's decision required that the Alabama state mental hospitals hire sufficient professional personnel to meet specific ratios, as recommended by the amici briefs. Stickney [29] feels that this part of the decision is a long step backward, since it does not address the need for additional community services and will inhibit the hospitals from attempting innovative and experimental treatment efforts and staffing patterns.

During the same period that Johnson was finding a constitutional basis for the right to treatment in *Wyatt,* another federal court heard a Georgia case and reached the opposite conclusion. [30] Judge Smith did not find a constitutional right to treatment in ruling on *Burnham* v. *Georgia,* and he suggested that the issue of treatment of involuntary patients in hospitals is not justiciable—capable of resolution by a court. The Supreme Court, in ruling on O'Connor's appeal, [31] found that the adequacy of treatment *is* justiciable, that a court is competent to decide whether treatment rendered a given person is adequate. Of course we can anticipate that judges will likely seek expert professional opinion on this matter before ruling in any given case. Perhaps the differences between the *Wyatt* and the *Burnham* decisions are entirely technical; perhaps they reflect differing views of the proper role of the judiciary in changing the social order.

Both *Wyatt* and *Burnham* were appealed, and the Fifth Circuit Court of Appeals assembled all of its justices to sit *en banc* to review the two cases jointly. Nearly two years later, in November 1974, the appeals court upheld Johnson in nearly every respect.[32] The Supreme Court has agreed to take the final appeal of *Wyatt* under consideration. The slowness of the highest courts to decide these cases invites speculation; one possibility is that the justices realize the enormous social and economic consequences of a constitutional guarantee of the right to treatment. As pragmatic evaluators of the current social order, and of the citizenry's readiness to fund and accept changes in it, they may feel that an official and definitive decision would be socially premature. Whatever the reason, the Supreme Court's reluctance to rule on the constitutional issue of the right to treatment stands in the record, as will be seen in the next section.

Sue the Doctor.   Kenneth Donaldson was forty-eight years old in 1957 when his father petitioned the Florida authorities; a county judge found him to be paranoid schizophrenic and committed him to Florida State Hospital. Despite repeated attempts by Donaldson and his friends outside the hospital to secure his release, the hospital authorities retained him, even though he had never been considered dangerous to self or others. He had refused drug therapy because of religious belief (Christian Scientist), and had not been offered other forms of therapy. Over the years he complained to various state and federal courts, but none accepted jurisdiction until 1971. At that time he succeeded in bringing a class action complaint to the United States District Court. The court, while ordering his release, denied the class action aspect of the complaint. Donaldson then filed an amended complaint, asking money damages from two doctors he named as defendants. The first had been one of his supervising physicians; the second, Dr. J. B. O'Connor, had originally supervised Donaldson's care and had served as superintendent of the hospital for a number of years, retiring shortly before Donaldson's suit was filed.

After a four-day trial the judge instructed the jury to find that the doctors had violated Donaldson's constitutional right to liberty if they had known "he was not mentally ill or dangerous, or knowing that if mentally ill, he was not receiving treatment for his mental illness. . . ." The trial judge also instructed the jury that an involuntary patient has "a constitutional right to receive such treatment as will give him a realistic opportunity to be cured or to improve his mental condition." [33] This instruction was *not* upheld by the Supreme Court on review, as will be discussed below.

It is noteworthy that the jury awarded Donaldson $38,500 in damages, $10,000 of which were *punitive* damages. This followed an instruction from the judge that the doctors were immune from any money damages if they "reasonably believed in good faith that detention of [Donaldson] was proper for the length of time he was so confined. . . ." The jury was instructed to levy punitive damages only if the defendant's actions were "maliciously or wantonly or oppressively done." [34]

Following the trial in the federal district court, the doctors went to the United States Court of Appeals, which affirmed the judgment against them in a far-reaching decision.[35] The appellate court held that when the rationale for confinement is the need for treatment, the Constitution requires that minimally adequate treatment actually be provided. They further found that, regardless of the reason for involuntary hospitalization, any such patient has "a constitutional right to receive such individual treatment as will give him a reasonable opportunity to be cured or to improve his mental condition." By implication, the court of appeals held that it is constitutionally permissible for a state to confine a mentally ill person who is not dangerous to anyone, in order to provide treatment.

The United States Supreme Court accepted Dr. O'Connor's request for a review of the appellate court decision and came forth with its unanimous opinion in June 1975, making headlines across the nation.[36] While many mental health authorities first acclaimed this as a landmark victory for the rights of the mentally ill, careful analysis of the decision leaves us with more questions than answers. Many of the findings of the court of appeals, including the existence of a constitutional right to treatment for those involuntarily hospitalized, were *not found* (but not necessarily denied) by the Supreme Court. In a masterpiece of judicial avoidance of central issues, Justice Potter Stewart, writing for the entire court, simply found that a mentally ill person who is not dangerous to himself or others has a constitutional right to *liberty*, and cannot be simply confined by the state. However, Steward lays open the possibility that a person might be dangerous to self if helpless to avoid the "hazards of freedom." No definition of this term was offered. Donaldson's release was upheld solely on the grounds that his involuntary stay was a violation of his constitutional right to liberty.

Importantly, the Supreme Court found that the court of appeals made findings which were broader than necessary.

> Specifically, there is no reason now to decide whether mentally ill persons dangerous to themselves or to others have a right to treatment upon compulsory confinement by the State, or whether the State may compulsorily confine a nondangerous, mentally ill individual for the purpose of treatment. . . . We need not decide whether, when, or by what procedures, a mentally ill person may be confined by the State on any of the grounds which, under contemporary statutes, are generally advanced to justify involuntary confinement of such a person—to prevent injury to the public, to ensure his own survival or safety, or to alleviate or cure his illness.[37]

Justice Stewart summarized the Supreme Court's decision as follows: "In short, a state cannot constitutionally confine without more a nondangerous individual who is capable of surviving safely in freedom by himself or with the help of willing and responsible family members or friends." The meaning of the term "without more" is quite unclear: Without more than mere custodial care? Without treatment?

In a surprise ending the Supreme Court vacated the money damages levied against the doctors and sent the case back to the court of appeals for further study, to determine the doctors' liability for money damages in the light of a recent Supreme Court opinion redefining the liability of public officials.

One can surmise that the Supreme Court avoided a split decision in *O'Connor* v. *Donaldson* by ruling very narrowly, solely on the issue of deprivation of liberty. Evidence for this comes from the fact that the chief justice of the Court, Warren Burger, wrote a separate concurring opinion which no other justice chose to cosign. Burger made clear that he does not support the existence of a constitutional right to treatment. He supports the historic authority of the state to confine the mentally ill without providing treatment, based on the continued use of *police power* or *parens patriae:* "The existence of some due process limitations on the parens patriae power does not justify the further conclusion that it may be exercised to confine a mentally ill person only if the purpose of the confinement is treatment." [38]

At this time, then, the Supreme Court has not yet ruled for or against the existence of a constitutional right to treatment for involuntarily hospitalized patients, whether confined because of dangerousness to self or others, or because of a need for treatment. Nevertheless, the court has taken the appeal of *Wyatt* v. *Stickney* under consideration. That right-to-treatment case, when it is decided, will probably reveal more of the thinking of our highest court on this matter.

The Right to Community Treatment.   The last several years have seen many thousands of long-term patients from state hospitals for the mentally ill and mentally retarded being discharged to communities, often with inadequate provision for continued care and treatment. The causes of this trend include:

1. Current professional treatment methods often recommend that hospitalization be as brief as possible, with treatment to be continued in the community after discharge (Chapters 15 and 28).
2. Challenges to involuntary commitment laws and procedures have made it more difficult for the hospitals to admit and retain patients.
3. The budgets of many state mental hospitals have not increased in proportion to inflation in recent years; decreasing the patient population has been a remedy used by administrators for making necessary fiscal adjustments.
4. Higher standards of care and treatment have been pushed by licensing and accrediting bodies, such as the Joint Commission on the Accreditation of Hospitals. One way of improving the staff:patient ratio in order to secure or retain accreditation when the hospital lacks funds to hire additional staff is to treat fewer patients.

These factors have increased enormously the pressure on community treatment resources to deal with greater numbers of seriously ill clients. Nevertheless, the executive branch of the federal government adopted a policy in 1969 to eliminate federal support for community mental health centers. In addition, state funds have not been increased in proportion to the vastly increased demands for community services. As a result, larger numbers of partially recovered patients have been competing for the short supply of existing community treatment and residential services.

A coalition of mental health professional and legal-civil libertarian groups, similar to the one that was referred to earlier in the *Wyatt* case, has decided to use the judicial approach to attack the problem of inadequate community treatment. It has brought the *Robinson et al.* v. *Weinberger et al.* suit against several defendants: the United States Department of Health, Education, and Welfare, the District of Columbia government, and St. Elizabeth's Hospital. The plaintiffs [39] argue that it is the responsibility of the defendants to provide the least restrictive environment in which each patient may be provided adequate treatment. They are asking the federal court to require that the District of Columbia government create an adequate system of sheltered care, foster care, halfway houses, and treatment services to meet the needs of patients being discharged from St. Elizabeth's Hospital:

> What we want to do is create a precedent about the right to treatment which requires an improvement in the provision of mental health care, which requires that community mental health concepts that have been offered as a reason for abandoning state hospitals be a reality and not just an excuse for precipitous deinstitutionalization.[40]

Issues in the Judicial Approach to Improving Mental Health Services

It seems fair to say that society is altering the rules of the social order which govern mentally disabled persons by incorporating both professional advances and changing general standards governing the responsibilities of society toward handicapped persons. A necessary step in the process of changing the social order includes incorporation into the rules of law. However, the laws are a stabilizing device for the social system, intended to maintain homeostasis by allowing only incremental changes in the law over time, in a continuing attempt to remain in balance with traditional and historical social standards and expectations. It should not surprise us, then, that Birnbaum's attempt to rewrite the legal contract between society and mentally disabled persons—by finding a constitutional basis for a right which was never considered by the drafters of the Constitution—is not accomplished quickly.

It is interesting to note, as we focus on the forms of emerging social trends, that Thomas Szasz (Chapter 17) and Morton Birnbaum,[41] two men whose views are considered to be generally divergent, published their landmark articles in the same year—1960. Do these two streams perhaps emerge from a common social source?

From the perspective of those who treat mentally ill persons, the emphasis on the right to treatment of only *involuntarily* committed patients is unfortunate and unrealistic. While the courts have focused on the difference between the rights of voluntary and involuntary patients, the distinction is generally irrelevant in actual hospital practice. Both classes of patients tend to be mingled in care and treatment activities. Programmatic groupings for care and decisions about treatment tend to classify and cluster patients more by age, diagnostic, behavioral, and functional factors. It might represent a significant setback for voluntary patients if court decisions should require hospitals to discriminate in the allocation of scarce treatment resources toward committed patients.

The Right to Refuse Treatment. Szasz, who has opposed the concept of the right to treatment, has proposed instead that we concern ourselves with the right to refuse treatment.[42] From the few cases which have already been decided it appears that the courts will often support the right of patients to refuse treatment under various circumstances.[43] Hospitals may be faced with situations in which some patients refuse all forms of active treatment, but may require indefinite hospitalization or care in an alternative institutional setting.[44]

Who Will Pay the Bill? Since the existence of a right implies the reciprocal existence of a duty, recognition of a right to treatment for patients implies that society has a duty to implement it. The next question is: Which elements of society have the duty? Mental health professionals in public service are assigned the *direct* duty, while the present facilities and resources, supplied by society through government, are simply inadequate to the task. Mental health personnel may thus bear an impossible burden, and those who leave public service because of it will increase the burden on those who remain. Do hospital staffs have a right to refuse to provide *inadequate* care and treatment? How can mental health professionals, naturally somewhat concerned about outcomes like the *Donaldson* case, assure that the duty to provide resources is properly placed on society and its appropriate agents—the executive and legislative branches of government? These and related questions have been considered by Pepper.[45]

If our society is visualized as a planet with a molten center contained by a thin, fragile crust, there is much pressure just beneath the crust for change in the way that we deal with those socially different persons we call "the mentally ill." The pressure is now being relieved by a variety of volcanic eruptions, earthquakes, and smaller shifts. Some patients—and some staff—will doubtless get burned, and others may fall into chasms before the crust settles into a new configuration which will serve society and the individual in the years ahead.

NOTES

1. Edwin M. Lemert, *Social Pathology* (New York: McGraw-Hill, 1951).

2. Erving Goffman, *Asylums* (Garden City, N.Y.: Doubleday, Anchor Books, 1961).

3. Thomas J. Scheff, "The Societal Reaction to Deviance: Ascriptive Elements in the Psychiatric Screening of Mental Patients in a Midwestern State," *Social Problems* 11, no. 4 (Spring 1964): 401–413.

4. A. Deutsch, *The Mentally Ill in America* (New York: Columbia University Press, 1949).

5. Pliny Earle, *The Curability of the Insane* (1876).

6. Isaac Ray, "Project of a Law for Determining the Legal Relations of the Insane," *American Journal of Psychiatry* 7 (1851).

7. William J. Curran, "Legal Psychiatry in the 19th Century," *Psychiatric Annals* 4, no. 8 (August 1974): 8–13.

8. Hugh Allen Ross, "Commitment of the Mentally Ill: Problems of Law and Policy," *Michigan Law Review* 57 (May 1959): 945–1018.

9. Scheff, "Societal Reaction."

10. *Sounder v. Brennan*, 367 F. Supp. 812 (1973). The Department of Labor lost this suit; it did not wish to enforce the Federal Fair Labor Standards Act in mental hospitals, but was ordered to do so by the court.

11. Stonewall B. Stickney, "Problems in Implementing the Right to Treatment in Alabama: The *Wyatt v. Stickney* Case," *Hospital and Community Psychiatry* 25, no. 7 (July 1974): 453–460.

12. *Lessard v. Schmidt*, 349 F. Supp. 1078 (E. C. Wisc., 1972). Specifically, the federal court guaranteed the Fifth Amendment's protection against self-incrimination, and noted that an individual's right to be heard at a commitment hearing could be prejudiced by incapacity caused by medication or lack of counsel. The standards set by the court also include: notice of the hearing must specify the basis and standard of detention; right to a jury trial; names of examining physicians and other persons testifying in support of continued detention and the substance of their proposed testimony; a hearing within fourteen days of the onset of detention.

13. *Jackson v. Indiana*, 406 U.S. 715 (1972).

14. *O'Connor v. Donaldson*, 43 U.S.L.W. 4929 (June 24, 1973).

15. Regulation 10.04.03 Governing Involuntary Admission to Mental Health Facilities Under the Jurisdiction of and/or Licensed by the Department of Health and Mental Hygiene. Amended 6/73; effective 10/1/73. State of Maryland.

16. Since this regulation was instituted, slightly less than 50 percent of the two-physician certificated commitments have been denied at the hearings, usually because the third condition—dangerousness—is not met. Roughly 25 percent of the hearings have resulted in forthwith release, while a similar number have led to the person agreeing to stay in the hospital for treatment on a voluntary basis. These results seem to support the thesis that *dangerousness*—the police power—is often overused to bring about hospitalization for other reasons, good or bad.

17. Code of Virginia, Section 37. 1–67.1 (1974).

18. Prior Virginia law permitted a judge to commit an individual involuntarily merely by having sufficient cause to believe that the person was mentally ill. In contrast, under the new law a judge must find that the defendant "presents an *imminent* danger to himself or others as a result of mental illness, or has *seriously* threatened or attempted to take his own life *just prior* to the hearing, or has otherwise been proven to be so seriously mentally ill as to be substantially unable to care for himself [emphasis added]." Further, the judge must find that there is no less restrictive alternative to hospital confinement and treatment.

19. Alan A. Stone, "The Right to Treatment and the Psychiatric Establishment," *Psychiatric Annals* 4, no. 9 (September 1974): 21–42.

20. Morton Birnbaum, "The Right to Treatment," *American Bar Association Journal* 46 (1960): 499–505.

20a. Bruce Ennis and Loren Siegel, *The Rights of Mental Patients* (New York: Avon Press, 1973), p. 13.

21. *Rouse v. Cameron*, 373 F. 2d 451 (1966).

22. Literally, "you have the body." Issuance of writ of habeas corpus results in release from confinement or other restraint of liberty.

23. *Basic Rights of the Mentally Handicapped* (Washington, D.C.: Mental Health Law Project, 1973).

24. In writing his decision, Bazelon speculated broadly and noted that failure to provide treatment raised significant constitutional questions regarding *equal protection under the law, due process,* and *cruel and unusual punishment.* However, he did not decide that there was a constitutional basis for the right to treatment; he did not need to, since the D.C. statute specifically required that treatment be provided: "A person hospitalized in a public hospital for mental illness *shall,* during his hospitalization, be entitled to medical and psychiatric care and treatment [italics added]." [D.C. Code, Title 21, sec. 562 (1967)]. Following standard judicial practice, Bazelon ruled as narrowly as possible in basing his decision on the specific statute. rather than finding a more basic, constitutional justification for his decision. This is reflective of the judiciary's conservative social role—to slow the rate of change.

25. *Wyatt v. Stickney*, 344 F. Supp. 373 (1972).

26. The American Psychiatric Association declined to participate as an amicus in *Wyatt v. Stickney*, and in the course of the complex and lengthy litigation, Birnbaum withdrew from participation. Over the years of this litigation—it was still on-

going late in 1975—social and professional issues have waxed and waned, and participants have come and gone accordingly.

27. Mental Health Law Project, *Basic Rights*, pp. 15–16.

28. *Wyatt* v. *Stickney.*

29. Stickney, "Problems in Implementing."

30. *Burnam* v. *Georgia*, civil action no. 16385, N.D. GA.

31. *O'Connor* v. *Donaldson.*

32. *Wyatt* v. *Stickney*, vol. 503, Federal 2d, p. 1305.

33. *Donaldson* v. *O'Connor*, 493 F. 2d 507, 5th Cir. (April 26, 1974).

34. *O'Connor* v. *Donaldson.*

35. *Donaldson* v. *O'Connor.*

36. *O'Connor* v. *Donaldson.*

37. Ibid.

38. Ibid.

39. The plaintiffs in *Robinson et al.* v. *Weinberger et al.* include the Mental Health Law Project, along with the American Orthopsychiatric, Psychiatric, Psychological, and Public Health Associations. The role of co-plaintiff in a suit of this kind represents a new departure for the American Psychiatric Association and continues to be the source of much unrest and tension within the governing councils and membership of the Association.

40. Stone, "Right to Treatment."

41. Birnbaum, "Right to Treatment."

42. Thomas Szasz, *Law, Liberty and Psychiatry* (New York: Macmillan, 1963), pp. 214–216.

43. *New York City Health and Hospital Corporation* v. *Stein*, 335 NYS 2d 461 (New York); *Winters* v. *Miller*, 446 F. 2d 65 2d Cir. (1971).

44. An ethical, professional, and economic question may then arise: should a bed and other resources of the facility be utilized indefinitely for such patients, with a consequent diminution of available beds and resources for others? Should such patients be cared for in residential settings other than hospitals, if dangerousness prevents outright discharge or community placement?

45. Bert Pepper, "The Right to Treatment and the Future of Psychiatry" (Paper presented to the annual meeting of the American Psychiatric Association, Anaheim, California, May 1975).

COMMENTARY

Pepper's paper has reviewed public, legislative, and judicial attitudes over the last century toward the rights of mentally ill persons to care, treatment, and freedom. He believes that a longstanding set of social and legal structures is now giving way to tides of change, and suggests that the movement to release nondangerous patients from involuntary hospital confinement and the right-to-treatment movement are inextricably intertwined. One can, however, argue that these are quite separate social and professional movements, a position taken by the Supreme Court in its decision on Donaldson.

The shape of mental health services to come seems likely to be significantly altered by court decisions on the rights of mental patients. Will state mental hospitals as we have known them survive? If they do, will they be active treatment institutions integrated with community services, or will they be more bureaucratized and beset with court-determined procedures and hearings? Will civil liberties groups succeed in legally eliminating involuntary commitments to mental hospitals, or at least making such procedures so cumbersome as to eliminate commitments in most cases? Above all, what will be the effect on seriously ill patients who could benefit from treatment but who, because of their impaired judgment, tend to avoid it?

The right to refuse treatment is particularly nettlesome. Many mental health professionals and lawyers will continue to argue this matter, with treatment-oriented individuals feeling that the very illness either minimizes or negates the patient's ability to decide on accepting treatment in his or her own best interest, and lawyers generally taking an opposite view and placing a higher priority on "freedom." What advice can be offered to a judge when a patient refuses treatment, and the refusal is apparently based on false belief apparently arising from the illness?

The Social Role of Professionals

In Chapter 3 the editors offered the hypothesis that the mental health system is an integral element of the general social system and, as such, is shaped by changing societal values and expectations. When a profession leads the way for change in the mental health system, it is doing so as society's agent—being moved into an active stance by general social pressure for change acting on the profession as a component of society and on its members as individual citizen-professionals.

Each health profession plays out its social role according to the length and content of its social history. The older professions are likely to represent social stability and conservatism; the younger professions are likelier to offer themselves as tools for change. The American Medical Association (AMA), for example, represents an older profession and speaks for the traditional values of society. It has opposed the development of a right to health care and treatment—although, of late, some of its leaders have advocated biting the bullet and accepting the clear demands of contemporary American society for recognition of this right. The AMA has, in the past, opposed federal payments for health services to citizens. It favors the older fee-for-service payment system over payment for health maintenance. It has opposed plans for the organized redistribution of health manpower, fearing interference with the established social order which gives the doctor the right to practice where he pleases. It has opposed the entry of new professions into the health services field, or the addition of new duties and roles for those other health professionals who have traditionally been classified by physicians as *allied, para-, or sub*professionals.

The American Psychiatric Association (APA), in slight but distinct contrast to the AMA, is an organization representing a newer specialization within the field of medical practice. Many individual psychiatrists, and the APA as their spokesman, have enjoyed taking on the roles of "Young Turks" in their jousts with the AMA and medicine in general. They have felt comfortable lobbying for federal payments for mental health services, have cautiously supported the concept of the right to adequate mental health care and treatment, and have moderately encouraged the development of increased responsibilities for nonmedical professionals. However, as a transitional profession, psychiatry has often represented an ambivalent and vacillating tool in the carving out of a new social order in the health and mental health field. To illustrate: The APA *opposed* Judge Bazelon's decision for the right to treatment in 1966 in *Rouse* v. *Stickney;* put together and took apart various task forces on the subject of the right to treatment in the following years; and suffered severe internal schisms and strains in 1974 when the trustees who governed the association voted to act as co-plaintiffs in a right-to-treatment suit (*Rosenberger et al.* v. *Weinberger et al.*, discussed earlier in this chapter).

The younger mental health professional groups, such as the American Psychological Association and the American Orthopsychiatric Association (AOA), have been active in supporting right-to-treatment cases since *Wyatt* v. *Stickney.* The American Psychological Association generally takes a "liberal" posture with regard to the right to treatment and other public policy issues bearing on mental health care.

The AOA represents a somewhat different clientele. Unlike the groups discussed earlier, its members come from various mental health professions and are drawn together by treatment and philosophical ideologies, rather than by training in the same discipline. A twentieth-century organization, AOA was organized to represent radical or liberal interests in mental health; those who joined were professionals who wanted to work in an *interdisciplinary* manner, rather than in structures which would recognize them by their particular profession. Those who have chosen to be active in AOA may have done so in some measure because of their personal identification with movements for change. Clearly, then, individuals may decide to act *as individuals in society* as they seek to alter the social order in accord with personal ideology. However, the continuing reciprocal interplay which brings the individual to bear on society at the same time that society brings itself to bear upon the individual cannot be forgotten. The initial choice of a profession is not culture-free, although it usually represents a major attempt at individuation. Once the choice is made, to a certain degree, the die is cast: Socialization to the profession proceeds to modify the trainee's value-belief complex, while the trainee, in turn, strives to influence the value-belief complex of colleagues and professional bodies.

The movement toward the development of a right to adequate health care and treatment, the movement toward the least restrictive treatment alternative, and the movement toward community-ambulatory rather than institutional-hospital care for the mentally ill can all be seen as parts of general social developments in the United States in the third and fourth quarters of the twentieth century.

Our society is now balancing the equities between the individual and society somewhat more in favor of the individual, apparently believing that our human, technological, social, and natural resources are sufficient to support the shift.

NAME INDEX

*denotes author of selection in this volume.

SUBJECT INDEX